KNOWLEDGE INTENSIVE COMPUTER AIDED DESIGN

IFIP - The International Federation for Information Processing

IFIP was founded in 1960 under the auspices of UNESCO, following the First World Computer Congress held in Paris the previous year. An umbrella organization for societies working in information processing, IFIP's aim is two-fold: to support information processing within its member countries and to encourage technology transfer to developing nations. As its mission statement clearly states,

IFIP's mission is to be the leading, truly international, apolitical organization which encourages and assists in the development, exploitation and application of information technology for the benefit of all people.

IFIP is a non-profitmaking organization, run almost solely by 2500 volunteers. It operates through a number of technical committees, which organize events and publications. IFIP's events range from an international congress to local seminars, but the most important are:

- The IFIP World Computer Congress, held every second year;
- open conferences;
- working conferences.

The flagship event is the IFIP World Computer Congress, at which both invited and contributed papers are presented. Contributed papers are rigorously refereed and the rejection rate is high.

As with the Congress, participation in the open conferences is open to all and papers may be invited or submitted. Again, submitted papers are stringently refereed.

The working conferences are structured differently. They are usually run by a working group and attendance is small and by invitation only. Their purpose is to create an atmosphere conducive to innovation and development. Refereeing is less rigorous and papers are subjected to extensive group discussion.

Publications arising from IFIP events vary. The papers presented at the IFIP World Computer Congress and at open conferences are published as conference proceedings, while the results of the working conferences are often published as collections of selected and edited papers.

Any national society whose primary activity is in information may apply to become a full member of IFIP, although full membership is restricted to one society per country. Full members are entitled to vote at the annual General Assembly, National societies preferring a less committed involvement may apply for associate or corresponding membership. Associate members enjoy the same benefits as full members, but without voting rights. Corresponding members are not represented in IFIP bodies. Affiliated membership is open to non-national societies, and individual and honorary membership schemes are also offered.

KNOWLEDGE INTENSIVE COMPUTER AIDED DESIGN

IFIP TC5 WG5.2 Third Workshop on Knowledge Intensive CAD
December 1-4, 1998, Tokyo, Japan

Edited by

Susan Finger
Department of Civil Engineering
Carnegie Mellon University
USA

Tetsuo Tomiyama
Research into Artifacts, Center for Engineering (RACE)
The University of Tokyo
Japan

Martti Mäntylä
Laboratory of Information Processing Science
Helsinki University of Technology
Finland

SPRINGER-SCIENCE+BUSINESS MEDIA, B.V.

Library of Congress Cataloging-in-Publication Data

IFIP TC5 WG5.2 Workshop on Knowledge Intensive CAD (3rd : 1998 : Tokyo, Japan)
Knowledge intensive computer aided design : IFIP TC5 WG5.2 Third Workshop on Knowledge Intensive CAD, December 1-4, 1998, Tokyo, Japan / edited by Susan Finger, Tetsuo Tomiyama, Martti Mäntylä.

Includes bibliographical references and index.

DOI 10.1007/978-0-387-35582-5
1. Design, Industrial—Congresses. 2. Computer-aided design—Congresses. 3. Expert systems (Computer science)—Congresses. 4. Product life cycle—Congresses. I. Finger, Susan. II. Tomiyama, T. (Tetsuo), 1957– . III. Mäntylä, Martti, 1955– . IV. Title.

TS171.A1 I39 1998
620'.0042'0285—dc21 99-048311

Originally published by Kluwer Academic Publishers in 2000
MyCopy version of the original edition 2000

Printed on acid-free paper.
www.springer.com/mycopy

Contents

Preface

Computer Aided Design (CAD) technology plays a key role in today's advanced manufacturing environment. To reduce the time to market, achieve zero defect quality the at first production, and use available production and logistics resources effectively, product and design process knowledge covering the whole product life cycle must be used throughout product design. Once generated, this intensive design knowledge should be made available to later life cycle activities. Due to the increasing concern about global environmental issues and rapidly changing economical situation worldwide, design must exhibit high performance not only in quality and productivity, but also in life cycle issues, including extended producer's liability.

This requires designers and engineers to use various kinds of design knowledge intensively during product design and to generate design information for use in later stages of the product life cycle such as production, distribution, operation, maintenance, reclamation, and recycling. Therefore, future CAD systems must incorporate product and design process knowledge, which is not explicitly dealt with in the current systems, in their design tools and design object models.

Between 1987 and 1989, the IFIP Working Group 5.2 organized a series of three workshops on "Intelligent CAD," which were followed by a working conference on the same subject in 1991. This new series of workshops extends the concept of intelligent CAD to the concept of "knowledge intensive engineering." The concept advocates that intensive life cycle knowledge regarding products and design processes must be incorporated in the center of the CAD architecture. The concept focuses on the systematization and sharing of knowledge across the life cycle stages and organizational boundaries. The first workshop was held at Helsinki University of Technology, Espoo, Finland in September 1995. The second workshop was held at Carnegie Mellon University, Pittsburgh, USA, in September 1996. The aim of the workshops is to clarify and elaborate the concepts of knowledge intensive design and CAD by providing an international forum for mutual discussions and exchange of opinions of experts of the field. The first workshop focused on exploring the concept of knowledge intensive design as a part of knowledge intensive engineering activities. The second workshop examined architectures and methodologies for "knowledge intensive CAD" based on the results of the first workshop. The third workshop looked at implementations and applications of knowledge intensive CAD systems. The scope of the third workshop included:

- Ontology
- Knowledge intensive CAD (KIC)
- Knowledge intensive design (KID)
- Knowledge representation for KIC

All in all, 17 papers were presented at the workshop, of which 13 were accepted for this volume after a review. The selected papers provide a vivid discussion to encapsulate particular aspects of the central themes. For example, Ontology and Knowledge Representation streams cover some of the fundamental issues associated with these subjects and the KIC and KID streams begin to introduce the applications. We included a keynote speaker paper to discuss the knowledge life cycle and a report about the past, present and future research directions of KIC.

Together with the proceeding of the previous workshops, the volume presents an overview of an important novel area of research for researchers, graduate and postgraduate students, system developers of advanced computer-aided design and manufacturing systems, and engineers involved in industrial application of KIC. It discusses not only theoretical aspects but also practical systems and experiences gained from these, and aims to provide a multi-disciplinary view of the subject both from computer science and engineering research angles.

The workshop was organized by the IFIP Working Group 5.2 and co-sponsored by the following bodies.

- Japan Society of Precision Engineering.

- The "Modeling of Synthesis" Project, funded by the Japan Society for the Promotion of Sciences' Program for Research for the Future, JSPS-RFTF 96P00701.
- Research into Artifacts, Center for Engineering, the University of Tokyo.

As the co-chairs of the workshop and co-editors of this volume, we should like to thank all authors for contributions to the workshop and to the volume. We also thank the members of International Program Committee for their reviews during the preparation of the workshop and the volume. Last but not least, a special thanks is due to Dr. Ken Ping Hew and Dr. Akira Tsumaya for their excellent organization of the workshop, the volume, its program, and special events.

Susan Finger
Tetsuo Tomiyama
Martti Mäntylä

PART ONE

REPORT ON WORKSHOP

1

Knowledge Intensive Computer Aided Design: Past, Present and Future

Tetsuo Tomiyama[1] and Ken Ping Hew[2]
[1]*RACE, The Univeristy of Tokyo, Japan*
[2]*JSPS-RFTF-The Modeling of Synthesis Project, The Univerity of Tokyo, Japan*

Key words: Knowledge Intensive CAD, Knowledge Management, Life Cycle Knowledge

Abstract: This paper is a report of the past, present and future research in knowledge intensive computer aided design (KIC). This paper reports the two previous workshops on KIC and provides the discussions and conclusions reached by the present KIC workshop (KIC-3). Three working groups and one invited paper that were formed from the attendees at KIC-3 are briefly discussed. The groups were assigned to discuss knowledge life cycle, ontology, knowledge intensive design (KID) and knowledge representations. Finally, we provide some guideline for the future research in KIC. It discusses the challenges and opportunities involved in KIC research, such as strategy and technology of knowledge management, system implementation for integration under design support systems, practical applications and evaluation of KIC, and life cycle knowledge as the focused content of KIC.

1. INTRODUCTION

Computer Aided Design (CAD) technology plays a key role in today's advanced manufacturing environment. To reduce the time to market, achieve zero defect quality at the first production, and use available production and logistics resources effectively, product and design process knowledge covering the whole product life cycle must be used throughout product design. Once generated, this intensive design knowledge should be made available to later life cycle activities. Due to the increasing concern about global environmental issues and rapidly changing economical situation worldwide, design must exhibit high performance not only in quality and productivity, but also in life cycle issues, including extended producer's liability.

This requires designers and engineers to use various kinds of design knowledge intensively during product design and to generate design information for use in later stages of the product life cycle such as production, distribution, operation, maintenance, reclamation, and recycling. Therefore, future CAD systems must incorporate product and process knowledge which are not explicitly dealt with in the current systems, in their design tools and design object models. This paper reports the past, present and future research in KIC. We outline the key discussions and conclusions reached in the KIC-3 workshop.

2. THE PAST

Between 1987 and 1989, the IFIP Working Group 5.2 organized a series of three workshops on "Intelligent CAD," which were followed by a working conference on the same subject in 1991 (Yoshikawa *et al.*, 1989, 1990, 1991, Brown *et al.*, 1992). This new series of workshops extends the concept of intelligent CAD to the concept of "knowledge intensive engineering." Knowledge Intensive CAD has multiple type of knowledge regarding products and design processes. The concept advocates that intensive life cycle knowledge regarding products and design processes must be incorporated in the center of the CAD architecture. The concept focuses on the systematization and sharing of knowledge across the life cycle stages and organizational boundaries. It concerns product knowledge management, formalization and sharing knowledge across the life cycle stages and organizational boundaries. KIC workshops aim at clarifying and elaborating the concepts of knowledge intensive engineering and CAD by providing an international forum for mutual discussion and exchange of opinions of experts of the field.

The first IFIP Working Group 5.2 Workshop on "Knowledge Intensive CAD" (KIC-1) was held at Helsinki University of Technology, Finland, on 26-29 September 1995. KIC-1 was the first workshop that extended the concept of intelligent CAD to the concept of "knowledge intensive engineering." This workshop discussed a variety of issues related to KIC; *knowledge intensive CAD frameworks, product and design process modeling, and methodologies, tools and techniques for knowledge intensive CAD.* The result of the first KIC workshop appeared as a book in 1996 (Tomiyama *et al.*, 1996).

The second workshop (KIC-2) in the series was held at Carnegie Mellon University in Pittsburgh, PA, USA, on 16-18 September 1996. This workshop dealt with the issues in *system architectures*, *representations* and *delivery systems*, as well as addressing topics from the point of view of research achievements, research issues and industry needs. The result of the second KIC workshop appeared as a book in 1997 (Mäntylä *et al.*, 1997).

The third workshop (KIC-3) in the series was held in Tokyo, Japan, on 4-7 December 1998. Based on the achievements made in the previous two workshops, it was aimed at identifying critical issues in *ontology, KIC and knowledge intensive design, and knowledge representations.* These issues later formed three working groups for the KIC-3 workshop. This paper reports the key discussions and conclusions made by these three working groups that were formed from the attendees at the KIC-3 workshop. The workshop's papers presented the current achievements and research issues in KIC.

3. CURRENT ACHIEVEMENTS AND RESEARCH ISSUES IN KIC-3

The section is about the current achievement using the discussion results from the KIC-3 workshop. The workshop has all together seventeen papers and one invited paper. Thirteen papers were accepted for KIC-3 volume after a review. The workshop was assigned into three discussion groups: ontology, knowledge intensive design and knowledge representation, and a keynote paper discusses knowledge life cycle. Key discussions from the invited paper and discussion groups are presented as below.

3.1 Knowledge Life Cycle

The present industry is focused on increasing the volume of projects and customers (and, therefore, revenue), reducing costs and shortening the delivery time and product life cycle. These are the forces that drive the companies throughout the world investigating, assessing, and reengineering their operations to reduce risk, to increase productivity, to streamline the design processes, and to improve their performances through automation and information technology. Effective management of life cycle knowledge is a key element in these activities. In the future, in order for the companies to keep the excellency of business, they must "reuse of existing knowledge" and make sure all knowledge created or learned is just-in-time for later use in a correct, accessible, and trusted manner from the very early stages of design (Mäntylä, 1996).

Blessing and Wallace introduce a conceptual system that supports the knowledge life cycle called process-based support system (PROSUS). In the PROSUS system, the flow of knowledge life cycle is accessible, relevant and trusted by the designers. The authors give an observation about the problem of mismatch between the available information resources and the sources of information that are accessed by designers. The authors give a discussion on the challenge of KIC development to capture this life cycle knowledge and its context, in the way that knowing where and when to apply it, as this knowledge constitutes expertise and is needed to determine relevancy and to build trust. The authors first characterize the intensive knowledge in engineering design as *wide variety of issues, complex relationship between issues, and dynamic nature of the knowledge*. The later focuses their work, in particular on capturing the knowledge that is being created and used in a project, as and when it is being created or used. Design Matrix is used as an approach to group together various types of design issues and life cycle knowledge. The most important contribution of this work is the new way of capturing and indexing life cycle knowledge based on the *context* as and when it is generated, and make it immediately available to other project members.

3.2 Ontology

Current CAD systems support complex tasks but they do not possess the body (intended meaning) of knowledge necessary for generating adequate design solutions. The designer has to take this burden. This burden should be shifted as much as possible back to the CAD systems. Ontology is a promising candidate to help to achieve this. Thus, ontology is a tool that captures the intended meaning of concepts and statements in a domain. Ontology has been studied and developed in artificial intelligence and have been proposed as a specification mechanism for knowledge sharing and reuse across different applications in KIC. A better understanding both of its roles in KIC and of its complex problems was discussed in KIC. Three papers focused on ontology issues in KIC have been presented at the KIC-3 workshop.

Salustri gives a discussion on formalizing a language for a product model considering the basis of the concept of "ontological commitments." The author argues why a totally new representation language is needed. He gives an explanation on how the "ontological commitments" can be constructed to map logical structures to the domain of design knowledge. He then goes on to explain how the commitments are necessary to establish a language for product modeling.

Sekiya, Tsumaya and Tomiyama give a discussion on formalizing structure of knowledge in an integrated manner for a modeling process. They present a Knowledge Intensive Engineering Framework to analyze and validate a design object by integrating various computational tools such as Finite Element Analysis (FEM) and its knowledge. The authors break the design of a FEM model in four stages: a design stage, where the phenomena to be studied via FEM are extracted and identified; an analysis stage, where relevant parameters of the artifact being studied are selected; modeling theory stage, where the artifact and FEM-related knowledge are combined to select a focus for the analysis and choose an appropriate analysis method; and tool stage where a FEM network is generated. The most important contributions of this work are the representation of designer's thought process and the formalization of knowledge in model building.

Shah, Rangaswamy, Qureshi and Urban present a system based on an ISO/STEP compatible data model that has two components: a product and process model. The system aims at supporting the design process by acting as a design history system. The authors concentrate on models of design rationale and suggest implementation using STEP-related tools. The most important contributions of this work are the information model of design rationale and the demonstration that it can be mapped to implementation structures to create a prototype design information capture system.

3.3 KIC and Knowledge Intensive Design

It was not until the mid-1990s that intensive knowledge started to be introduced into CAD, and since then new CAD theories and design concepts have been introduced in line with knowledge management results. KIC is a field of study that focuses on developing computational techniques for performing complex design tasks. The designed product of these processes takes advantage of intensive knowledge flows at different stages. One of the important aspects of addressing intensive knowledge for CAD is to create a design tool that would effectively make reuse of product information at many levels, starting with the functional specifications and overall design rationale and ending with individual product modules, components, and their technical and geometric details. Seven papers were included in this workshop and they presented the most up to date concepts of KIC and knowledge intensive design (KID). Papers of *Xue, Ozawa et al., Rosen, and Yoshioka et al.* discuss the issue of KIC and papers of *Susca et al., Chan et al., and Bok et al.* discuss the issue of KID.

Xue discusses the issues in modeling product life cycle knowledge and data for an intelligent concurrent engineering design system. The author reports on the design and implementation of a concurrent design system that maintains several aspects of a design under development using AND-OR tree structure and feature concepts. The approaches suggested provide a basis for building a KIC system with concurrent design capabilities.

Ozawa, Cutkosky and Howley give an overview of the work done on an agent-based concurrent engineering system and model sharing in a collaborative CAD. The focus of this paper is the development of methods for capturing and exchanging the information that agents need to share in a machine-readable form. The authors first review the design information sharing problem and examine the different levels of abstraction and detail at which such information is represented and shared. They then introduce a representation language and information-sharing infrastructure that was employed in the agent-based concurrent engineering system. The authors describe how this approach can be used to redesign an optical pick-up head for DVD (digital versatile disk) player. The benefits using this approach facilitate (design) model sharing and execute more design tasks in parallel and evaluate design trade-off from the very early design stages.

Rosen discusses integration of product realization processes in RTTB, a system based on decision-based design, which is an approach using explicit problem-solving models created separately by "meta-design" activities. The author also discusses a typical prototyping case study.

Yoshioka, Shamoto and Tomiyama describe the use of KIEF (this concept already appeared and discussed in the previous KIC workshops) environment in a new domain of building foundation design and engineering. The authors usefully illustrate a knowledge intensive CAD system that is capable of describing the casual relationships among physical phenomena and relationships between physical phenomena and analysis methods.

Susca, Mandorli, Rizzi and Cugini describe an application of a commercial knowledge-based configurator to the problem of designing a racing car in a limited problem domain. The authors use knowledge-based engineering technology to represent design information of a car body-weight. The information related to design of a car body, such as design specifications, engineering rules, component shapes and design constraints, is captured in a knowledge-based system. This information is arranged in a polymorphism manner that the digital car model can actually respond in different ways and take many forms driven by the configuration values.

Chan and Finger introduce the concept of "reflective-interactive" design aiming at representing not only the artifact being designed, but also designer's "situation" with respect to the design process, i.e. the design context. They suggest a design artifact model composed of "concepts" and "relationships"; concepts are composed of "phases" related to function, behavior, and form. A rough proof-of-concept implementation is also outlined.

Bok, Myung, Han, Moon and Park describe an experimental system that permits a connection between a commercial CAD system (Solid Edge) and an expert system shell to be created across Internet using distributed object technologies (OLE/DCOM and COBRA). The authors give useful details on the implementation of a KIC system to support commercial product design.

3.4 Knowledge Representation for KIC

Knowledge representation (KR) is a set of syntactic and semantic conventions for describing designer's know-how information. KR syntax specifies on symbols used and the ways they arranged. The study of semantics in KR is mainly focused on how the meaning is attached to the syntax. The sorts of things what need to be represented are design problems, knowledge and reasoning and range from objects, (sequences of) design processes/events, human know-how and what we do not know (human learning). For reasoning, the representations are focused on deductive (inferring new knowledge from old), inductive (inferring generalization from known instances), by analogy (inferences based on similarities), and meta-reasoning (inferences based on meta-knowledge; knowledge about decision making strategies and knowledge about information/raw data). We believe that to create and use a large-scale domain theories with multiple axioms will require concepts such as *machine learning*, advanced *reasoning methods and integrated life cycle knowledge* media and framework. Two papers were selected to discuss the above issues and they present the current state-of-the-art of KR in KIC.

Crecu and Brown focus on *machine learning* in a group of collaborative agents. They claim that agents in CAD have to display flexibility in learning like a human. They usefully discuss the need for *learning*, the parameters of *learning*, where and when to *learn*, and the possibility of refocusing on new *learning* tasks essential for multi-agent design systems. A method of guiding *learning* in multiple agents design systems is described. The basic idea in this method is to use deviations of "expectations" that agents have on each other to trigger a *learning* process. The *learning* itself is based on a "wrapper" that tries to choose the best way to maintain expectations so that unexpected responses of other agents can be accommodated.

Borg, Yan and Juster describe a system that supports the designer by providing knowledge about consequences of the decisions they take. These consequences cover the whole product life cycle. Their work deals with concepts, architecture, implementation and initial experience with a KIC system intended to offer a design environment that can provide a designer with pro-active help about life cycle consequences of design choices.

4. THE FUTURE DIRECTIONS

KIC research and development have undergone considerable changes and improvements over the last three years. KIC has become more complex using new technological developments, well-structured ontology, and better knowledge representation strategies. However, from the viewpoints of practical developments, there are also increasing competition, stronger customers' awareness and stricter regulations. This means that technical products and processes also become complex at the same time. Products have to be technically excellent in design as well as commercially successful. All of these have resulted in better quality, better value for money, shorter time to market and tighter requirements.

New directions to improve effectiveness and efficiency of KIC research and development are needed to cope with these changes and to support the product development in order to remain competitive. The basic needs of industry are making products better, faster, cheaper and meet all the safety regulations. According to Brown (1997), these needs remain the same in the last ten years and future KIC systems have to "satisfy the needs of industry" as one of the goals. There is a new recognition and need that the design process must consider; an effective knowledge management and knowledge life cycle, that can be examined and refined together with the KIC architecture. Knowledge is the key resource that is important to capture, maintain, improve and use within the KIC system. The problem and issue of knowledge management and implementation in KIC are complex. They must be understood both from the practical and the theoretical perspectives. The followings are some research directions that represent various combinations of the practical and theoretical aspects.

4.1 Strategies and Technologies for Knowledge Management

The overall aim of knowledge management (KM) is to *translate knowledge into value*. Technology is, of course, important. Without it, KM will be difficult to implement. This is a good reason to establish a better KIC technology for the future. It is arguable that businesses can only survive and thrive by exploring every possible advantage in an increasingly competitive market. The knowledge that an organization might have range from company's intellectual property (know-how, know-what, know-why and know-who) to the special skills and innovative engineering design processes. These are the assets worth capturing, keeping, sharing and nurturing. Here, the focus of KIC technology is to take a hard look at these sets of assets as the challenges and opportunities that drive the entire engineering design and business process towards better performances and best practices. New KIC research directions must consider the combination of KM with multiple disciplinary designers, strategies and technologies. Future KIC systems have to share knowledge to gain competitive advantages and also to be capable of feeding knowledge from those who have it to those who need it.

The above discussion raises a number of important questions for future KIC development within the scope of KM:

i. How to systematize knowledge?
ii. How to manage knowledge systematically?
iii. How to share knowledge systematically?
iv. How to translate knowledge into value systematically?
v. How to use knowledge?
vi. How to continually absorb and renew knowledge in a KIC system?
vii. How is a successful knowledge management established for a KIC system?
viii. What are the strategic problems that could be solved if knowledge about better performance and best practices were better managed, shared, translated and used systematically within a KIC system?

The first to forth questions lead to issues such as what techniques should be used to manage, share, translate and use knowledge, and what tools can be used to computerize this knowledge structure systematically. The techniques and tools must have these criteria: (i) a shared knowledge representation (language and vocabulary), (ii) protocols that can represent notification and subscription and exchange information, (iii) facilities for context and content-directed routing, and (iv) intelligent matching of information for getting knowledge from "producers" and delivering to "consumers" who need it. Merely archiving knowledge in itself is inadequate; knowledge has to be improved and this is learning. The sixth question leads to issues as what type of machine learning technique can be used to keep up-to-date knowledge systematically. The seventh question leads to issues such as what the influences and validations of successes are how these influences correspond to the engineering design's objectives, and how they are validated or measured. Validation is needed to determine whether our research has been successful. Investigation into these issues will increase our understanding of design as a knowledge-intensive process and that knowledge has to be managed to facilitate the entire design process. The last question gives rises to issues related to the translation of this understanding into new KIC methods and theories considering the KM's elements. It also focuses on tests about the impact of the adopted techniques and tools. The traditional KIC research must be improved to resolve KM issues.

4.2 Implementation of KIC Systems

Future research and development should consider the implementation of the concept of KIC. It is the essential stage in the development of KIC in which the conceptual frameworks, knowledge representation and knowledge-intensive design are modeled in a computer in an executable form, such as programming language or mathematical method. Many current research efforts have focused on giving a systematic conceptual framework and discussed the architectural of the KIC system. Future research should use it to develop a computer-based system in order to test the concept and the feasibility of the methodology. The test is performed by programming a KIC conceptual framework and following this with a computer simulation to implement the codes as a working system, which will facilitate the design.

According to Hew (1998), there are four key steps and checklists in setting up a strategy for KIC implementation using advanced technology. They are outlined below.

Step I: Define the purpose (ultimate design goal) and policy of a KIC system. The first step is to identify the purpose of the system, and the policy about how much information and knowledge to allocate into the system in order to meet the final design goal or business plan. *Checklist*: Have a plan. The plan is important to address a design strategy and find out the application of KIC techniques necessary for business and design goals. Without it, the system developer will simply waste the technology, investment and time. The plan should be a constantly evolving procedure taking account of all details of early design stages input, barriers and objections. Some of the related information and knowledge to be worked out:

i. Basic aim, expressed in term of what the overall functions of KIC system are.
ii. Scope, expressed in term of what the content and context of the knowledge for the KIC system are.

iii. Demand, expressed in term of how the designer would use the KIC system.
iv. Interactive multiple disciplinary knowledge resources for the design process.
v. Design constraints and integration, expressed in term of what the system can do and what it cannot do.
vi. Programming cost, time deadline, computer technology issues and modeling technique.

Step II: Re-design (program) the product in the KIC system. The second step is to know what the design scenarios, desired design activities, design functions, behaviors and states of the model are. It is also necessary to identify the integrated design methods for the multiple models in KIC considering the design scenarios, design activities, functions, behaviors, and states. *Checklist*: Keep it simple. KIC implementers should consider a simple solutions and systems for a complex design. Simply, the user has to be able to understand it. Some of the related information and knowledge to be work out:

i. What are the design activities, modules, design scenarios, functions, behaviors and states?
ii. Who is the user?
iii. How to divide each design activity, design scenarios, functions, behaviors, states into computer-based models in KIC and how many?
iv. How will the models be run and organized together, so that they can be interactively related each other?
v. What prototyping techniques and communication tools are required to program KIC and its design models?

Step III: Integrate knowledge using a synthesis and analysis design thought process. The third step is to consider an integrated design environment for KIC. Design is an interactive design process involving multiple disciplinary knowledge. It is important to identify a thought process to operate the knowledge in this interactive environment. According to Tomiyama (1998) and Hew *et al.* (1999), design knowledge operation can be systematically and mathematically defined by referring to analysis oriented and synthesis oriented thought processes. Elements of design knowledge that need to be interactively related and operated from one to another are know-how, rules, standards, design requirements and anticipated physical needs for the environment (such as stiffness, energy consumption, maintenance, green and environmental issues, etc.), down to the smallest conceivable detail. *Checklist*: Plan top down, but implement bottom up and avoid over-integration. Implementation as an inside-out or bottom-up approach builds from the smallest knowledge elements to form a larger component of the product. There must be a trade-off between flexibility and integration, in particular, it should not replace the creativity of designer, but support the designer with useable knowledge.

Step IV: Implement KIC techniques and solutions to achieve *Step I's* purpose and policy. At this stage, a KIC system will be implemented module by module, or model by model, and in stages. KIC is implemented only if it is needed to achieve business needs and engineering design goals. *Checklist*: Be committed. A move towards the development of a "good engineering design assistant system" for the design process is needed. It is important to believe that such assistance is achievable. Support from senior management is demanded, for, without this commitment, the project cannot in any case succeed. Some of the related information and knowledge to be work out:

i. What are the current industry barriers?
ii. What are the current designer objections?
iii. What are human factors in accepting change?
iv. How to achieve adequate investment?
v. What is the adequate computing technique for KIC?

The motivation for setting up this brief and implementation strategy is to make sure that the application of KIC and its technique will be right, because in the end, it does not depend on the technology alone, but on organization and multi-disciplinary factors. The KIC system must be applied in order to integrate under a design support system. For example, users and system developers must understand what information others need, when they need it, and how to control and distribute it. The KIC implementation, for every stage of engineering design process, can result in either a powerful enabling tool in improving the design process, or a burden of useless and costly complexity. Thus, the KIC integrated design concept, although easy in execution, must be subject to detailed scrutiny considering every aspect of the design activities and life cycle knowledge. In particular, it must be simple to use.

4.3 Practical Application of a KIC System

The working system of KIC in the industry should be further improved for commercial use and practical application, rather than remaining as a research tool. This would require the setting up of a strategy, software system and team. We suggest six practical design lessons for the basic and successful application of KIC systems.

i. It is needed to have a framework for underlying structure and classifying the terms for the knowledge as models.
ii. KIC systems must meet the daily needs of users/designers.

iii. It needs a clear strategy for KIC to contribute to optimize design and the business.
iv. The application should emphasize on what works, but not perfection. Practically KIC should be focused on knowledge structure, knowledge integration, function specification, desired behavior, and technology.
v. Is necessary to involve senior management in the initiative of KIC application.
vi. Measure the impact of KIC from the very beginning.

One of the successful criteria of KIC system is to solve the problem of knowledge archipelago (islands of knowledge). We point out that it is important to have a strategy, framework and computer-based models to support the practical application of the KIC system. It is because without these, the practical application process will end up in chaos. The computer-based models and the knowledge strategists need to work together. The focus must be getting the right information from the right resources at the right time for the potential users to meet the needs of works. The system must be able to improve the design processes and even can support the business plan. Contribution to the business is one way to market the system by fixing the organization's vision and values with the practical application of KIC. However, it is important to understand that KIC technology is pragmatism and it always has its limits. Thus, the application shall only "focus on what works, not perfection." We recommend that we should emphasize solving the strategic problems in knowledge structure, knowledge integration, function specification, desired behavior, resulting physical states and exploring the enabling technology. In order to apply KIC successfully, it is necessary to have the involvement of senior management, substantial funding and organization reformation or change. This is for removing barriers, making application a priority, and eliminate negative impacts on the gathering of knowledge from multiple disciplinary. Finally, measurement of the impact of KIC application in term of benefit, strength and weakness of the system must be carried out from the beginning. Someone will ultimately question whether benefits are derived from the investment cost on KIC. Thus, it is necessary to monitor the contributions and impacts of KIC applications that can spell out the "advantages" and "proof of the values." Further discussion related to measurement is discussed in the sub-sequence section.

4.4 Measuring and Evaluating the Impact of a KIC System: Verification and Validation

The KIC system must be attested. Verification and validation are the critical evaluation factors of a KIC project. In fact it is equally important to work out these KIC's measurers, as to celebrate the successes of the application. We strongly recommended that the measuring process should be planned from the very beginning of the research and figure out the contributions of the KIC system versus the measurement's factors. There are many other factors in measurement process, however it may be helpful to bear the following two factors in mind: verification and validation. Verification is the process which measures whether the KIC system conforms to the architectural framework and specifications developed as part of the computational methodology (Sriram, 1997). In the verification process, we suggest to measure the correctness and significance of the KIC after the system is implemented properly. Validation is the process which measures whether the implemented KIC system performs the functions that it is intended for (Sriram, 1997). In the validation process, we suggest to measure the application of KIC to see if the system can solve the right problem. Validation in KIC involves setting up criteria for success and measuring the success from these criteria after carefully studying the strength and the weakness features of the system.

The followings are some keys for success or milestone for the measurement phase:

i. Plan the measurement process as early as possible in the development and application of KIC, so that knowledge gathering can be organized around the system and any necessary strategy and technical skills can be appropriated for the research goals.
ii. It is important to be thoroughly familiar with the methods of measurement and must understand how to deviate from them.
iii. Test the contributions of KIC wherever possible using the measurement methods suggested.
iv. Present the finding to the industry experts (or targeting users) as you go so that it is clear what you are claiming.
v. Expose all the measurements to the scrutiny of the industry experts (or targeting users) and review them so as it progresses in order to make the system to stand for the "proof of the values."
vi. Respond to all the doubts expressed by the targeting users and senior management about the contribution of the KIC system, and check whether the measurement methods have the necessary depth for your level of research in KIC.
vii. It is always safe to do more than necessary.

There are several techniques that can be used in the measurement phase. It is suggested that the performance of the system can be measured up using:

i. Industry as a field trial.
ii. Test design scenario or protocol.
iii. Test design data.

4.5 Capturing the Life Cycle Knowledge as the Content of KIC

Future KIC systems must include the life cycle knowledge as the content of the systems, to generate more added-value. These values are, for instance, manufacturability, design for assemble ability, consumer serviceability, recyclability, reusability, and disposal ability. The goal of capturing the life cycle knowledge in KIC systems is to maximize these values in design, while minimizing its costs and environmental impacts. Developing a life cycle knowledge intensive system to support this is a challenging task because of the following characteristics:

i. Large quantity of life cycle knowledge.
ii. Wide diversity of values in life cycle knowledge.
iii. Fragmented relationship within the life cycle knowledge.
iv. Complexity in knowledge-creation from capturing and storing knowledge, to retrieving and reuse of knowledge.
v. Usefulness of the knowledge in the life cycle design stages.
vi. Dynamism of life cycle knowledge.

Future research directions in life cycle knowledge for KIC should encounter the following problems and research questions:

i. Systematic methodologies that can support the design easier as well as more complete using the life cycle knowledge.
ii. Implementation issues for the essential life cycle knowledge in a systematic manner.
iii. Where the life cycle starts and ends?
iv. Knowledge life cycle is triggered off by what factors?
v. How to maintain the cyclical and interactive nature of knowledge life cycle?

5 CONCLUSION

The papers presented in the KIC-3 workshop provided a vivid discussion on many other themes of interest in knowledge intensive CAD. This paper reported an overview of an important discussion from each individual paper. The papers discuss not only theoretical aspects but also practical systems and experiences. Overall, the workshop successfully provided the participants with multiple-disciplinary views of the subject both from computer science and engineering design research angles.

This paper also reported and contributed effectively to the future development and application of knowledge-intensive CAD. More research needs to be done in helping the research design, from life cycle knowledge, theory, implementation strategy, measurement, to practical application. The working system of KIC should be further improved for commercial use, rather than remaining as a research tool. This would require the setting up of a software production system (or team) which would involve considerable financial investment.

REFERENCES

Brown D.C., Waldron M.B., Yoshikawa H. (1992) *Intelligent Computer Aided Design*, North-Holland.

Brown, D.C. (1997) "Which Way to KIC?" *Knowledge Intensive CAD*, Vol. 2, (eds.) Mäntylä, M., Finger, S, Tomiyama, T., Chapman & Hall.

Hew, K.P. (1998) *A Knowledge-Based Electronic Prototype System (KEPS) for Building and Services Design Integration*, Ph.D. Thesis, The University of Reading, UK.

Hew, K.P., Washio, T., Tomiyama, T., Umeda, Y. (1999) "Mathematical Theory of Synthesis Design: Foundation, Framework and Method", *Proceeding of 4th International Design Thinking Research Symposium on Design Representation*, MIT, April 23-25, 1999, pp. II, 205-217.

Mäntylä, M., Finger, S, Tomiyama, T. (1997) *Knowledge Intensive CAD, Vol. 2*, Chapman & Hall.

Mäntylä, M. (1996) "Knowledge-Intensive CAD: Introduction and a Research Agenda", *Knowledge Intensive CAD*, Vol. 1, (eds.) Tomiyama, T., Mäntylä, M., Finger, S., Chapman & Hall, 1996.

Sriram, R.D. (1997) *Intelligent System for Engineering*, Springer.

Tomiyama, T., Mäntylä, M., Finger, S. (1996) *Knowledge Intensive CAD*, Vol. 1, Chapman & Hall.

Tomiyama, T. (1998) "An Overview of the Modeling of Synthesis Project", *International Symposium on Modeling of Synthesis*, The University of Tokyo, Japan, 5 December, 1998, pp. 3-12.

Yoshikawa, H., Gossard, D. (1989) *Intelligent CAD I*, North-Holland.

Yoshikawa, H., Holden, T. (1990) *Intelligent CAD II*, North-Holland.

Yoshikawa, H., Arbab, F., Tomiyama, T. (1991) *Intelligent CAD III*, North-Holland.

PART TWO

INVITED TALK

2

Supporting the Knowledge Life-Cycle

Luciënne Blessing and Ken Wallace
Engineering Design Centre, University of Cambridge, UK

Key words: Knowledge life-cycle, Product development, Design process

Abstract: This paper describes the mismatch between the information sources available to designers and the information sources accessed by designers. Possible reasons for this mismatch are accessibility, availability and trustworthiness. Current support for product development does not deal with this issue because only part of the knowledge life-cycle is addressed. A model of the knowledge life-cycle is introduced that focuses on knowledge generation. To support the knowledge life-cycle, a system is introduced based on a model of the design process. This system, PROSUS, is discussed and the issues needing further development identified.

1. INTRODUCTION

Engineering design is a knowledge-intensive activity. The knowledge used comes from a variety of sources, including those within the company as well as those outside, and those related to work as well as those not related to work. This knowledge includes that gained from positive and negative experiences. Knowledge is stored as information and data in handbooks, drawings, documents, electronic means and, in particular, in the heads of individuals. As products become more complex and competition intensifies, it is essential to make the maximum use of the available knowledge and to deliver that knowledge in the appropriate form at the right time in the product development process. Developing a knowledge-intensive system to support this is a challenging task because of the following knowledge-related characteristics of engineering design:

– wide variety of issues to be addressed;

– complex relationships between issues;
– dynamic nature of the issues.

These characteristics make the development of knowledge-intensive CAD a challenging task and are the reason why the design process will continue to be driven by human designers.

1.1 Wide variety

Knowledge of various technical and non-technical domains has to be combined when designing engineering products in order to address the multitude of life-cycle issues, and also the requirements and constraints of all business functions and external parties. This variety is expressed, or should be expressed, in the requirements specification. Several methods and models have been developed to help designers obtain an overview of the relevant issues. Examples include: checklists for formulating requirements, e.g. [Pahl and Beitz 1996]; QFD to assist designers with the translation of customer needs into technical demands [Clausing 1994]; Pugh's Information Input model [Pugh 1991]; and the overview of properties of technical systems and life-cycle demands from the environment as given by [Hubka and Eder 1988].

1.2 Complex relationships

Engineering design is knowledge intensive because of the wide variety of issues involved and because of the complex relationships between the issues. Hubka and Eder illustrate this by describing the multitude of relationships between design properties. According to Altschuller [1984] a design problem exists *because* of a contradiction between the requirements placed on two related properties, e.g. high stiffness and low weight.

The existence of these relationships requires the ability to make trade-offs. Some argue that design is essentially a process of trading off requirements and constraints. Every design project is different because at least some of the requirements or constraints have changed. This means that there is no unique route to a solution and no single solution to a design problem.

1.3 Dynamic nature

Engineering design is also knowledge intensive because of the dynamic nature of the knowledge applied. This is captured in the term experience: every step in a design project adds knowledge, at least to the individual involved. Design is a continuous learning process: the knowledge base changes continuously. For systems to be truly knowledge intensive, it is necessary for them to take into account the dynamic nature of the knowledge. This knowledge can relate to the *product* being designed as well as to the design *process* being undertaken. Currently most of the knowledge captured explicitly relates to the product.

1.4 Focus

Our work focuses on capturing the knowledge that is being created and used in a project, as and when it is being created and used. In this way the variety of knowledge and the "trade-off" knowledge is captured most comprehensively, whilst doing justice to its dynamic nature.

The next section discusses why capturing the knowledge that is being generated and used, rather than simply the product-related outputs of the design process, is the focus of our work. Section 3 introduces the knowledge life-cycle and provides an outline of the requirements of a support tool based on this life-cycle model. Section 4 gives a summary of the PROSUS system, which addresses the life-cycle issues we consider essential. Section 5 discusses PROSUS in the light of the knowledge life-cycle. The concluding section presents the issues that still need to be addressed.

2. KNOWLEDGE USE

The need to capture knowledge as it is being generated and used suggests that the knowledge currently captured in various forms is not sufficient. The wish of many companies to store more knowledge seems strange at a time when more knowledge and information than ever are available. However, comparing some research findings shows an interesting mismatch between what is available and what is being used.

2.1 Mismatch between availability and use

University libraries, such as those in Cambridge, need about 4 kilometres of shelving space to stock the most essential scientific literature generated in one year. About 1.5 million new books are published in the world each year [Ehrlenspiel 1997]. The amount of information stored within a company has also reached enormous proportions. For example, the development of an aero engine produces approximately 40,000 documents. At Rolls-Royce the technical library is reported to support 60 million sheets of A4 documentation per quarter [Marsh 1997]. New technologies are increasingly used to reduce storage space and increase availability. The large amount of shelving space needed for books and documents can be reduced to a few metres when CD ROMs are used as the storage medium. In 1997, around 200,000 new pages were installed on the Internet each day and the number is growing rapidly [Ehrlenspiel 1997]. Some are convinced that one day we will never need to visit a library because we will simply search the WWW and download the relevant information directly into our computers.

At the same time, observations in industry indicate that the single greatest factor (30% of cases) underlying wrong decisions is lack of information, rather than lack of experience [Frankenberger and Badke-Schaub 1997]. This is not due to the time researchers spent searching for information. Several researchers found the proportion of a designer's time absorbed by information acquisition activities to be between 20-30% [Court 1995, Marsh 1997]. Marsh also found that the majority of information is obtained from personal contacts, confirming earlier findings such as [Lera et al 1984, Hales 1987, Blessing 1994]. In 78% of cases these contacts retrieved the information from their memories. Formally recorded information was obtained on average twice each day, but was accessed directly in only 55% of cases observed, that is it is often obtained through others. This is interesting because the company studied by Marsh stores large amounts of information about past cases. It is also interesting to note that despite new technologies that should make retrieval easier and quicker, the percentages do not seem to have changed significantly.

The effect on the working environment of using personal contacts for obtaining information is large. Marsh [Marsh 1997] observed that there is less than a 50% chance of working continuously for longer than 8 minutes before an interruption occurs stemming from a designer's own requirements for information or those of colleagues. The chance of working for 30 minutes or more is less than 25%. Also, as most searches for information involve two people, the required effort could be reduced by up to 50% if a good non-human source of information was available.

On the one hand the findings suggest superabundant information, on the other hand a strong, almost sole, reliance on personal contacts. Three possible reasons are:

- accessibility of documented information;
- availability of relevant information;
- trustworthiness of information.

Supporting evidence for all three reasons is presented below.

2.2 Accessibility

Several studies have concluded that it is often difficult to find the relevant information. Earlier studies, summarised in [Lera et al 1984], have revealed that information was perceived as either inaccessible, unavailable or not in an applicable form, and that consulting written information was seen as time consuming. The latter perception was also observed in more recent experimental studies where the subjects relied on the experiment leader to answer questions. This was presumably because of the ease with which the information could be obtained, even though all the information was available to them in written form [Kuffner and Ullman 1991]. These findings were confirmed in the experiments described in [Blessing 1994] and [Klaubert 1998]. The studies discussed earlier in this section show similar results by indicating the large number of personal contacts used as information sources, despite the fact that more and more information is available in electronic format intended to accelerate access.

One of the problems appears to be that sources such as the Internet have grown so large and diverse that it is not unusual for a search to result in several thousand "hits", of which only a few are relevant. Commercial claims (KPMG consultants in [Marsh 1997]) are that 95% of filed documents are only ever retrieved once, and that is to discard them. A major problem of accessing existing databases is because their indexing systems were set up before knowing what information will eventually be requested. Research is ongoing into making large legacy databases containing product and process data more accessible, without resorting to keywords and predefined indices [Carlton 1998].

2.2.1 Availability

Relevant information is not always available. Marsh looked into the different types of information and their impact on the working time of designers. He showed that on average 24% of each designer's working day was spent obtaining or providing information. This 24% was made up as follows:

- 6% of time was spent on product-based information acquisition. This is anything relating directly to factual knowledge about the product, its description, specification, and associated design data.
- 11% of time was spent on process-based information. This information represents knowledge about how to perform tasks, approach problems, etc.
- 3% of time was spent on resource information. This includes knowledge about how to operate complex computer-based tools, the information provided by standards, formal representation of "know-how", etc.

- 4% of time was spent on miscellaneous information. This information is concerned with arranging meetings, organising information flow, etc.

In particular, process-based information was difficult to find in a generally accessible form. Product-based information was only partially available. The lessons learnt, the rationale behind the product, and the various alternatives that were considered but rejected, were normally only to be found in designers' notebooks, if at all. This, in particular, is the knowledge that builds up into experience: the information that makes designers "experts".

The knowledge of experts is considered difficult to capture. In addition, this knowledge can be contradictory, as research in the field of knowledge acquisition has clearly demonstrated. Marsh [Marsh 1997] concluded from his study that in the engineering environment he observed only a quarter of queries relating to design expertise, answered with reference to past experience, required the abilities of an expert to evaluate, interpret and explain. The single greatest use made of experts was to provide an awareness of alternatives, of concerns, of work carried out in the past, of problem symptoms, etc. It is significant that the contributions made by experts in the majority of cases was comparable to the type of support that *could* be provided by structured information management and knowledge capture, rather than the replication of human cognitive abilities.

The need for this knowledge to be more widely available has led to companies applying a variety of approaches to capture expertise. Rolls-Royce, for example, has started a "lessons learnt" database and is engaged in a project to capture knowledge from experts using novices to undertake the knowledge acquisition. British Gas, on the other hand, is employing knowledge engineers to capture the knowledge. The techniques used have one significant disadvantage, namely the retrospective nature of the resulting information. This issue is discussed in section 3.

2.3 Trustworthiness

Trust in the information supplied is an important reason why information sources, even those generated within a company, may not be accessed and why designers prefer to go to experts who are considered to be more knowledgeable and up-to-date. This factor should not be underestimated. Adding to a database the source, date of entry and, most importantly, the context in which the information was used, could help built trust and confidence.

3. KNOWLEDGE LIFE-CYCLE

The previous section suggests that much information is available, but what is requested most, namely expertise, is not available or difficult to access. As this is the knowledge generated during the design activity, knowledge-intensive CAD represents a challenging task.

A knowledge-intensive environment cannot rely on a *knowledge use-cycle*, that is Capture-Store-Retrieve-Reuse. Reuse is too limited because it suggests that the knowledge being used does not change. Our use of the word knowledge includes within it the knowledge of where and when it can be applied. As such, knowledge includes the expertise that is needed to determine relevancy and build trust. Using this concept of knowledge means that every time knowledge is used new knowledge is generated, even if it is only further detailed knowledge about how the knowledge was applied.

When developing any knowledge-based support for design it is important that the whole *knowledge life-cycle* is taken into account, see Figure 1. In order to know what to capture, it is important to investigate what is used. What is captured needs to be stored in such a way that it is easy to retrieve and is relevant to the situation in which it is going to be used. Use of knowledge may be successful, if, when it is retrieved and possibly adapted, it is useful in the new situation. Use of knowledge may also be unsuccessful, if when it is retrieved it is not useful. However, in both cases new knowledge is generated. This new knowledge may replace or refine old knowledge, or be a new addition. The knowledge base needs to be continually updated. This is like a basic learning process. A more sophisticated learning process involves generating meta-knowledge (knowledge about knowledge) or generic knowledge from what has been captured and stored. The dynamic nature of knowledge is determined by the generation of new knowledge as a result of knowledge use, that is a continual "learning process".

Figure 1 can be seen as the representation of the knowledge life-cycle of an individual, of a team, and of a company. In each of these cases, the term "outside sources" takes on a different meaning. The outside sources themselves have their own knowledge life-cycles. Knowledge from outside sources can be captured directly, for example at the start of building a knowledge base, or it can be captured indirectly, for example when certain knowledge elements are being used and are captured as a consequence of this use. The latter is the preferred route as the relevance to work in hand is guaranteed.

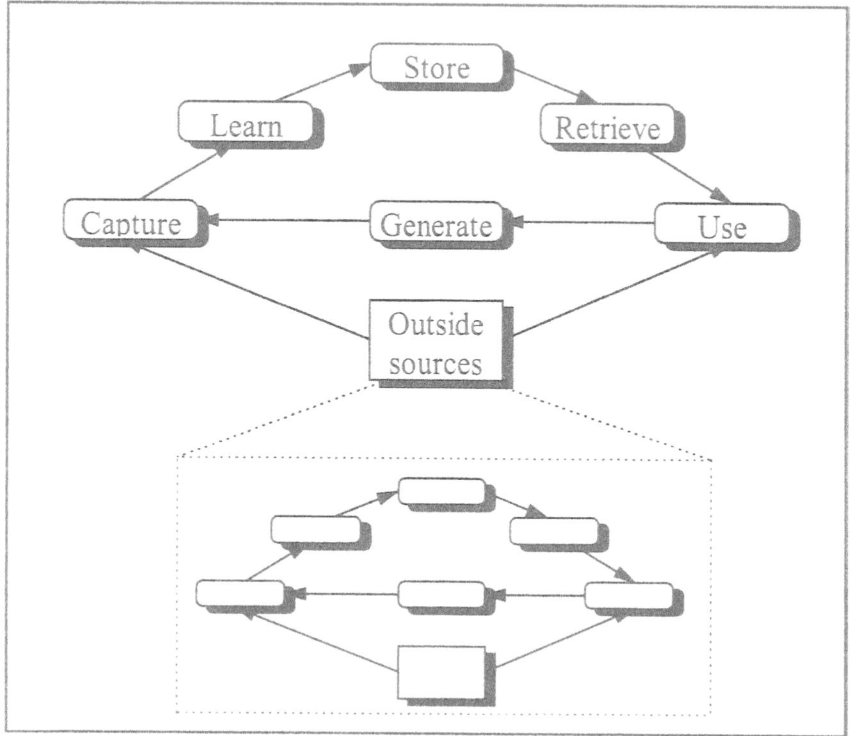

Figure 1. The knowledge life-cycle

Knowledge is *generated* throughout the design process, and in large quantities, by everyone involved. Capturing this knowledge after the event requires considerable additional effort and results in a retrospective account. Depending on the frequency of capturing, this may result in loss of important knowledge. Capturing knowledge therefore needs to be done in real time, that is as and when it is being generated and by the people who are generating it. Knowledge engineers can be involved at the start, to build the initial knowledge base, but subsequently their role should be no more than that of webmasters.

Capturing knowledge in real time has the advantage that knowledge can be made available soon after its creation. This improves the communication within a design team by having the latest information available on which to base decisions, in particular if these decisions require trade-offs between different aspects of the product.

The consequence of relying on a busy user to capture the knowledge means that it is unlikely that the generated knowledge will be abstracted or that a conscious effort to identify and extract reusable knowledge fragments will take place, as suggested in [Duffy et al 1995]. Instead, the knowledge-cycle will have to be based on a basic learning process. This learning includes comparing the newly-captured knowledge with the stored knowledge and deciding on the required updates. Techniques such as machine learning will have to be used to derive meta-knowledge and generic knowledge from the captured and stored knowledge. It has been suggested that to make knowledge useful, some abstraction and transformation is needed [Mantyla 1996]. We think that the knowledge as it is generated and captured by the user, supported by automated indexing based on the context in which the knowledge is generated, can make this knowledge useful for reuse. Any abstraction may enhance the usefulness of the knowledge, but is not essential.

Ideally a design support system is only populated with knowledge that might be retrieved, rather than that what is known. There is little use in capturing the knowledge every designer is familiar with, unless this knowledge is stored to automate certain design tasks. We are interested in the knowledge that differentiates experts from novices; the knowledge and experience generated during design projects. As we described earlier, most of this knowledge currently comes from memory. The knowledge captured in memory is context dependent, is based on personal beliefs and opinions, and is often heuristic in nature. The main challenge is to capture this knowledge along with its context.

New structures are needed to store the knowledge as current product models are unsuitable. A system has been developed that addresses the knowledge life-cycle with the aim of capturing a greater proportion of what is generated during a design process, the context in which it is generated, as well as the rationale and other process-related knowledge. The next section gives an outline of the structure of the system. A discussion of how the system addresses the various stages in the knowledge life-cycle can be found in section 5.

4. A PROCESS-BASED SUPPORT SYSTEM

The proposed system addresses the knowledge life-cycle in order to help improve the design process. Its main focus is on: capturing design data[1] resulting from design activities throughout the design process; and assisting

[1] The use of the term "data" rather than knowledge in this context is based on the definition that what is generated is data until linked to other contextual data and processed in some way, that is until it obtains meaning. This implies that design data contains knowledge for the experienced user of that data.

in the creation of this data. Design data contains the knowledge that is used and generated in a design project. As it is not possible to obtain a complete set of design data, it is important to ensure that one can represent and reason with what is captured, i.e. what one can expect the designer to make explicit within the constraints of an industrial context [Blessing 1996].

Design data includes:

- *product data* describing the product covering: all stages of development, including the requirements specification, functional diagrams, sketches, drawings, calculations, graphs, etc; the whole product-life cycle, including production plans, user manuals, maintenance instructions, etc; and all the alternatives that were considered at every stage of the process.
- *process data* including the rationale behind product data such as arguments and decisions related to the various stages of the product and the various alternatives that were considered; and the information to support the arguments, along with the various aspects of the business involved.
- *process administration data* including the planned and actually applied resources (who did what, when and how).

In particular, much process data is lacking in current project documentation, and so are descriptions of the various alternatives and the reasons why some of these were rejected.

Capturing design data is the most direct way of capturing knowledge and hence making it available. In an earlier paper [Blessing 1996] it was argued that:

- it would be ideal to capture all design data;
- only a small fraction is currently being captured;
- we cannot capture all data;
- we can capture more;
- a low level of indexing detail can be sufficient;
- capturing and indexing should be in real time;
- capturing and indexing should be based on the process.

4.1 The PROSUS concept

PROSUS, a PROcess-based SUpport System, is a workbench that aims to improve the design process by using a *process model* as its core to capture the data resulting from design activities, and to support the creation of these data throughout the process [Blessing 1994]. The process model:

- provides process-related guidance to the designer or design team, but allows different approaches;
- provides a structure for the design team to document and retrieve design data in all stages of the design process;

- provides the basis for the system to determine the context in which the data were generated and use this to automatically index the data;
- enables the system to suggest relevant knowledge, methods, tools, design histories throughout the design process because these can be linked to steps in the design process.

PROSUS enables a shift in the task distribution and different levels of implementation to adapt to developments in computer technology, to new software for particular design activities, and to specific company characteristics.

PROSUS has three levels:

- *primary level* containing the basic building block of PROSUS, the Design Matrix, which is the main working area for the design team based on the process model;
- *control level* to determine the strategy, that is the sequence of steps in the process model or matrix;
- *support level* to determine the best support (method, tools, history) to execute a step.

This paper concentrates on the primary level, the core of which has been implemented. For more details about the other levels see [Blessing 1994].

4.2 The core of PROSUS: the design matrix

The basic building block of PROSUS is the design matrix. This matrix is based on a combination and extension of two complementary models: Methodical Design, a problem-oriented approach to design [Pahl and Beitz 1996, van den Kroonenberg 1978]; and IBIS, an Issue-Based Information System based on the approach to design proposed by Rittel [Kunz and Rittel 1970, McCall 1986].

The design matrix represents the design process as a structured set of *issues* and *activities* and is the interface between the user and the system. Figure 2 shows a simplified design matrix. For reasons of clarity, the various issues following "Concept", including assembly, installation, material, geometry, etc, have been grouped under the heading "Detail design".

Each cell can be envisaged as an area in which designers can document the results, both final and intermediate, of executing that particular step. Specific tools are not available for every step in the design process (a cell in the matrix), particularly during the early stages of the design process. For this reason, a default text tool and graphics sketching tool are linked to every cell.

The rows of the design matrix cover the different issues that need to addressed during the design process[2]. The list of issues can be adapted to suit the approach of a specific company. The columns of the design matrix relate to the activities of the deliberation process needed to resolve an issue.

The left-hand column contains the relevant *issues*. Each issue can be addressed in three steps: Generate, Evaluate and Select. A Generate step results in *proposals*. This column may also contain data such as calculations or references to knowledge used to develop a proposal. Evaluation is the comparison of each proposal with the requirements and results in one or more candidate solutions, arguments and decisions. ***Arguments*** give the design rationale supporting or opposing a proposal. Arguments are the basis for taking decisions but can also lead to new issues or proposals. ***Decisions*** describe the status of a proposal. In the case of more than one candidate solution, a selection has to be made to decide upon the solution to pursue further by comparing the candidates. This activity results in a decision to select one or more solutions together with the arguments for this selection. Evaluation focuses to a large extent on the demands in the requirements list; selection focuses more on the wishes, and involves making trade-offs. As a consequence, different methods and tools are used for each of these activities.

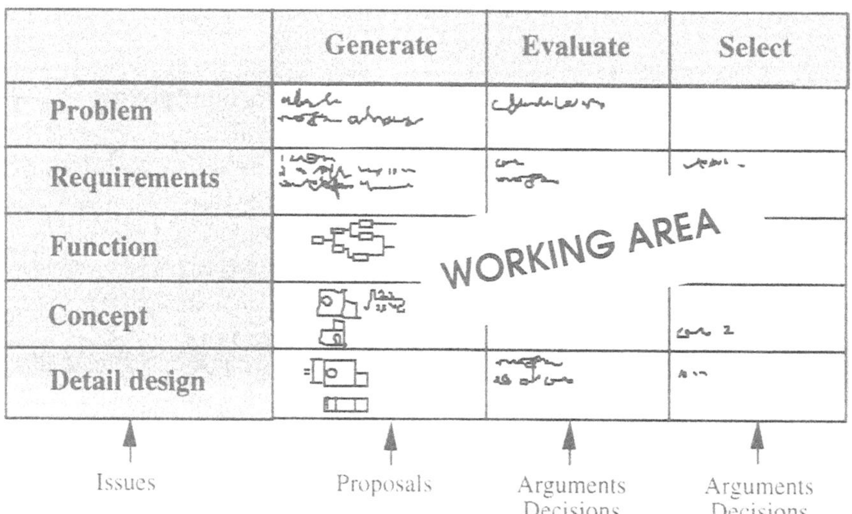

Figure 2. A simplified design matrix

[2] The word "issue" is often used to refer to a (potential) problem that needs attention, such as "reduce noise". In this context, problems such as "reduce noise" are considered to be aspects, probably formulated as requirements that are dealt with during evaluation or selection.

The process model repeats itself in a slightly modified form for every assembly and component in the product. To support indexing and retrieval of the documented data, a separate matrix is used for each assembly (including the overall product) and component. Every design project therefore consists of a set of matrices, all linked together. The product and assembly matrices are identical. They only differ from the component matrices in the detail design issues they address. The matrix for standard components differs also in the first few issues.

4.3 Capturing design data

Data can be entered into the design matrix in any order; no sequence of addressing the cells is prescribed, nor do all cells have to be filled in. The cell in which the data is entered provides the context for the system to "understand" what the data is about and attach the relevant indices. These indices include the step in the process (the cell index), the user, the date and the time.

All data are captured in units called events. Every event is uniquely numbered within a project. An event relates to a specific combination of product element, issue, activity, method, tool, person and time. In terms of the matrix, this means that a move to another cell will start a new event, as does the use of a new method or tool, or another designer beginning to work on the project. In addition, designers can decide to start a new event, for example to generate a new alternative. Events can "live" in parallel.

When designing it is often not possible to know whether a product element will be an assembly or a component. The designer can choose to postpone this decision and start working on a matrix containing only the first four issues, which are identical for every matrix.

The system captures the various versions of the proposals that are generated to maintain a track record. In addition the system actively supports the generation and capture of alternatives.

Once completed, a design matrix contains a description of the design process for a specific product element. The description is structured around the rationale applied and may not be chronological. It is considered more important to see, for example, the various alternatives that were generated for a particular component clustered together, and the order in which they were generated, than to know exactly when they were generated. Each matrix structures the (intermediate) results of the process independently of the sequence in which they were generated, but, as each piece of data is automatically time-stamped, the chronological order can be retrieved when required.

4.4 Supporting the generation of design data

A design matrix is more than a structured and passive notebook. The use of a process model allows PROSUS to suggest relevant knowledge, methods, tools and design histories, as these aids can be linked to specific activities, that is to one or more cells. When the designer is generating requirements, for example, the system is aware of this because it can detect the cell in which the designer is working. As a consequence the system can suggest to the user checklists and specification building tools, or the requirements list set up for the assembly one level up in the product hierarchy. The links between matrix cells and tools are currently structured as a direct links though the intention is to make them agent driven.

4.5 Initial evaluation

An initial evaluation of the use of the matrices in a design process focused on the applicability and usefulness of the design matrix concept [Blessing 1994, 1996]. The evaluation involved experienced designers and was based on a comparison of the design processes of two groups of designers: one working with the design matrices and one working without them. The findings were promising and justified further development. Since then a prototype has been implemented [Ball et al 1998] and is currently being evaluated.

5. PROSUS AND THE KNOWLEDGE LIFE-CYCLE

5.1 Capture

The use of the design matrix provides a way of capturing and indexing based on the context in which the data were generated. The context is defined by: the project; the product element and its relation to the rest of the product; the issue; the activity; the time; and the date. In addition, the author and the means used are captured. The event number (see 4.3) relates each data element to data captured in other events. This context is captured together with the data itself, which is only possible because the system is based on a process model.

PROSUS thus allows the capture of knowledge and its context as and when it is generated, and makes it immediately available (read-only) to other project members. It captures the dynamic and opportunistic nature of the design process, which is necessary to understand the decisions taken and the data that is used and generated. Obviously this requires the collaboration of the users, but the hope is that using PROSUS will encourage designers to document more of their processes. The initial evaluation of the matrix concept provided support for this hope.

5.2 Learn

Currently all that is captured is stored directly without any checks. The database is up-to-date because it contains the latest data. The users do consistency checks. The availability of all data, including the context, makes this task easier. Immediate availability, including the results of all the steps in the process, whether erroneous or not, are the primary drivers behind PROSUS.

It is assumed that it is better to have the various opinions stored next to each other with context, author and date, than to try to find the best opinion, even if this exists. This allows future users to determine what is relevant in their own situation. The fact that negative experiences are also captured is very important, as these constitute a large part of the lessons learnt. Nevertheless, more attention needs to be paid to the aspect of updating and real learning from the captured data as discussed in section 3.

5.3 Store

Data elements are indexed and stored as and when they are generated. Retrospective capturing and indexing is not considered to be a feasible alternative given the enormous time pressures in industry and the potentially biased nature of recollecting events and decisions. The indexing system is based on what can be expected from the designers while working on developing a product, and on what indices could be captured automatically.

To enable the variety of captured data to be stored, a product model has been developed in which product as well as process data can be stored [Ball 1998].

5.4 Retrieve

PROSUS is based on the assumption that the whole knowledge life-cycle is essentially in the hands of the users, that is the design teams. This led to the decision to use the same indices for capturing and retrieving, and base these on the design process as well as the product. Typical search queries might be: show all concept alternatives that were generated for assembly X in project Y; provide the reasons why a particular material was chosen;

present the use and safety considerations of a particular component; and indicate the complete set of requirements used in a particular project.

The concept of events allows the replay of the history of an individual's activities; the activities related to a particular project or to a particular product element within a project; and also the events related to an earlier retrieved event. This linking of activities provides some understanding of the rationale in so far as this is not captured.

It would be useful if knowledge could be derived from what is captured and stored to support the retrieval of relevant data in projects with which the designer is unfamiliar. This is likely to require transformation and abstraction. Care should be taken that the context and any existing differences in opinion remain available, or at least accessible.

5.5 Use

Using PROSUS as a workbench would allow direct access to available methods, tools, knowledge and design histories. This would:

- encourage the consideration of knowledge generated in previous projects;
- support the use of up-to-date project related data;
- increase documentation of a project (e.g. for liability cases or reuse);
- encourage a more systematic approach to the process (project management);
- support teamwork by providing a communication aid.

In addition it could increase familiarity with and use of the various existing design tools in industry.

5.6 Generation

The use of PROSUS, and the supporting tools it suggests to the designer, supports the generation of new data, and allows this to be captured. Part of the newly created data will immediately be captured if a computer tool is used. However, most tools do not normally produce intermediate results and process-related data. Accessing the tools via PROSUS allows the system to capture at least some of the intermediate results and process-related data.

6. CONCLUSIONS

A mismatch has been observed between the information sources available to designers and the information sources accessed by designers. Possible reasons for this mismatch are lack of accessibility, availability and trustworthiness. Current support for product development does not appear to deal with this issue, because it only addresses part of the knowledge life-cycle A knowledge life-cycle was introduced that emphasises the generation of knowledge as the consequence of using knowledge.

The proposed design support system, PROSUS, was not developed to explicitly address the knowledge life-cycle. However, the concept is suitable to form the basis for knowledge life-cycle support because it is a way of indicating context, which is the basis of understanding. The system needs further development, in particular the issue of updating and extending the knowledge base by learning from the captured and stored data needs addressing.

ACKNOWLEDGEMENTS

The development of PROSUS has been undertaken in the Cambridge Engineering Design Centre supported by a grant from the Engineering and Physical Sciences Research Council (EPSRC). Further development and testing of PROSUS is one of the tasks of the new British Aerospace/Rolls-Royce University Technology Partnership (UTP) for Design. This is a partnership between the two companies and the Universities of Cambridge, Sheffield and Southampton. The focus of the Cambridge UTP is on research into engineering knowledge management throughout the product life-cycle, the results of which will influence the future direction of the PROSUS system.

REFERENCES

Altschuller, G.S. (1984) *Erfinden: Wege zur Lösung technischer Probleme*, VEB Verlag Technik, Berlin.

Ball N.R., Matthews P.C. and Wallace K.M.(1998) Managing Conceptual Design Objects: An Alternative to Geometry, *Proceedings AID98* (Eds. Gero, J. and Sudweeks, F.), Lisbon, 67-86, Kluwer, Dordrecht.

Blessing, L.T.M. (1994) *A Process-Based Approach to Computer Supported Engineering Design*, PhD Thesis, University of Twente, The Netherlands, published Cambridge.

Blessing, L.T.M. (1996) Design Process Capture and Support, *Proceedings of the 2nd Workshop on Product Structuring* (Eds. Tichem, M. et al), Delft, 109-121.

Carlton, C.(1998) *The Retrieval of Mechanical Design Information*, PhD Thesis, University of Cambridge.

Clausing, D. (1994) *Total Quality Development*, ASME Press, New York.

Court, A. (1995) *The Modelling and Classification of Information for Engineering Designers*, PhD Thesis, University of Bath.

Duffy, S.M., Duffy, A.H.B. and MacCallum, K.J. (1995) A Design Reuse Model, *Proceedings of ICED 95*, Prague, 490-495, Heurista, Zurich.

Ehrlenspiel, K. (1997) Knowledge Explosion and its Consequences, *Proceedings of ICED 97*, Tampere, Vol. 2, 477-484, Heurista, Zurich.

Frankenberger, E. and Badke-Schaub, P. (1998) Integration of Group, Individual and External Influences in the Design Process, *In Designers: The Key to Successful Product Development* (Eds. Frankenberger, E., Badke-Schaub, P. and Birkhofer H.), 149-164, Springer-Verlag, Berlin.

Fricke, G. (1993) *Konstruieren als flexibler Problemlöseprozeß: empirische Untersuchung über erfolgreiche Strategien und methodische Vorgehensweisen beim Konstruieren*, Dissertation, University of Darmstadt, VDI Fortschrittberichte 1.227,VDI Düsseldorf.

Hales, C. (1987) *Analysis of the Engineering Design Process in an Industrial Context*, PhD Thesis, University of Cambridge, Gants Hill Publications, Hampshire.

Hubka, V. and Eder, W.E. (1988) *Theory of Technical Systems*, Springer-Verlag, Berlin.

Klaubert, H.L. (1998) *Tiny Design: A Study of the Design of Microelectromechanical Systems*, PhD Thesis, University of Cambridge University.

Kroonenberg, H.H. van den (1978) *Methodisch Ontwerpen*, Diktaat, University of Twente, Enschede, The Netherlands.

Kuffner, T. and Ullman, D.G. (1991) The Information Requests of Mechanical Design Engineering, *Design Studies*, Vol. 12, No. 1, 42-51.

Kunz, W. and Rittel, H. (1970) *Issues as Elements of Information Systems*, Center for Planning and Development Research, University of California, Berkely.

Mantyla, M. (1995) Knowledge-Intensive CAD: Introduction and a Research Agenda, *Proceedings of IFIP WG 5.2* (Eds. Tomiyama, T., Mantyla, M. and Finger, S.), Finland, Chapman & Hall, 3-12.

Marsh, J.R. (1997) *The Capture and Utilisation of Experience in Engineering Design*, PhD Thesis, University of Cambridge.

McCall, R.J. (1986) Issue-serve Systems: A Descriptive Theory of Design, *Design Methods and Theories*, Vol. 20, No. 3, 443-458.

Lera, S.G., Cooper, I. and. Powell J.A. (1984) Information and Designers, *Design Studies*, Vol. 5, No. 2, 113-120.

Pahl, G. and Beitz, W. (1996) *Engineering Design*, 3rd Edition, Springer-Verlag, London.

Pugh, S. (1991) *Total Design*, Addison-Wesley, Wokingham, UK.

PART THREE

ONTOLOGY

3

Ontological Commitments in Knowledge-Based Design Software: A Progress Report

Filippo A. Salustri, P.Eng.

Department of Mechanical Engineering, Ryerson Polytechnic Institute, 350 Victoria Street, Toronto, ON, M5B 2K3, Canada

Keywords: logic, ontological commitment, knowledge representation, design

Abstract: The increased sensitivity of engineered products to external forces requires new computer-based design tools that can express the richness and complexity of product knowledge. This paper is a progress report of the author's research towards the development of such a knowledge-based design tool, called the Design Knowledge Specification Language (DKSL). A key goal is to ensure the maximum possible logical rigor. In order to do this, *ontological commitments* are constructed to map logical structures to the domain of design knowledge. The first part of the paper discusses a number of ontological commitments the author has discovered for design. The second part of the paper presents the current, incomplete implementation of DKSL. An example of the structural and steady-state thermal analysis of a wall is used to present DKSL's capabilities. Although much work remains to be done, it appears that DKSL may be able to accurately and rigorously describe any design knowledge.

1. INTRODUCTION

As engineered products and engineering processes become more sensitive to economic, social, and technological forces, CAE tools must be made to express the richness and complexity of the information used in engineering environments. To treat the complexity, CAE systems are moving towards a knowledge-based approach, that is distributed transparently over intranets and the Internet. One of the author's on-going research projects is the design and implementation of a network-centric knowledge-based system (KBS) for engineering design applications.

There are many other research efforts aiming at the same or similar goals. For general knowledge representation (KR) applications, KIF, Ontolingua, and KQML (Genesereth and Fikes, 1992; Gruber, 1992), developed at Stanford University, and the KL-ONE family of languages (Brachman et al., 1991) are the most well-developed. These are very large systems able to represent general knowledge in a number of domains. In engineering domains, KIF has found some applications (Hurst, 1991; Hakim and James H. Garrett, 1993). Systems specific to engineering have also been developed (Alberts, 1994; Eastman et al., 1991b).

In the author's view, there are two problems with these approaches. Those efforts aimed at general KR (such as KIF) have to manage "common sense" knowledge, which is substantially different than the technical knowledge typical in engineering environments. On the other hand, those efforts specific to engineering tend to have relatively informal foundations. The author believes that it is possible to develop logical systems for CAE tools that are more rigorous than those currently available, yet are targeted specifically to engineering. The key to achieving this is in developing a proper set of *ontological commitments*, which formalize the correspondence between logical structures and the domain of engineering design.

This paper gives an overview of the current status of the project, starting with a discussion of the ontological commitments that have been established to date. The second part of the paper covers the implementation of DKSL (Design Knowledge Specification Language), which embeds those commitments in a frame-based KR system.

2. BACKGROUND

The author's research involves the development of logical theories of the various aspects of engineering design. The author's current focus is in the development of a language for the description of products. In the previous KIC workshop, the author presented a formal theory of product description, called AIM-D (Salustri, 1996). This paper will discuss the ongoing development of a specification language, DKSL, which implements AIM-D in the form of a programming language environment with knowledge base (KB) capabilities. Because DKSL depends on AIM-D, a brief summary of the theory is presented here.

AIM-D is an interpretation of ZF[1] axiomatic set theory (Copi, 1979). Set theory is a basic tool of logic, used in fields like number theory to prove the existence of the integers (Bernays, 1968). Though its validity is not provable due to Godel's Theorems, it is quite robust – robust enough, the author contends, to provide a degree of rigor for design theories that has heretofore been lacking.

Specifically, AIM-D uses the ZF axioms to define formally the information needed to model products. Currently, AIM-D covers quantities, features, parts, and assemblies, as well as sub-assemblies and systems, and types of all these entities. It does so by imposing a fixed semantics on the ZF axioms. This kind of interpretation amounts to making *ontological commitments* about the nature of designed products. Insofar as the author is ultimately interested in implementing a KBS for designed products, it is not so much the axioms as the ontological commitments that must be embedded in the KBS; the axiomatic theory demonstrates the (degree of) validity and rigor.

In closing, there are two particular points of interest about AIM-D that are noteworthy here. First, not all the axioms of ZF were used in developing AIM-D. This opens the interesting possibility that there is a logic, simpler than set theory and perhaps even demonstrably valid, that may be sufficient for design purposes.

The second point regards the ease with which ZF can formalize otherwise intuitive notions universal to design, leading to more robust computable algorithms. For example, the ZF Axiom of Foundation limits the notion of a set to those entities for which set membership is antisymmetric. That is, if A contains a set B, then A can only be a set if B does not contain A. This has a clear correspondence to the intuition that an assembly a cannot have b as a subassembly if b already contains a as a subassembly.

3. ONTOLOGICAL COMMITMENTS

An *ontological commitment* is a mapping between a language and a structure that systematically axiomatizes the forms and modes of being in a domain; this allows only certain *intended* meanings of models to be captured (Guarino et al., 1994). In other words, an ontological commitment is a decision to adhere to a certain interpretation of a language in a some domain; it is a mechanism to help ensure that a given model written in a given language communicates exactly and only what was intended by the model developer. For example, mathematical algebra includes ontological commitments regarding what variables such as x and y mean, what operators such as $+$ do, etc. Meaning can be ascribed to algebraic statements only when there is agreement on its underlying ontological commitments. Similarly, in design, there exist ontological commitments regarding the meaning of the various symbols used in blueprints. The meaning of the blueprint is lost if ontological commitments are missing or inconsistent.

The general problem of KR is that it admits a domain so broad that it is considered inappropriate to make ontological commitments about it. This is especially difficult in representing "common sense" knowledge held by the average individual, which is often incomplete, inconsistent, or even incorrect. This means that such KR systems must be able to treat the incompleteness, inconsistencies, and outright errors, which in turn greatly complicates the whole problem.

On the other hand, in the highly technical and relatively restricted domain of engineering design, we strive to minimize these problems. Here, some ontological commitments can be used as *simplifying assumptions* to improve the robustness, complexity, and computability of knowledge representations of designed products.

Though this occurs at the expense of expressiveness, a restricted solution today is in some ways better than the promise of a more general solution tomorrow; also, such a solution for design may provide a stepping stone to more general solutions by providing experience needed to develop more powerful KBSs in the future.

In developing any KBS, some ontological commitments must be made to limit the models possible in the system to only those models *intended* by the developers of the models and the users of the KBS. Often, these commitments are only implied, opening the possibility of *mis*interpretation. A fundamental goal of the author's work is to find the basic ontological commitments needed to define product models. To this end, the ontological commitments made in the development of DKSL are discussed in this section. So far, only some arise directly from AIM-D, which is a work-in-progress; some other, more tentative commitments must be made to allow continued development of DKSL while the theory is being developed. These other commitments deal specifically with modeling aspects of product function, of the various kinds of part-whole relationship (*mereology*), and of contexts.

3.1 COMMITMENTS ARISING FROM AIM-D

AIM-D maps ZF set theory to the domain of product modeling via ontological commitments that constrain DKSL. These ontological commitments result in a hierarchy of fundamental types. At the most primitive level are *quantities*, which are tuples of a value and a dimensional metric; *5 ft*, *100 N* are examples of quantities. A *feature* defines a geometrically and functionally relevant entity that is not necessarily realizable (e.g. a hole, or a fillet); features are compositions of interrelated quantities. *Parts* are aggregates of interrelated features, that are realizable through non-assembly manufacturing processes (casting, machining, etc.). Finally, an *assembly* is an aggregate of interrelated parts that are realizable only through assembly processes. These four domains of entities are disjoint, and are fundamental for product modeling because each domain covers a unique and distinctive class of entity in a designed product.

Additionally, AIM-D supports the concepts of both sub-assemblies and systems, but as entity domains existing outside the hierarchy described above. While sub-assemblies are essential *conceptual* entities in any design or manufacturing process, the author does not believe they constitute "real-world" entities. For example, an automobile engine may be considered an assembly by the engineers that design the engine, but as a subassembly by the engineers that design the whole automobile. But whether the engine is actually in an automobile (i.e. a subassembly) or not (i.e. an assembly) does nothing to alter the essential nature of the engine. If the notion of subassembly is context-dependent, then it cannot be fundamental to AIM-D, which is intended to capture the essential nature of the product. Thus, assemblies in AIM-D are composed of manufactured (non-assembled) parts; sub-assemblies are useful, perhaps even essential, constructs for both *designing* and *manufacturing* processes, but are only *ancillary* with respect to description of products as real objects.

This approach contradicts the relatively common intuition exemplified by statements such as *"The automobile is an assembly of the following sub-assemblies. . . "*, which suggests that sub-assemblies have a substantive nature. However, once assembled, the distinction between sub-assemblies disappears without prior knowledge of the assembly process. This argument should not be taken as one diminishing the importance of sub-assemblies in engineering; it is intended only to distinguish the notion of subassembly as an artificial one, and to incorporate and formalize that distinction into AIM-D.

The more generic notion of a *system* is also formalized in AIM-D, due to its relevance in engineering. But, as with sub-assemblies, systems are ancillary. Indeed, it was found during the development of AIM-D that the only substantive difference between sub-assemblies and subsystems was that system components need not be in direct contact with each other, whereas direct contact is required for sub-assemblies; otherwise, the formalizations for systems and for assemblies are the same.

Another aspect of the ontological commitments of AIM-D regards the representation of *type* information. An extremely popular commitment is to the existence of explicit *classes* (as in object-oriented languages) or *concepts* (as in description logics such as CLASSIC). Classes and concepts are meta-level information units; this raises issues of reflection and its computational counterpart, recursion.

While there are modeling problems that can be solved efficiently with classes, there is also evidence that the human mind works more "by example" than by abstraction (Jaynes, 1976; Damasio and Damasio, 1992), and that design is one area where the generally accepted semantics of classes and types can impede the development of accurate, flexible, and robust models (Johnson and Zweig, 1991; Eastman and Fereshetian, 1994). For example, there is a tendency in automotive engineering to regard a blueprint of an automobile as a model of a *typical* automobile and not as the *set or class* of automobiles of a certain make and model. Also, the tolerancing of dimensions can be viewed as the definition of a "vaguely" defined prototype: any item whose dimensions fit within the limits described by the tolerances can be thought of as a specific version of the more general prototype. That is, designers tend to use an exemplar-based, rather than a class-based, approach to model products. In keeping with this observation, AIM-D admits no notion of class or concept, but rather uses the notion of an *exemplar*, an entity typical of items in a collection. Collections themselves exist only intentionally. (It is noted that it is possible to develop class-based systems from prototype-based ones.)

In order to structure collections of entities, AIM-D uses notions of generalization of entity attributes. Generalization occurs in AIM-D by *ignoring* certain aspects of entity attributes. Specifically, three kinds of generalization are defined within AIM-D: ignoring whole attributes, ignoring the values of attributes, and ignoring the number of values of attributes.

3.2 COMMITMENTS DUE TO PRODUCT FUNCTION AND BEHAVIOR

There is a difference of opinion in the research community regarding the meaning *function* and *behavior*; no standardized, consistent model of these terms exists. Some researchers consider function as a description of the actions a product can perform (e.g. (Qian and Gero, 1996)), while others treat it as a description of a subset of *behaviors* (i.e. intended behavior or "purpose", as in (Sturges et al., 1996)). Various other definitions are given in (Chittaro et al., 1994; Chakrabarti, 1993).

The current author defines *behavior* as the response of a system to predefined inputs which are not necessarily quantified; it describes the *role* played by a product in a larger system. The behavioral perspective takes the product being designed to be a "black box" whose internal function is not visible (or even known); the inputs, outputs, and operational environment of the product, on the other hand, are "transparent" (see Figure 3.2b). Insofar as behavior describes the response of a product, it is seen as answering the question *"What does the product do?"* Behavior is described without commitment to the form of the product.

Function, on the other hand, is a description of *how* a product works rather than what it does (Figure 3.2a), where the environment is now opaque, and the product is "transparent," and is composed of a series of black box subsystems whose interaction describes how the product comes to exhibit a certain behavior, but without necessarily making commitments about product form.

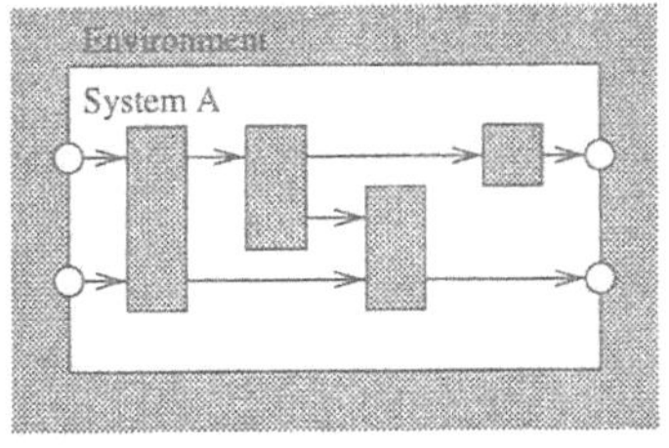

Figure 3.1a Example of the functional perspective.

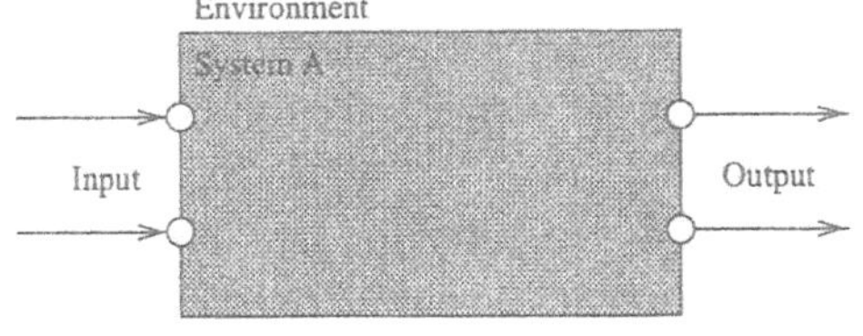

Figure 3.1b Example of the behavioral perspective.

These perspectives are meant to demark the different kinds of tasks that can be performed with functional/behavioral information. At the behavioral level, design is systems-based, concerned with identifying functional requirements to be met by a product. At the functional level, on the other hand, design consists of a configuring components and their interrelationships. So-called "top-down" design proceeds by alternating between behavioral and functional perspectives at ever increasing levels of details. Identifying these perspectives is used below to demonstrate that behavioral and functional descriptions are essentially the same; they are just viewed in different contexts.

It is noted here that the definitions of function and behavior adopted by the other are the opposite of those commonly used in the literature. While the need for terminological consistency is aknowledged, the author believes his definitions are more in keeping with those conventionally implied by practicing engineers. In any event, it matters little in the long run since the distinction between function and behavior is shown (below) to be an artificial one only.

In order to explore this matter further, consider the following three statements:

1. The refrigerator keeps food cold.

2. The refrigerator keeps things cold.

3. The refrigerator preserves food.

Any of these statements in isolation can be considered a *behavior* of a refrigerator. If statement 1 is considered a behavior, then we may ask *How is this behavior achieved?* The answer involves the functions of a refrigerator (isolating a region of space, transferring heat from that space by some means, etc.). However, we may also ask *Why does the refrigerator keep food cold?* One answer to this question is statement 3. Now, considering statements 1 and 3 together, statement 1 is a *function* rather than a behavior. Thus ,whether the statements are taken as functional or behavioral, *context* plays a crucial role in (a) providing terminological information about the words appearing in the statements, and (b) implying information about the operating environment. For example, in statement 1, the terms "cold" and "keeps" are relative to the context of refrigerators.

Function and behavior are thus *relative to the reference frame of an agent* making assertions about a product; that is, they are not intrinsic properties of designed products. Nonetheless, functional and behavioral information about a product is very important, especially during the product's design. Therefore it is essential that it be representable in the author's system.

It is often possible to represent both functions and behaviors in single natural language clauses that seem quite intuitive to humans (e.g. "...to support a load in bending...."); both behavior ("to support a load") and function ("in bending") are intimately connected in a single phrase. The fact that both the behavior and function can be described in a single natural language statement only obscures their distinction. This constitutes, in the author's opinion, a significant problem with the use of natural language, or any other *in*formal language, to precisely define the nature of designed products. Natural language is used herein only for expository purposes; the author intends this research to lead eventually to a more formal specification of functional/behavioral information.

In order to avoid this confusion while maintaining a sense of connection between them, the author uses the term *predicative description* to include both function and behavior descriptions. This term captures the sense of activity, as well as the complexity of the concepts.

The basic relation that connects function and behavior is the "how/why" relation: given a function, the *why* relation describes its behavior; and given a behavior, the *how* relation describes the function that results in it. The how/why relations are disjoint and intransitive with other relations, particularly with respect specialization. In figure 3.2 four predicative statements about a refrigerator are given, and both the how/why and specialization/generalization relations are shown. It may be argued that the *why* relation is a kind of generalization: in comparing statements 1 and 3 in the figure, it is sensible to think of "preserving food" as a generalization of "keeping food cold". But this is a generalization based on the intent the statement as a whole, rather than one associated with the *components* of the statements. A similar argument can be made about the specialization and *how* relations. The key differences between function and behavior in the author's work can be summarized as in the table in Table 3.1.

Predicative descriptions are *complex* in that their expression tends to be formed as *predicate* clauses consisting of verb/object pairs (VOPs). That is, they describe actions performed by an entity upon some other entity, independent of the phrasing in natural language.

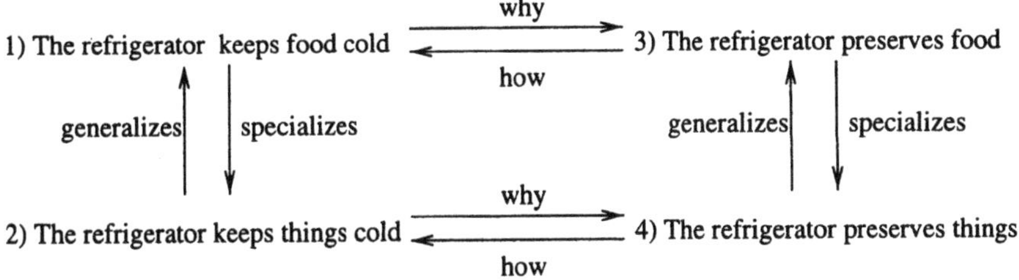

Figure 3.2 Example of abstraction of predicative descriptions. Numbered statements are assertions about a product. Labeled arrows indicate predicative and taxonomic relations between assertions.

This apparent verb/object structure of both functions and behaviors has been used as the root of various formalizations, such as in (Umeda et al., 1996); the current author also employs this approach. Consider again the statements in Figure 3.2: statements 1 and 3 are related through how/why relations. Statement 2 is related to statement 1 by generalization on the object of the VOP. A similar generalization carried out on statement 2 (yielding statement 4) is virtually meaningless. The author believes that generalizations will not generally transfer through how/why relations; in other words, abstraction relations and predicative relations are not transitive. Also, that the abstraction occurred only on the object part of the VOP suggests that in the general case, abstraction can occur on either the verb or the object parts independently.

Table 3.1 Differences between Function and Behavior

Behavior	**Function**
role-dependent	operational
goal-oriented	process-oriented
what a system does	how a system does it
based on purpose/usage	based on physical properties

The key to abstraction of predicative relations is the verb part of the VOPs. But since a VOP can be *both* a functional and a behavioral description (depending on the context), any generalization rules for the verb parts of VOPs must be based on the definition of the verb term itself rather than on its functional or behavioral connotations.

Finally, these definitions of function and behavior deal only with the reactions expected of products for given sets of inputs; that is, no notion of *intended*, or designed-in, function or behavior, or of *purpose* is implied.

3.3 COMMITMENTS DUE TO MEREOLOGY

Mereology is a branch of logic that uses part-whole relationships to describe entities. For example, in a conventional ontology, one might model an automobile as having the property of having four wheels; in a mereological perspective, a relation is defined between the automobile and the wheels themselves. Obviously, in engineering design, both the conventional and the mereological approaches are relevant. Surprisingly, little work appears in the recent literature outside Europe on mereology in AI, and there is almost no work on mereology as such in the engineering literature.

The basic problem of mereology as a field of study is that there appear to be various, often inconsistent, semantics associated with the term "part of". For example, consider the following three statements.

1. A piston is a part of an engine.
2. An engine is a part of an automobile.
3. An automobile is a part of a fleet.

Each statement, on its own, is perfectly reasonable. Furthermore, from the first two statements, we can reasonably deduce that *"A piston is a part of an automobile."* But from all three statements, can we reasonably deduce that *"A piston is a part of a fleet"*? The problem is that there are two different meanings of the term "part of," and that transitivity is not preserved between them. Mereology's main concern is establishing an overall structure to reason reliably with all the possible part-whole relationships.

There appear to be two schools of thought regarding the treatment of mereology. One school advocates a single, universal, and transitive part-of relation, based on the assumption that all distinctions about types of parts are really conceptualizations and are not rooted in reality. In order to address the paradoxes that result, first-order predicate calculus is used to introduce sufficient predicates to distinguish between kinds things. This approach is taken by the developers of Ontolingua and KIF (Gruber, 1992) and the logics of Lesniewski (Srzednicki et al., 1984).

The other school of thought contends the cognitive distinctions must be represented; in other words, a proper mereology must handle the transitivity problem directly by admitting distinctions between different part-of relations. This approach is supported by the work of Artale et al. (Artale et al., 1996b; Artale et al., 1996a) and Simons (Simons, 1987). In this approach, different part-of relations are explicitly defined to handle different conceptualizations (e.g. assembly/component versus space/region), and transitivity is not preserved across them. Also, the part-of relation is seen as complex, rather than primitive, which requires the development of specialized logics that integrate mereology with topology and morphology as in, for example, (Borgo et al., 1996).

A fundamental problem with this approach is that there is no way to enumerate all the different "primitive" part-of relations. For example, in (Winston et al., 1987) six primitive part-of relations are defined; they are summarized in Table 3.2. It has been shown ((Artale et al., 1996b)) that (a) it is impossible to decide if these constitute a complete set of part-of primitive relations, and (b) some of these relations (such as stuff/object) are more linguistic artifacts than actual cognitive or other constructs of knowledge.

Table 3.2 Summary of part-of relations in (Winston et al., 1987).

RELATION	EXAMPLE
component/integral-object	"wheels are parts of cars"
member/collection	"a product is part of a batch"
portion/mass	"3 ft. of stock rod"
stuff/object	"a car is partly aluminum"
feature/activity	"grasping is part of carrying"
place/area	"the front of the car"

Rather than siding with one school or the other, the author proposes a new mereological framework, wherein the part-of relation is a well-defined function mapping triplets of arguments to the boolean values. That is:

$$P(p, W, \pi) \Rightarrow \{\mathcal{T}, \mathcal{F}\} \tag{3.1}$$

where p is a part, W is a whole, and π is a property or properties used by the P part-of function.

This approach is based on the observation that parthood is related to some sort of *overlapping* between the values of at least one property of a part on the values of the same properties of a whole. For example, to establish a part-of relation for regions of a space, π is the set of properties defining the size and position of a spatial region. P, then, asserts that p is wholly contained by W if its volume is contained in W's volume.

This approach addresses a variety of open issues. First, by "deferring" uniqueness of different part-of relations to the properties π, P itself remains a single universal, ternary predicate, which is logically elegant. Second, primitive part-of relations can be defined as those whose properties π are fundamental in AIM-D (e.g. properties of length, mass, time, etc.); complex part-of relations are constructed by composing primitive ones; this suggests an abstraction hierarchy of part-of relations which would be useful for automated reasoning processes, such as case-based reasoning and decision support. Third, transitivity is preserved to the degree that different properties are used in different part-of relations.

This last point deserves some explanation. Transitivity is preserved entirely in reasoning processes where different instances of P use the same properties π. On the other hand, different instances of P that use properties that have no commonality in the abstraction hierarchy are not transitive at all. These two cases correspond to the typical behavior of other approaches. For example, transitivity is preserved over different instances of the group/member relation, but not between a group/member relation and an assembly/component relation.

However, the author's approach allows *partial* transitivity to be recognized. In the example at the beginning of this section, it was shown that one may reason that a piston is a part of a rental fleet of automobiles if there is only one part-of relation. While there is clearly something wrong with such a conclusion for most conventional uses, there is still a certain sense in which it is reasonable. The author believes that this "partial" sense of the conclusion results from the partial subsumption of the properties with which part-of is used in the example. Being able to represent this kind of partial parthood opens the possibility of substantially different reasoning processes that can be automated in a KBS, and should allow for a richer representation of design knowledge.

Specific mereological axioms using the formalism presented above are currently under development for the next "version" of AIM-D. The current version of AIM-D (Salustri, 1996) contains only an implied notion of mereology as captured by the four levels of product composition defined therein. That is, AIM-D has specific axioms for the construction of assemblies from parts, parts from features, and features from quantities. Equation 3.2 gives an example: the axiom relating parts and assemblies. It states that a part p consists of features f that are in the set of all features F, and that satisfy a predicate ϕ, which is taken to be any possible mereological relation between features f.

$$\exists p \, [\forall f \, [(f \in p) \equiv (f \in F) \bullet \phi(f)]] \tag{3.2}$$

Each axiom implies a different parthood relation between the whole (e.g. assemblies) and its parts (e.g. parts). The next version of AIM-D will have a more explicit formulation of parthood relations based on the material presented herein.

3.4 COMMITMENTS FOR CONTEXT-SENSITIVITY

Engineering terms can often have different meanings depending on the various *contexts* in which they are used. A context is essentially a mapping between terms and denotations. An assertion may be found true in one context but false in another. Contexts may also include special rules for carrying out those reasoning processes. For example, consider: *"the block deck height of the engine includes the thickness of the engine gasket."* If the designer in charge of the engine block believes this assertion, but the designer in charge of the cylinder head does not believe it, the designers will disagree about the answer to the question *"What is the total height of the engine?"*; the two designers are working in two slightly different contexts. Contexts have various uses ranging from encapsulation of parts of a KB, to providing a shorthand notation for omitting common arguments (such as location, time, etc.) and separating meta levels of languages (Sowa, 1992). Contexts are currently a topic of significant interest, especially in the KR community, where the issues raised in their treatment impacts on distributed computing and AI. Some of the possible uses of contexts include (Sowa, 1992):

- partitioning a knowledge base into more manageable modules;
- encapsulating parts of a knowledge base, as in so-called object-oriented systems;
- providing a shorthand for omitting common arguments, such as location, time, etc.;
- providing a way to resolve indexical referents, such as "this", "I", and definite noun phrases beginning with "the;"
- representing environments whose modality, level of certainty, or hypothetical existence is different from that of other environments;
- supporting propositional attitude verbs, such as "believe;" and
- separating a meta level of language that is used to talk about the language in a nested context.

There are also several ongoing efforts to formalize notions of context. Akman and Surav (Akman and Surav, 1996) give an excellent overview of the various approaches.

Contexts are clearly relevant to product modeling, since typically many designers are involved in concurrently developing a single product. In this kind of environment, an unintentional contextual difference can lead to disastrous results.

The author is currently working to incorporate contexts into AIM-D. The general approach is most similar to that of McCarthy and Buvac (McCarthy and Buvac, 1994), wherein contexts are essentially namespaces binding terms to semantics. Contexts can be nested, and various predicates are provided to test the truth value of a statement in a particular context, and to "lift" terms commonly defined in different contexts to higher, more universal contexts.

One very important aspect of contexts in AIM-D regards the terms used to name entity attributes. This is best illustrated with a simple example.

Consider the statements: (a) *"The color of the car is green,"* and (b) *"Green is a color."* Linguistic idiosyncrasies aside, the term *color* is used in two distinct, but related, ways: as the name of an entity attribute, and as a generalized relation entity. It is possible to capture the relation between the various uses of a term without recourse to linguistic constructs.

In AIM-D, the names of entity attributes are the names of relations between entities, and are themselves terms defined in some context. This means that a term such as *color* must be used consistently throughout a given context where it is defined, and in all its sub-contexts. This is different from the approach taken in object-oriented modeling, where the semantics of an instance variable are consistent only across the instances of a given class. By making the universality of attribute name definitions explicit, (semi-)automated reasoning about attributes, and the relations they represent, is now possible.

Contexts also matter in terms of managing mereological relations. For example, (Gerstl and Pribbenow, 1996) suggest that a primary characteristic of item that leads to different mereological relations is whether the item is homogeneous (having no parts), uniform (consisting of like parts only), or heterogeneous (having various different parts). However, it depends on the context of a particular task how a particular item will be regarded. For example, in the context of engine assembly, an aluminum part may be regarded as a homogeneous item; but from a context of materials engineering, aluminum is at least uniform if not heterogeneous. Clearly, the interactions between context and mereology still need further exploration.

3.5 SUMMARY

Ontological commitments can be regarded as decisions about the interpretation of statements in a given language. A variety of commitments have been presented in this section that pertain to the description of designed products. Clearly, significant work remains to be done; there are many other commitments about designed products that can be found or deduced from other research efforts. However, to help ensure rigor, the only commitments currently part of AIM-D are those that apparently allow a consistent logic to exist.

4. IMPLEMENTATION OF DKSL

In this section, the design and implementation of DKSL is discussed, including how the ontological commitments made thus far have been, or are being, embedded within it. Generally, the commitments amount rules that DKSL must satisfy in order to preserve logical rigor: no model should be representable in DKSL if the model violates the ontological commitments.

For example, AIM-D defines sub-assemblies in terms of subsets of the set of all parts of a product, rather than as parts of those products. This implies that DKSL must be able to distinguish automatically between parts, sub-assemblies, and product assemblies. Furthermore, DKSL has restrictions on how assemblies are formed through the merging of defined sub-assemblies.

The author has not yet investigated the changes that would have to occur in DKSL if different ontological commitments were made; this issue remains an open one for future research.

4.1 UNDERLYING KNOWLEDGE REPRESENTATION

The current implementation of DKSL is as a small, stand-alone program with a text-based user interface. It is a "concept-proving" implementation, to allow the author to study internal structures and algorithms needed to represent and manipulate design information effectively.

SCM, an implementation of the Scheme programming language by Aubrey Jaffer, is currently used to implement DKSL. SCM is small, robust, and true to the IEEE standard for Scheme (IEEE, 1991); it also has a number of extensions that facilitate rapid software prototyping (e.g. POSIX-compliant file I/O operations).

DKSL is implemented using a *frame-based* KR scheme. Frame systems are similar to object-based systems, but introduce a finer level of representation. Object systems are based on object-attribute-value triplets: objects contain attributes which have values. Frames, on the other hand, use frame-slot-facet-value quadruplets. Slots are composed of possibly many facets, which allows a richer representation of attributes. Furthermore, functions called *procedural attachments* can be associated with slot facets. These functions may be triggered automatically or at a user's request to carry out various management tasks such as constraint checking and inverse relation maintenance. A procedural attachment that fires automatically is called a *demon.* Generally, demons execute in three cases: when a new value is (a) added to or (b) removed from a slot, and (c) when a slot's value needs to be calculated rather than retrieved.

Frame systems as described above are common in KR systems such as CLASSIC (Brachman et al., 1991). However, the system implemented in DKSL is substantially different from these others. These differences arise from the ontological commitments, and are presented here.

Context-sensitivity. Conventional frame systems make no particular commitments about the contexts in which terms are resolved into frames. However, DKSL supports the notion of a context as a "dictionary" mapping terms to frames, implementing the ontological commitments regarding context sensitivity (Section 3.4). Contexts in DKSL may be created by the user, and may be nested. A System Context contains basic definitions needed by DKSL, and a User Context, which is a sub-context of the System Context stores user-defined frames. Other application-specific contexts are under development. Lifting of terms (per (McCarthy and Buvac, 1994)) is achieved by a simple comparison of different frames with the same name in different contexts. Furthermore, a slot is viewed as a relation having a uniform semantics over a whole context.

No Classes. There are no explicit classes or "meta-frames" in DKSL. Rather, a prototype-based approach is used, wherein any entity can be an *exemplar* with which other frames can be *cloned.* The use of prototypes is consistent with the ontological commitments made in Section 3.1: AIM-D entity types are not explicit, and neither are those in DKSL.

Inheritance through specialization. Without classes, a different kind of inheritance mechanism is needed. *Specialization* of individual frames is used: an exemplar generalizes its clones. Specialization information is used only during frame construction; no specialization information is kept in frames. The most important reason for this is that it allows an exemplar and its clones to change with time without requiring complex change management to preserve that relation beyond a frame's construction.

Calculated type compatibility. Type similarity between frames is calculated as needed. Two frames are type-compatible if there are some slots in one frame with the same names as some slots in the other frame. Since slot names have uniform semantics in a given context, no checks are needed once a value is added to a slot. A frame is a *specialization* of another if the one has at least as many slots as the other, and if every slot in the other has a type-compatible correspondent in the one. Generalization is just the converse of specialization.

Although this clearly imposes a heavier computational load than conventional type systems, it also increases the expressiveness of the language to represent *varying degrees* of type similarity. For example, it is possible to determine if one frame *could be* a specialization of another. This allows the system to "guess" type compatibility of frames, which could be very useful for exploratory algorithms such as case-based reasoning. Also, it is possible to develop automatically *normalized* abstraction hierarchies of arbitrary collections of frames. This raises the possibility of transmitting KBs between systems or agents in forms that are reliably re-constructible in different environments. This kind of type-compatibility is consistent with the ontological commitments in AIM-D.

Location and Names of Demons. DKSL supports two kinds of `if-added` demons, called `pre/put` and `post/put` demons. The `pre/put` demons are predicates that check the validity of the new values before they are added to slots. If a `pre/put` demon fails, either a warning message is displayed and the assignment continues, or an error is triggered and the assignment does not occur; which of these actions occurs depends on whether the demon is *hard* or *soft* (discussed below). The `post/put` demons are run after new information is inserted into a KB; these demons perform conventional management tasks such as maintenance of inverse relationships.

The location of demons is standardized in DKSL, and takes advantage of the uniform semantics rule for slots. This allows a well-defined, yet extensible technique for searching, storing, and checking the validity of data, as well as maintaining interrelationships between the data. Demons may be stored in the frame that defines the semantics of a slot, in which case they will be triggered wherever that slot is used; they may alternatively be stored in facets of a particular instance of a slot, in which case they are only triggered for that slot instance.

Hard and soft constraints. Demons can implement constraints on the knowledge stored in the system. These constraints can be either *hard*, violation of which causes an error to be triggered, or *soft*, in which case a warning message is displayed for the user only. This distinction accounts for the different implications of a constraint violation with regards to KB integrity. Hard constraints preserve the basic integrity of the KB, whereas soft constraints indicate an inconsistency in the product being modeled. Since design can be regarded as driven by the need to eliminate such inconsistencies, it is important to represent them differently than those arising from the KBS itself.

Partial meta-information. DKSL also allows some kinds of *meta*-level information about entities to be stored. For example, one constrain the number of values that a slot can have, and the types of values that a slot can contain by associating exemplars representative of those types with particular facets. This kind of information can be used by `pre/put` and `post/put` demons to perform a variety of checks and other operations automatically.

There is other useful meta-information that could be stored, but one must be careful when adding meta-level information to a KBS: one may create *terminological cycles* and other semantic artifacts for which even simple computations are intractable. Work on DKSL is intentionally proceeding slowly in this regard, so that sufficient care is taken to avoid these problems.

5. DKSL FOR ENGINEERING DESIGN

An example of a simple DKSL product model is introduced to demonstrate its applicability. The example involves the structural and steady-state thermal modeling of a wall. It is based on one presented in (Eastman et al., 1991a), but is lacking in some details. Its use will facilitate a comparison of DKSL to various other modeling schemes discussed in (Eastman et al., 1991a).

We begin with an overview of the model's structure; this will be followed by a description of some of the frames needed to describe the model in DKSL, and some of the operations possible on that model.

5.1 STRUCTURAL MODELING CONSIDERATIONS

The reader is referred to Figure 3.3, which shows schematically a wall, labeled with the major structural components as described below.

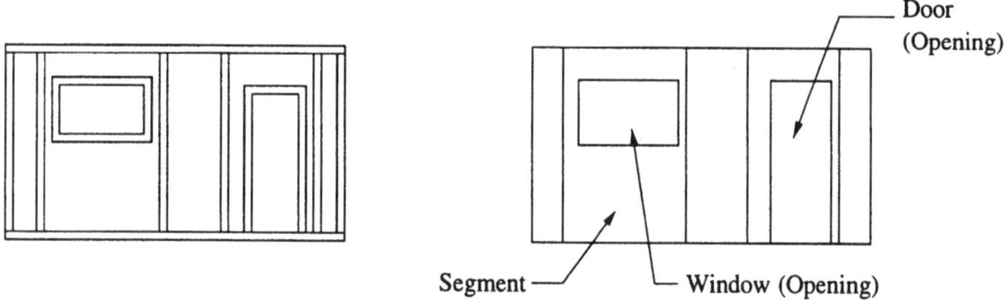

Figure 3.3 Structure of a wall.

In order to model a wall's structure and steady-state thermal behavior, both the geometry and composition of the wall must be considered. Since the example only models an isolated wall, the width and height of the wall are arbitrarily defined values. Had the model included many attached walls, width and height would have been determined by the overall structures of which they were a part. Wall thickness, however, depends on the wall's composition. A wall is composed of various *layers*, each serving a specific purpose – load bearing, insulation, covering, and so on. Each layer consists of a single material, is of constant thickness, and contributes to the overall thickness of the wall.

Complex wall shapes can be described as compositions of area-wise *segments*; a small collection of regular planar shapes can be combined to produce quite complex geometries. Each segment is composed of layers, and all layers in a segment have the same surface area.

Finally, a wall may contain various kinds of *openings* or passages. In this model, openings lie within single wall segments and must pass entirely through the wall. For simplicity, only windows and doors are considered. An opening is a kind of segment: it occupies an area and may be composed of many layers (e.g. multi-paned windows); however, openings are not allowed to contain other openings.

5.2 STEADY-STATE THERMAL MODELING CONSIDERATIONS

The following mathematical model of the steady-state heat behavior of a wall is assumed. The physical relationships are drawn from (Eastman et al., 1991a) and a standard thermodynamics text (Reynolds and Perkins, 1977).

The steady-state heat flow through a wall is given approximately by the following equations, where ΔT is the change in temperature through the wall,

t_w and A_w are the thickness and area of the wall respectively, and k_w is the overall of coefficient thermal conductivity of the wall (calculated by analogy with electrical systems). The thermal resistance of the ith layer of the wall is by r_i.

$$\dot{Q}_w = \frac{k_w A_w}{t_w} \Delta T, \quad k_w = \frac{1}{\sum_i r_i}, \quad r_i = \frac{t_i}{k_i}. \tag{3.3}$$

5.3 DEFINITION OF WALL EXEMPLAR OBJECTS

Given this conceptual model, DKSL frames can now be constructed to represent it. The frames defined here are simplified versions, intended to focus only on the particular example being presented. In a "real" implementation, many more slots and facets would be defined. All quantities are in SI units.

First, we establish a context for this application; this is shown in Figure 3.4. The `simple-walls` context is defined as a sub-context of contexts for 2.5D geometry, SI units for physical systems, and physical assemblies. Setting the context to `simple-walls` ensures that all subsequent assertions are made in that context; this information becomes persistent so that future queries to the information defined in this context will be evaluated within it. (It is assumed that a user intends for knowledge to be used always in the same context, unless that knowledge is intentionally "lifted" into other contexts.) Setting the value of `coordinate-type` establishes a term in the new context that will be used by other frames related to geometry to determine the kind of coordinates to be used in this context.

```
(define-context simple-walls
  (2.5d-geometry
   si-physical-units
   physical-assemblies))
(set-context!  simple-walls)
(set!  coordinate-type
      cartesian-coordinate-system)
```

Figure 3.4 A context for the example wall model.

A `material` exemplar is defined in Figure 3.5; for brevity, only one necessary property, thermal conductivity, and one instance is included. Thermal conductivity data is from (Reynolds and Perkins, 1977).

Wall layers are modeled in Figure 3.6.

A derived attribute (one whose value is calculated from other attributes) for thermal resistance is also included. The `region` exemplar, defined in

```
(define-frame material
  (new (the-frame)
       (thermal-conductivity
        (watt/meter-degree 1.0))))
(define-frame glass,window
  (new (material)
       (thermal-conductivity
        (watt/meter-degree 0.78))))
```

Figure 3.5 Material exemplar and instances.

the `physical-attributes` context, indicates that `layer` can take part in region/space mereological relationships.

```
(define-frame layer
  (new (region)
       (material (new material))
       (thickness (centimeter 1.0))
       (thermal-resistance
         (derived-from (thickness material)
           (/ thickness
              (material 'thermal-conductivity))))))
```

Figure 3.6 Layer objects.

A `wall-atom` frame is defined to model the kinds of properties common to both openings and wall segments (see Figure 3.7). It too is a kind of region. The `(all layer)` construct returns all slot values in the current frame that are of type `layer`. The `thermal-conductivity` slot models the overall coefficient of thermal conductivity per unit area, calculated according to the mathematical model in Section 5.2.

Now `wall-atom` can be used to define exemplars for openings and segments (Figure 3.8). The *specific heat flow* of an opening is the rate of heat flow per degree of temperature difference at steady-state. Also, a distinction is made between the solid wall area of the segment and the area of any openings in the segment. The specific heat flow of a segment is the sum of the specific heat flows of the openings and of the rest of the segment. Finally, the `heat-flow` slot models the heat flow through a wall segment for a given temperature difference (`delta-t`).

No geometric (shape) information has been embedded in `segment` and `opening`; shape information will be provided when specific segments and

```
(define-frame wall-atom
  (new (region)
       (thickness
         (derived-from ((layers (all layer)))
           (apply + (for ((l layers))
                          (l 'thickness)))))
       (thermal-conductivity
         (derived-from ((layers (all layer)))
           (/ 1.0
              (apply +
                (for ((l layers))
                  (l 'thermal-resistance))))))))
```

Figure 3.7 Atomic wall components for openings and segments.

openings are created (see below). This does not, however, prevent us from referencing attributes such as `area` when defining frames so long as they are defined by the time they are used.

The `opening` frame is specialized for doors and windows (Figure 3.9). The `door` exemplar specializes both `opening` (for composition and thermal analysis) and `rectangle` (for geometric characteristics). It also specializes `part`, provided by the `physical-assemblies` context, to signify that it can enter into a part/assembly relation (which is different from a region/space relation). The `rectangle` exemplar and other geometric information is defined in the `2.5d-geometry` context.

The `window` exemplar is further specialized into one- and two-paned windows. Finally, two specific kinds of windows are created: a single-paned window with a 5 millimeter pane of glass, and a double-paned window with two 5 millimeter panes separated by a 4 millimeter air gap. Note that shape has not yet been assigned to the window objects. The `cardinality` facet is used to limit the number of panes in each kind of window.

The last exemplar, for the wall itself, just gathers `segments` (see Figure 3.10), since all the important functions for thermal analysis have been defined elsewhere. The `heat-flow` slot calculates the total heat flow through a wall for a given temperature difference. The `wall` enters into both part/whole and region/space relations.

This completes the DKSL model. It is not a model of a *particular* wall, but a template from which various models can be built. The model is intended to be as general as possible, so that it may be used for other purposes that just steady-state thermal analysis. It would have been substantially simpler had we targetted it specifically and exclusively for thermal analysis, but it would also have been of very limited use.

```
(define-frame opening
  (new (wall-atom)
       (specific-heat-flow
         (derived-from (thermal-conductivity area)
           (* thermal-conductivity area)))))
(define-frame segment
  (new (wall-atom)
       (opening-area
         (derived-from ((openings (all opening)))
           (apply + (for ((o openings))
                          (o 'area)))))
       (segment-area
         (derived-from (area opening-area)
           (- area opening-area)))
       (specific-heat-flow
         (derived-from ((openings (all opening))
                          thermal-conductivity
                          segment-area)
           (+ (apply +
                  (for ((o openings))
                    (o 'specific-heat-flow)))
              (* thermal-conductivity
                 segment-area))))
       (heat-flow
         (derived-from (specific-heat-flow)
           (using (delta-t))
           (* specific-heat-flow delta-t)))))
```

Figure 3.8 Exemplar for wall openings and segments.

```
(define-frame door
  (new (part opening rectangle)
       (layer (new layer))))
(define-frame pane
  (new (part layer)
       (material glass,window)))
(define-frame window
  (new (part opening)
       (pane (new pane))))
(define-frame window,1pane
  (new (window)
       (pane cardinality 1)))
(define-frame window,2pane
  (new (window)
       (pane cardinality 2)
       (gap (new (layer) (material air)))))
(define-frame window,1pane,5
  (new (window,1pane)
       (pane (thickness (centimeter 0.5)))))
(define-frame window,2pane,5-4-5
  (new (window,2pane)
       (pane (new (layer)
                  (thickness (centimeter 0.5)))
             (new (layer)
                  (thickness (centimeter 0.5))))
       (gap (thickness (centimeter 0.4)))))
```

Figure 3.9 Exemplars for doors and windows.

```
(define-frame wall
  (new (part region)
       (segment (new (segment)))
       (area
         (derived-from ((segments
                          (all parts segment)))
           (apply + (for ((s segments))
                      (s 'area)))))
       (opening-area
         (derived-from ((segments
                          (all parts segment)))
           (apply + (for ((s segments))
                      (s 'opening-area)))))
       (heat-flow
         (derived-from ((segments
                          (all parts segment)))
           (using (delta-t))
           (* (apply +
                (for ((s segments))
                  (s 'specific-heat-flow)))
              delta-t)))))
```

Figure 3.10 Exemplar for walls.

The goals for developing the model this way are: (a) for demonstration purposes, to showcase the flexibility of DKSL, and (b) to define a model that is not necessarily restricted to thermal analyses only.

5.4 USAGE OF THE WALL MODEL

This section defines a particular wall and calculates the heat flow through it. The sample wall (Figure 3.11); consists of two segments, a large rectangular segment with a door and a window, and a triangular segment with no openings. Figure 3.12 defines the necessary `segment` and `wall` frames.

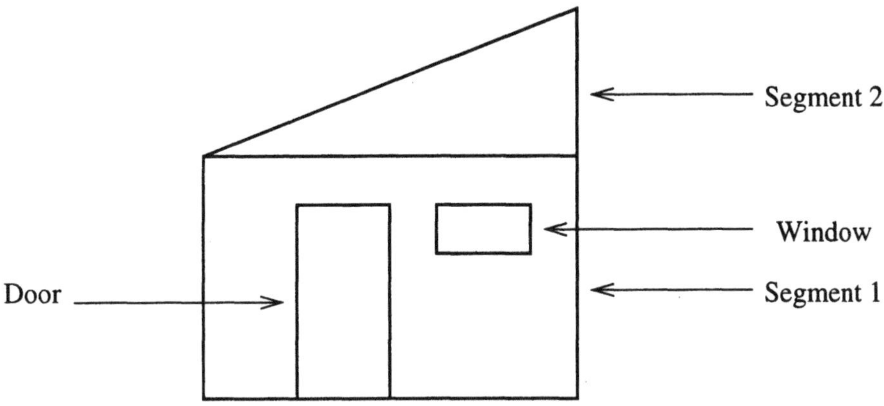

Figure 3.11 Geometry of sample wall.

Figure 3.13 shows three messages sent to the wall w, and the values that are returned. The third message returns the heat flow through the wall for a temperature difference of 20 degrees.

The specific wall model defined here contains all the information needed for a preliminary thermal analysis, even though the geometric relationships between the components have not yet been specified. For example, the door and window have not been positioned in `segment1`; nor have the segments been positioned with respect to each other. The operations to do this are shown in Figure 3.14. The forms in the figure take advantage of methods defined in the `2.5d-geometry` context that translate and scale objects.

Topological relations, such as the physical connection between wall segments, are not yet supported by DKSL. These kind of relations are currently a topic of study of the author.

Let us say that too much heat was being lost through the wall as defined above. One alternative is to change the single-paned window to a double-paned window. This is shown in Figure 3.15. We find that a double-paned window improves the overall thermal insulation of the wall.

```
(define-frame segment1
  (new (segment rectangle)
       (width (meter 4.0))
       (height (meter 2.5))
       (door (new (door)
                  (layer (material wood,pine,white)
                         (thickness (meter 0.06)))
                  (width (meter 1.0))
                  (height (meter 2.0))))
       (window (new (window,1pane,5 rectangle)
                    (width (meter 1.0))
                    (height (meter 0.5))))
       (outer (new (layer)
                   (material brick,face)
                   (thickness (meter 0.1))))
       (core (new (layer)
                  (material wool,rock)
                  (thickness (meter 0.1))))
       (inner (new (layer)
                   (material plaster,gypsum)
                   (thickness (meter 0.01))))))
(define-frame segment2
  (new (segment triangle)
       (width (meter 4.0))
       (height (meter 1.5))
       (outer-face (new (layer)
                        (material wood,pine,white)
                        (thickness (meter 0.005))))
       (outer (new (layer)
                   (material brick,common)
                   (thickness (meter 0.1))))
       (core (new (layer)
                  (material wool,rock)
                  (thickness (meter 0.1))))
       (inner (new (layer)
                   (material wood,pine,yellow)
                   (thickness (meter 0.005))))))
(define-frame w
  (new (wall)
       (segments segment1 segment2)))
```

Figure 3.12 Synthesis of sample wall.

```
(w 'area)              ⇒ 13
(w 'opening-area)      ⇒ 2.5
(w 'heat-flow 20)      ⇒ 1712.554
```

Figure 3.13 Queries and actions for the sample wall.

```
;;; position window and door within segment 1.
(((w 's1) 'wdw) translate 0.75 1.5 0)
(((w 's1) 'door) translate 2 0 0)
;;; position segment 2 with respect
;;; to segment 1 in the wall.
(((w 's2) 'scale 0 -1 0) 'translate 4 2.5 0)
```

Figure 3.14 Positioning objects in the sample wall.

```
((w 's1) 'wdw (combine ((w 's1) 'wdw)
                       Wdw,2Pane,5-4-5))
(w 'heat-flow 20)       ⇒ 213.065
```

Figure 3.15 Altering the window.

The `combine` form creates a new frame that is a clone of its first argument (the window in `segment1`) with any extra slots in its other arguments (`wdw,2pane,5-4-5` in this case). The resulting window has the same position and orientation as the original window, but will have two panes instead of one.

We close this section with two examples of *assertions* (see Figure 3.16), which can be regarded either as constraints on data, or as the statement of *facts* from which reasoning may then proceed. The first assertion may be read as "*For all segments in wall* w, *the heat flow through the segment for a temperature difference of 20 degrees is less than 300*". Similarly, the second example may be read as "*There exists at least one door in wall* w". The `forall` and `exists` constructs correspond to the two logical quantifiers in propositional logic.

5.5 EVALUATION OF DKSL

Only a preliminary evaluation of DKSL is possible at this time, since it is still under development. However, it appears that DKSL has the potential to compare favorably to other approaches.

```
(forall s (all w segment)
  (< (s 'heat-flow 20) 300))
(exists p (all w part)
  (is-a? p door))
```

Figure 3.16 Two examples of assertions.

Table 3.3 Evaluation criteria of Eastman and Fereshetian

full abstract data types	multiple specializations
composite objects	relations within compositions
relations on object structure	relations between variables
variant relations defined operationally	variant relations
external applications integrity mgmt	management of partial integrity
schema evolution	refinement versus classes/instances

Currently, the author uses the criteria established by Eastman and Fereshetian (Eastman and Fereshetian, 1994) to evaluate DKSL; they are summarized in Table 3.3. These criteria were established to compare data models rather than KR schemes, so some mismatches are expected. In particular, the *external applications integrity management* criterion is inappropriate for DKSL. Also, there are other efforts to establish criteria (such as Ward's criteria of precision, density, and naturalness (Ward, 1992)) that are worth pursuing. The author is currently working towards a set of criteria for KR systems that incorporate these efforts and others.

Abstract data types are supported in that (a) frame interfaces are implementation independent, (b) the type comparison predicates operate uniformly on all frames, and (c) frame behavior is specified via methods. *Multiple specializations* (without name-clash resolution) and *composite frames* are obviously supported. Since compositions are inherent to DKSL, relations both *within compositions* and *on object structure* are supported. *Relations between variables* can also be represented, but due to the strictly representational nature of DKSL, the dynamics of manipulating those relations are not treated. Nonetheless, a user is free to develop Scheme procedures that use the relational information for any purpose.

DKSL is deficient with respect to the last three criteria: *variant relations*, *schema evolution*, and *management of partial integrity*. Since DKSL is intended to be representational only, it does not directly support the *active*, dynamic management of the information it represents. In real design situations, the management of change, of which these three criteria are all examples, is essential. But before these issues can be addressed, the author must generate suitable theory to supplement the current formal underpinnings of DKSL; this is a point of on-going research.

6. FUTURE WORK

There are many aspects of DKSL and its underlying ontological commitments that remain to be explored. This section mentions a few of the more important ones.

Only the ontological commitments made by AIM-D are currently supported by a formalization. Other commitments mentioned in this paper are currently the subject of formalization efforts by the author. It is unclear that DKSL will not require alteration as those formalizations are achieved.

DKSL currently only advises the user about violated constraints that do not jeopardize the integrity of the KB. However, it is exactly the need to resolve such constraints that drives design processes. Therefore, some way of representing the status of constraints must be added to DKSL.

Function modeling has not been incorporated into DKSL yet.

Although an algorithm for automatic categorization of DKSL entities has been devised, it is of little usefulness in "real" application domains. Automatic categorization allows a user to develop DKSL models in isolation, yet allows the system to normalize those models with respect to other contexts. This removes the onus from the user to understand fully the potentially extensive libraries that may be available, yet still allows the system to take advantage of them to organize design knowledge. Automatic categorization may also be very relevant to certain reasoning systems, such as case-based reasoning, in that it facilitates comparing user-provided entities to case libraries.

The user interface to DKSL clearly needs to be made substantially more usable by people unfamiliar with Scheme or Lisp. Currently, the author is considering a combined graphical/textual interface written in Java to take advantage of web-based functionality. The use of Java is also expected to bear on the ability to distribute DKSL entities on the Internet. Comparatively little work has been done in this regard so far, but it seems clear that substantial performance and functionality improvements may be possible.

7. CONCLUSIONS

This paper has presented a progress report on the author's efforts to construct a KBS for engineered products that is rooted in logical foundations. Various ontological commitments have been suggested. These commitments are necessary to establish a fundamental basis for the development of the system.

An overview of the Design Knowledge Specification Language (DKSL) has also been presented. Though still under development, DKSL appears to provide a sufficiently rich representational form for product knowledge can be stored so as to be useful in design, analysis, and even manufacturing areas. Significant work remains to be done to more fully demonstrate the system's adequacy, and to provide an interface that is useful to typical practicing designers. However, the author believes that, based on the contents of the paper, there is reason to be optimistic that these goals can be achieved.

Acknowledgments

The author gratefully acknowledges the National Sciences and Engineering Research Council of Canada for funding this work under grant number OGP0194236.

Notes

1. The name ZF comes from its originators, Zermelo and *F*raenkel.

References

Akman, V. and Surav, M. (1996). Steps toward formalizing context. *AI Magazine*, 17(3):55–72.

Alberts, L. K. (1994). Ymir: A sharable ontology for the formal representation of engineering design knowledge. In Gero, J. S. and Tyugu, E., editors, *Formal Design Methods for CAD*, IFIP Transactions, pages 3–32, Amsterdam. North Holland.

Artale, A., Franconi, E., and Guarino, N. (1996a). Open problems with part-whole relations. In *Proceedings of 1996 International Workshop on Description Logics*, pages 70–73, Boston, MA.

Artale, A., Franconi, E., Guarino, N., and Pazzi, L. (1996b). Part-whole relations in object-centered systems: An overview. *Data and Knowledge Engineering*, 20:347–383.

Bernays, P. (1968). *Axiomatic Set Theory*. North-Holland Publishing Company, Amsterdam.

Borgo, S., Guarino, N., and Masolo, C. (1996). A pointless theory of space based on strong connection and congruence. In Aiello, L. C. and Doyle, J., editors, *Principles of Knowledge Representation and Reasoning - KR96*. Morgan Kaufmann.

Brachman, R. J., McGuinness, D. L., Patel-Schneider, P. F., and Resnick, L. (1991). *LIVING WITH CLASSIC: When and How to Use a KL-ONE-Like Language*, chapter 14, pages 401–456. Morgan Kaufmann Series in Representation and Reasoning. Morgan Kaufmann Publishers, Inc., San Mateo.

Chakrabarti, A. (1993). Towards a theory for functional reasoning in design. In Roozenburg, N. F. M., editor, *Proceedings of ICED 93, 9th International Conference on Engineering Design*, volume 1, pages 1–8, Zurich, Switzerland. Heurista.

Chittaro, L., Tasso, C., and Toppano, E. (1994). Putting functional knowledge on firmer ground. *Applied Artificial Intelligence*, 8:239–258.

Copi, I. M. (1979). *Symbolic Logic*. Macmillan.

Damasio, A. R. and Damasio, H. (1992). Brain and language. *Scientific American*, 267(3):89–95.

Eastman, C. M., Bond, A. H., and Chase, S. C. (1991a). Application and evaluation of an engineering data model. *Research in Engineering Design*, 2:185–207.

Eastman, C. M., Bond, A. H., and Chase, S. C. (1991b). A formal approach for product model information. *Research in Engineering Design*, 2:65–80.

Eastman, C. M. and Fereshetian, N. (1994). Information models for use in product design: a comparison. *Computer-Aided Design*, 26(7):551–572.

Genesereth, M. R. and Fikes, R. E. (1992). Knowledge interchange format reference manual, version 3.0. Technical Report Logic-92-1, Computer Science Department, Stanford University, Stanford, California.

Gerstl, P. and Pribbenow, S. (1996). A conceptual theory of part-whole relations and its applications. *Data and Knowledge Engineering*, 20:305–322.

Gruber, T. R. (1992). Ontolingua: A mechanism to support portable ontologies. Technical report, Knowledge Systems Laboratory, Stanford University, Stanford, CA.

Guarino, N., Carrara, M., and Giaretta, P. (1994). Formalizing ontological commitments. In *Proceedings of the 12th National Conference on Artificial Intelligence*, volume 1, pages 560–568, Seattle, WA, USA. AAAI Press.

Hakim, M. M. and James H. Garrett, J. (1993). A description logic approach for representing engineering design standards. *Engineering with Computers*, 9(2):108–124.

Hurst, T. N. (1991). Automated model generation using the kif declarative language. In Gupta, G. and Shoup, T. E., editors, *Proceedings of the 1991 ASME Computers in Engineering Conference*, pages 137–144. ASME, American Society of Mechanical Engineers.

IEEE (1991). Ieee standard for the scheme programming language. IEEE Std 1178-1990. Institute of Electrical and Electronic Engineers.

Jaynes, J. (1976). *The Origin of Consciousness in the Breakdown of the Bicameral Mind*. University of Toronto Press.

Johnson, R. E. and Zweig, J. M. (1991). Delegation in c++. *Journal of Object-Oriented Programming*, 4(7):31–34.

McCarthy, J. and Buvac, S. (1994). Formalizing context (expanded notes). Technical Note STAN-CS-TN-94-13, Computer Science Department, Stanford University, Stanford, CA.

Qian, L. and Gero, S. (1996). Function-behavior-structure paths and their role in analogy-based design. *Artificial Intelligence for Engineering Design, Analysis and Manufacturing*, 10:289–312.

Reynolds, W. C. and Perkins, H. C. (1977). *Engineering Thermodynamics*. McGraw-Hill.

Salustri, F. A. (1996). A formal theory for knowledge-based product model representation. In *Knowledge-Intensive CAD II: proceedings of the IFIP WG 5.2 workshop*. Chapman & Hall.

Simons, P. (1987). *Parts, A Study in Ontology*. Clarendon Press, Oxford.

Sowa, J. (1992). Discussions about kif and related issues. Interlingua Mailing List, 20 July.

Srzednicki, J. T. J., Rickey, V. F., and Czelakowski, J., editors (1984). *Lesniewski's Systems: Ontology and Mereology*. Nijhoff International Philosophy Series 13. Martinus Nijhoff Publishers, The Hague.

Sturges, R. H., O'Shaughnessy, K., and Kilani, M. I. (1996). Computational model for conceptual design based on extended function logic. *Artificial Intelligence for Engineering Design, Analysis and Manufacturing*, 10:255–274.

Umeda, Y., Ishii, M., Yoshioka, M., Shimomura, Y., and Tomiyama, T. (1996). Supporting conceptual design based on the function-behavior-state modeler. *Artificial Intelligence for Engineering Design, Analysis and Manufacturing*, 10:275–288.

Ward, A. C. (1992). Some language-based approaches to concurrent engineering. *International Journal of Systems Automation: Research and Applications*, 2(4):335–351.

Winston, M. E., Chaffin, R., and Herrmann, D. (1987). A taxonomy of part-whole relations. *Cognitive Science*, 11:417–444.

4

Classification of Knowledge for Generating Engineering Models

-A Case Study of Model Generation in Finite Element Analysis-

Takayuki Sekiya, Akira Tsumaya, and Tetsuo Tomiyama

Research into Artifacts, Center for Engineering (RACE), The University of Tokyo, Japan

Key words: Model Generation, Engineering Model, Ontology, Knowledge Intensive Engineering

Abstract: During design, a designer uses various computational tools, such as a geometric modeling system, analysis tools, and databases. To support these design processes, a system that can integrate such computational tools and support him/her to use the tools and to build, operate and modify models is required. For this purpose, we have been developing the Knowledge Intensive Engineering Framework (KIEF) system. This paper describes the structure of knowledge model used in a modeling process of engineering models. We analyzed engineering knowledge used for Finite Element Analysis (FEA), categorized it, and finally built an environment to support FEA on KIEF.

1. INTRODUCTION

Recent progress of both software and hardware technologies made computational tools, such as geometric modeling systems and analysis tools, popular. Although we have already various convenient tools, a designer sometimes realizes that he/she does not have powerful ways to transfer data from one software to another and that he/she has to input a similar data again and again.

To solve this problem, integrated CAE (Computer Aided Engineering) systems were developed. Most commercial CAE systems allow the designer to transfer CAD data to a numerical analysis tool such as an FEA system, based on product modeling technologies and STEP (Fowler, 1995). They support designers' engineering activities including design and analysis. Typically automotive and aircraft industries heavily use such systems for their engineering activities.

However, model construction is a quite intellectual process and requires the designer's appropriate judgement, including questions like which part of a product must be modeled and which kind of conditions must be applied to the model. This signifies that to develop a system which integrates various design tools, and that supports only data exchange is not enough.

When building a model, the designer uses a wide variety of engineering design knowledge, from common sense knowledge about the physical world to domain specific knowledge about how to use tools. The Knowledge Intensive Engineering Framework (KIEF) (Tomiyama, 1994b, Tomiyama, 1995) is our attempt to provide designers with such modeling knowledge in an integrated manner.

In this paper, we describe the structure of engineering knowledge required for model building. First, we analyze modeling processes, and extract modeling knowledge used in these processes. Next, we categorize it and propose its knowledge structure represented on KIEF. Finally, we illustrate an example to represent modeling knowledge.

2. THE MODELING KNOWLEDGE OF THE KNOWLEDGE INTENSIVE ENGINEERING FRAMEWORK

We have been developing KIEF that enables the designer to integrate existing design tools, and supports him/her in such processes as building, operation, and modification of models. There are similar approaches to our study and some of them aim at full automation of modeling.

2.1 Modeling Automation Approaches

One of our research interests is to represent the designer's thought process in model building. Research in automated modeling in AI is based on the notion that the computer solves a modeling problem. In automated modeling, there are several approaches such as model composition and model selection.

The model composition approaches construct a model by combining predefined model fragments. A designer specifies a scenario description and some queries to be answered by the system. A scenario description describes the object to be modeled in terms of components and their connections. The model construction system then uses a library of model fragments to construct a model. For instance, Falkenhainer's Compositional Modeling (Falkenhainer, 1991) and Nayak's approach (Nayak, 1996) fall into this approach.

The model selection approaches prepare several types of models beforehand for a physical domain, and each model has conditions to be satisfied. The designer specifies conditions to hold for the model. The system searches an appropriate model in the library of models. For instance, Addanki's Graphs of Models (Addanki, 1991) is a typical one.

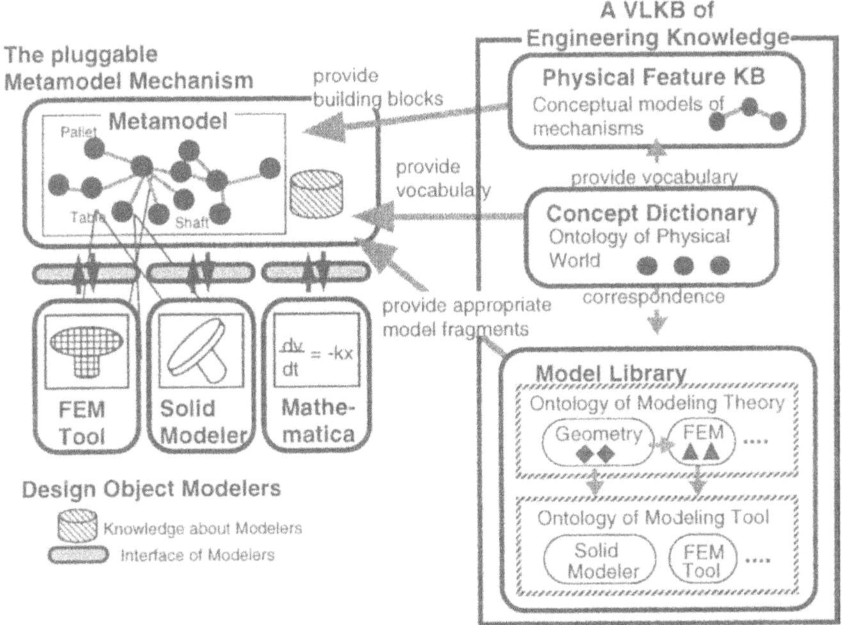

2.2 Knowledge Intensive Engineering Framework

KIEF is a system that integrates existing design tools and supports the designer's activity on the tools, such as model building, model-based reasoning, and model validation. Figure 1 depicts the architecture of KIEF.

The main features of KIEF are the **pluggable metamodel mechanism** (Yoshioka, 1993) that is a mechanism for integrating design tools and the

Very Large-scale Knowledge Base (VLKB) (Ishii, 1995) which supports the metamodel mechanism by supplying primitive knowledge about the physical world.

The metamodel mechanism has symbolic representation of concepts about physical phenomena and mechanical components. A **metamodel** of a design object is represented as a network of relationships among concepts that appear in aspect models. Types of relationship include causal dependency among physical phenomena, arrangements of components, and quantitative relationships. These concepts and relationships constitute the ontology of KIEF. An existing external modeler however, usually deals with an aspect model. Therefore it is desirable that we could plug such existing modelers into KIEF. The **pluggable metamodel mechanism** allows easily plugging in external modelers into KIEF (Yoshioka, 1993). Each external modeler can access data defined in other modelers through the pluggable metamodel mechanism.

VLKB for KIEF supplies fundamental knowledge about the physical world. VLKB consists of the three primary knowledge bases, **concept dictionary, model library**, and **physical feature knowledge base**. The concept dictionary contains the fundamental and general ontology of KIEF, such as physical concepts and relationships among concepts. The ontology is used for building a metamodel and representing engineering knowledge. The model library stores ontologies specific to external modelers, such as model fragments of external modelers and correspondence between them and physical concepts the concept dictionary provides. The physical feature knowledge base contains **physical features** that are combinations among physical concepts. The physical features are the statements that describe physical situation, and the designer constructs a metamodel with physical features.

Roughly speaking, a model building process on KIEF consists of two steps. The first step is to extract a part of the conceptual network in the metamodel that is related to the tool that the designer wants to use, and to convert each concept to a tool-specific concept. We call the network of concepts extracted in the first step, an **aspect model**. The second step is to add quantitative information to an aspect model, and then to prepare data for further numerical analysis.

Through these modeling steps, the designer makes decisions for modeling, while the system just presents possibilities (such as tool-specific concepts) to him/her by automatically retrieving data from appropriate tools and calculates it after the designer specifies necessary data.

2.3 Our Approach

There is a gap between the AI approaches reviewed in Section 2.1 and what we aim at. These AI approaches are based on the idea of automating the entire model building process for a specific domain, and require the existence of a library which stores well-prepared knowledge. However, from an engineering point of view, there are too many design objects and too many ways to analyze design objects. This means that it is quite impossible to prepare a complete library. The designer does not necessarily expect the system to build a model fully automatically.

To integrate design tools on KIEF, the system has to tell the designer which tool can be used for a certain design object, for a certain goal, and in a certain situation. Therefore, what we first need is to understand how the designer builds a model and to systematically represent the designers' knowledge.

3. KNOWLEDGE REQUIRED FOR A MODELING

This section describes an analysis of model building knowledge based on observation of an actual modeling process.

3.1 The Modeling Process for Structural Analysis of a Turntable Mechanism

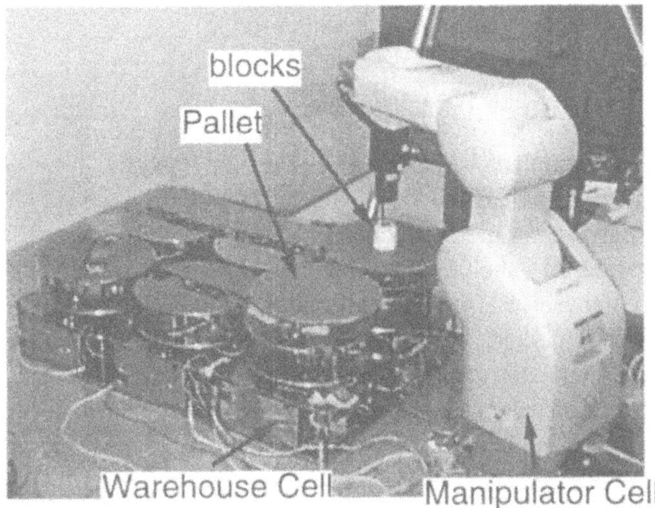

Figure 2: The Cellular Automatic Warehouse

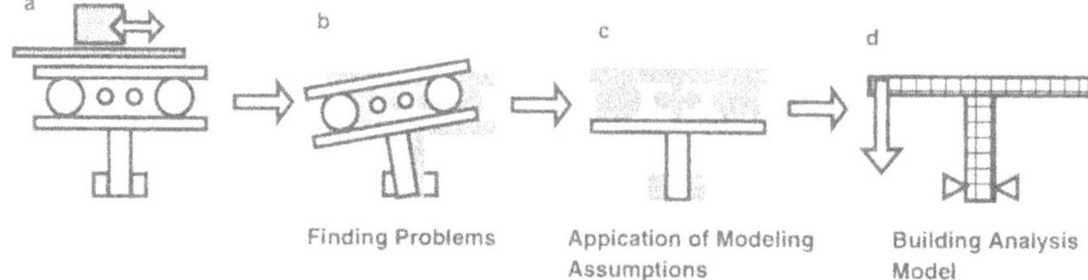

Figure 3: The Structural Analysis of a Cell

Our group has been developing a mechanical system called "Cellular Automatic Warehouse" which consists of homogeneous intellectual autonomous cells arranged in a two dimensional space (Sakao, 1996) (See Figure 2). Each cell has its own CPU and a turntable with rollers, and can transfer a pallet to neighboring cells.

We observed structural analysis of the turntable mechanism that is a part of a cell and identified information required for modeling. The whole modeling process from finding problems to building an FEM model is illustrated in Figure 3. First, we roughly classified the information required for this modeling process into engineering knowledge, a description of a design object itself, and reasoning results derived from them. The followings are the all information explicitly observed.

1. Engineering Knowledge
   (a) Phenomenon Related to Analysis
   - If a heavy object on another object is moving, then the load applied to the latter object will always be changing.
   - If an object is loaded, then it will deform.

   (b) For General Analysis
   - Simpler model is preferred.
   - If the stiffness of material is low, it is easy to bend.
   - Deformation can be detected by structural analysis.

   (c) Knowledge about FEM
   - If a twisting moment does not work on an object, it can be regarded as a shell.
   - (In many cases), minor details are negligible.
   - Simpler models, such as those consisting of simpler elements and fewer elements, can save analysis costs and time.
2. Descriptions of a Design Object
   (a) Functions, structures, and behavior of the turntable mechanism
   - The table is thin.
   - A shaft supports the table.
   - A heavy load on the table moves.
   - The cells are spread on a plane.

- The table rotates with a pallet.
- The machine delivers a pallet to neighboring cells.

(b) Goal of Analysis

- Estimate approximately how much the table will deform.

3. Reasoning Results

(a) Necessity of Analysis

- To check if the deformation of the table and the shaft prevent the machine from working as the designer expects.

(b) Reasoning Result for Structural Analysis

- The detailed structure of the table is neglected, because the goal of analysis is to estimate approximately how the table will deform and because simpler models save cost and time for analysis.

3.2 Findings in the Model Building Process

We analyzed the process of building an FEM model of the turntable mechanism and found out the following issues important.

3.2.1 Relationships between the Goal of Analysis and the Information of Design Object

Most AI approaches to automated modeling are appropriate for dealing with modeling process after a modeling goal is defined. In an engineering modeling process, a designer usually starts the modeling process with an informal problem statement (Pos, 1997). On the other hand, an experienced designer knows what kind of problems should be considered for design. He/she has knowledge about correspondences between design objects and such problems, and the knowledge about information of the design object, such as function, behavior, and structure. In case of the turntable design, the designer analyzes deformation of the table, because it works against one of the fundamental functions to deliver a pallet, or the structure of the turntable has little resistance against load. It will be helpful for less experienced designers to detect problems that occur to the design object.

3.2.2 Selecting an Analysis Method and Determining of Conditions Required for Analysis

During the design process, the designer repeats analysis of the same design object while he/she changes parameter values, according to the result of the analysis. So it is important to save cost and time for one analysis step as much as possible. The designer always has to select an appropriate analysis method and appropriate modeling conditions for a modeling goal.

4. CLASSIFICATION OF ENGINEERING KNOWLEDGE REQUIRED FOR ANALYSIS

In Section 3.1, we analyzed an analysis process from finding a problem to building an analysis model on KIEF. We classify the modeling process into the following four stages (see Table 1). In the following sections, we consider what the designer is doing and how to support him/her at each stage.

4.1 Design Stage

First, the designer specifies a domain of the modeling problem and a goal of modeling in this stage, and considers what problems will occur to a design object after that. Skilled designers can guess problems to be considered by looking at the design object, because they can compare the situation with their experiences and imagine how the design object works.

Table 1: Steps of Modeling Process

	Description	Model Representation for Reasoning	Knowledge
Design Stage	Choose Problem and Derive Unexpected Phenomenon	Part Relationship Network	Relationships between Function and Problem
Analysis Stage	Select Tools and Determine Conditions	Parameter Network	Related Parameters to Physical Phenomenon Model Modification Rules
Modeling Theory Stage	Map to Modeling Theory	Model Specific Representation	Theory specific Rules
Tool Stage	Convert Data for Modeling Tool	Parameters	Tool Specific Rules

Theoretically, if our knowledge is perfect, it is possible to derive every phenomenon that may occur to the design object. It is not realistic to do so, but the designer still somehow has to select relevant phenomena. Therefore, we will look for a mechanism to highlight only necessary phenomena.

As mentioned in Section 3.2.1, the goal of analysis has some connections with information of the design object. Therefore, in this research we build a knowledge base that contains correspondences between function, behavior, structure and problems that should be considered. The designer selects some problems to be solved after the system proposed problems to be considered with the knowledge base.

```
Procedure extract-related-rules(phenomenon, answer)
   /* extract reasoning rules related with the specified physical phenomenon
    phenomenon */
   phenomenon, conditionPP : physical phenomenon;
   collectionPP : collection of physical phenomenon;
   pf : rule of reasoning phenomenon;   pfCol, answer : collection of rule;
   RuleBase : all reasoning rules;
begin
   for every pf stored in RuleBase do
   begin
    collectionPP = get-all-phenomena-reasoned-out-by(pf);
    /* get all physical phenomena reasoned out by applying a rule pf */
    if (collectionPP includes phenomenon) and not (answer includes pf) then
    begin
       add pf to answer;
       for every conditionPP in (get-all-phenomena-to-reason-out(pf)) do
           /* get all physical phenomena required to apply a rule pf */
               extract-related-rules(conditionPP, answer);
    end;
   end;
end;
```

Figure 4: The Algorithm to Extract Related Rules

Next, the system reasons out physical phenomena that may occur to the design object, and that are relevant to the problems to be considered. Supposing that the system stores a large number of reasoning rules, a lot of phenomena, some of which may be fatal, and others of which may be trivial, are derived. They may prevent the designer from understanding important problems to be considered for design. Therefore we implemented an algorithm to extract rules related only to the phenomena which are specified beforehand as unrelevant phenomena that cause problems (see Figure 4). The procedure, "extract-related-rules," recursively searches rules used for reasoning out a specified phenomenon, "*phenomenon*." The designer moves to the next step, after the system proposes unexpected phenomena that occur to the model.

4.2 Analysis Stage

In this stage, the designer selects an analysis method and determines conditions required for analysis. In order to support the designer to select an appropriate analysis method, it is necessary to prepare knowledge about analysis methods themselves as follows.

- Inputs to analysis methods

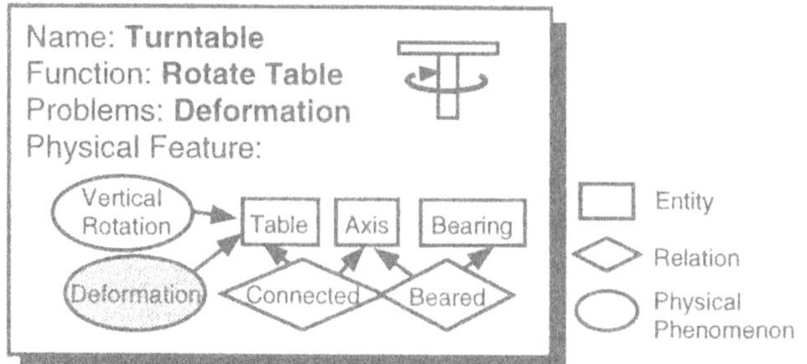

Figure 5: Knowledge about a Goad of Analysis

- Outputs from analysis methods
- Required conditions to execute the analysis

Determining the extent and conditions for analysis is as important as selecting an analysis method. For example, in case of FEM, it is seldom to generate mesh data from original CAD data without processing it. Detailed data is negligible because of Saint Venant's principle. Usually, the designer judges whether or not each geometric data can be regarded negligible when building an FEM model. It is also important to set constraints in the model. There might not be a general way to represent such designer's knowledge as rules.

However, for example, consider a case that the allowable maximum stress is given, and the goal of analysis is to confirm if applied stress never excesses the maximum value. However, the value of stress calculated by analysis will be larger than the true value even if the designer neglects the parts for reinforcement. Therefore, the true values will not excess the maximum value if the value with the simplified model does not excess it. In short, "The detailed data does not have to be paid attention to when neglecting it affects a simulation result and it falls into the safe side comparing the result with the goal of analysis." We call this heuristic rule the reliable minimum one. In order to use such a kind of rules, we will build a parameter network representing that parameters are proportion to one another.

In our KIEF system, we have a qualitative reasoning tool to analyze a qualitative behavior of a design object. To build a model for this tool, the system provides knowledge about correspondence between physical phenomena reasoned out at a previous stage, and qualitative relationships among parameters that are related to the phenomena. In this research, we will use this type of knowledge to build a parameter network.

4.3 Modeling Theory Stage and Tool Stage

General concepts are converted into concepts specific to the modeling theory. There must be a domain specific theory and a domain specific ontology, and a domain specific way to support modeling. The ontology in the modeling theory stage is dependent on a modeling theory, but independent of a modeling tool. In case of FEM, the ontology of FEM includes such elements for FEM as beam, shell, constraints, and materials. These elements are general to any FEA system, but each system uses is own representation and data format for these elements.

The primary work on the tool stage is to prepare the data required for executing the analysis process with a specific tool.

5. SYSTEM ARCHITECTURE AND AN EXAMPLE

This section presents an overview of the system architecture (see Figure 1) and discusses in detail various system components using an example.

5.1 System Overview

In this research, we add some knowledge bases and tools to our existing KIEF system to support model building based on the ideas described in the previous section. The following features are developed for this research.

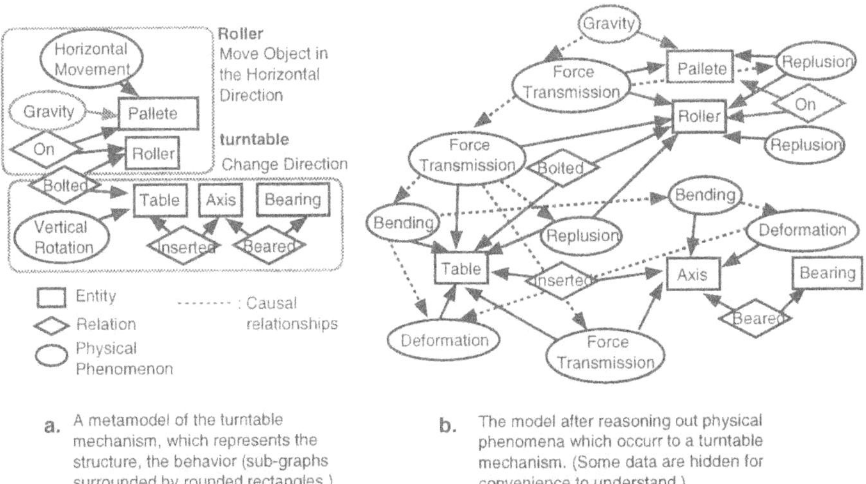

a. A metamodel of the turntable mechanism, which represents the structure, the behavior (sub-graphs surrounded by rounded rectangles.)

b. The model after reasoning out physical phenomena which occurr to a turntable mechanism. (Some data are hidden for convenience to understand.)

Figure 6: A Metamodel of the Turntable Mechanism

- Knowledge base about a goal of analysis (not yet implemented)
  We build a knowledge base that contains correspondences between function, behavior, structure, and problems that should be considered. Figure 5 depicts a turntable mechanism to realize the function, "To rotate a table," and a deformation of the table to be considered.
- External tools (A solid modeler and an FEM solver)
  As an example of model building on KIEF, we demonstrate how to build an FEM model of the turntable mechanism. For this purpose, we plugged a solid modeler and an FEM solver into KIEF, and prepared a model library for it.
- Modeling workspace
  In the modeling theory stage, general concepts are converted into concepts specific to the modeling theory. We developed a workspace for this process. In case of FEM, by referring to the ontology of FEM such as finite elements and constraints, the system supports a designer to build an FEM model on the workspace. The workspace is used as an interface between a pre-processor of FEM and KIEF.

The implementation is currently at an early stage. We demonstrate how the system will support the designer for building an FEM model of the turntable mechanism.

5.2 Example of Modeling Process

We assume that the following data about the turntable mechanism exists in the system, such as function, behavior, structure and geometric data.

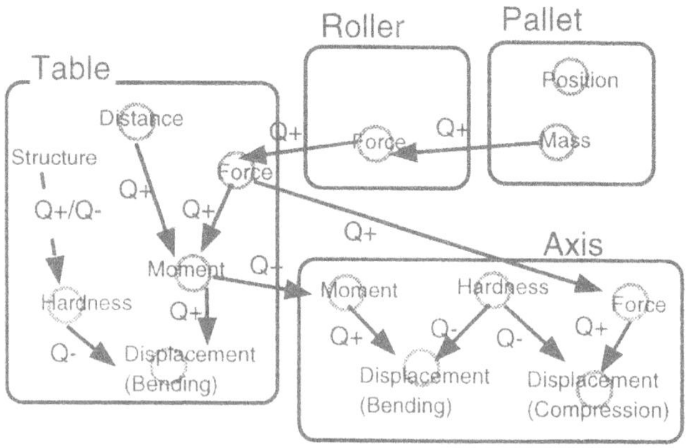

Figure 7: A Parameter Network related to "Displacement"

Figure 6 depicts the function, structure, and behavior of the turntable mechanism.

First of all, the system supports the designer to decide what kind of problem should be analyzed. The design object consists of a turntable mechanism and a roller mechanism (Figure 6a). The system searches each of them from the knowledge base about the goal of analysis, and tells the designer problems which should be analyzed. In this case, the designer pays attention to the problem that is deformation of the table. The system automatically prepares rules related to "Bending," and then reasons out that there is a possibility that table will "bend."

All of the derived phenomena are depicted in Figure 6b. For example, "Force Transmission" means that the load to one object is transmitted to another object.

Next, the designer selects an appropriate analysis method and decides the extent and assumptions for analysis. The definition of a physical phenomenon contains relationships among attributes of entities that the phenomenon occurs to. According to the metamodel with the derived phenomena in the previous stage, the system instantiates attributes related to the phenomena one by one, and derives possible relationships among those attributes by referring to the knowledge about qualitative relationships among the attributes. Figure 7 shows the parameter network generated by this process.

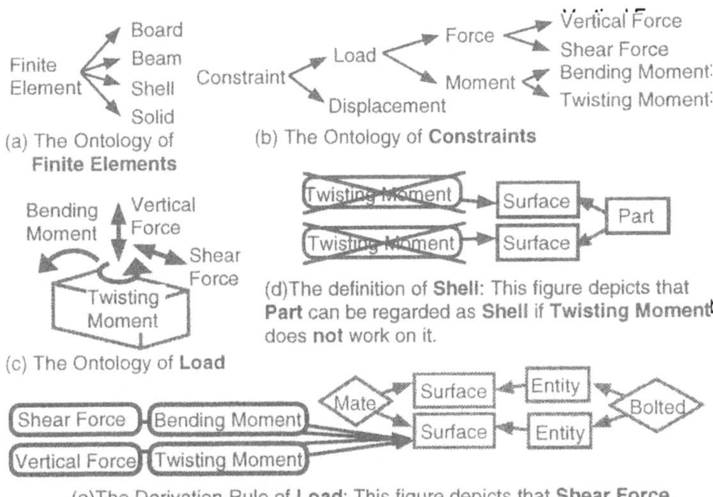

Figure 8: The Ontology of FEM

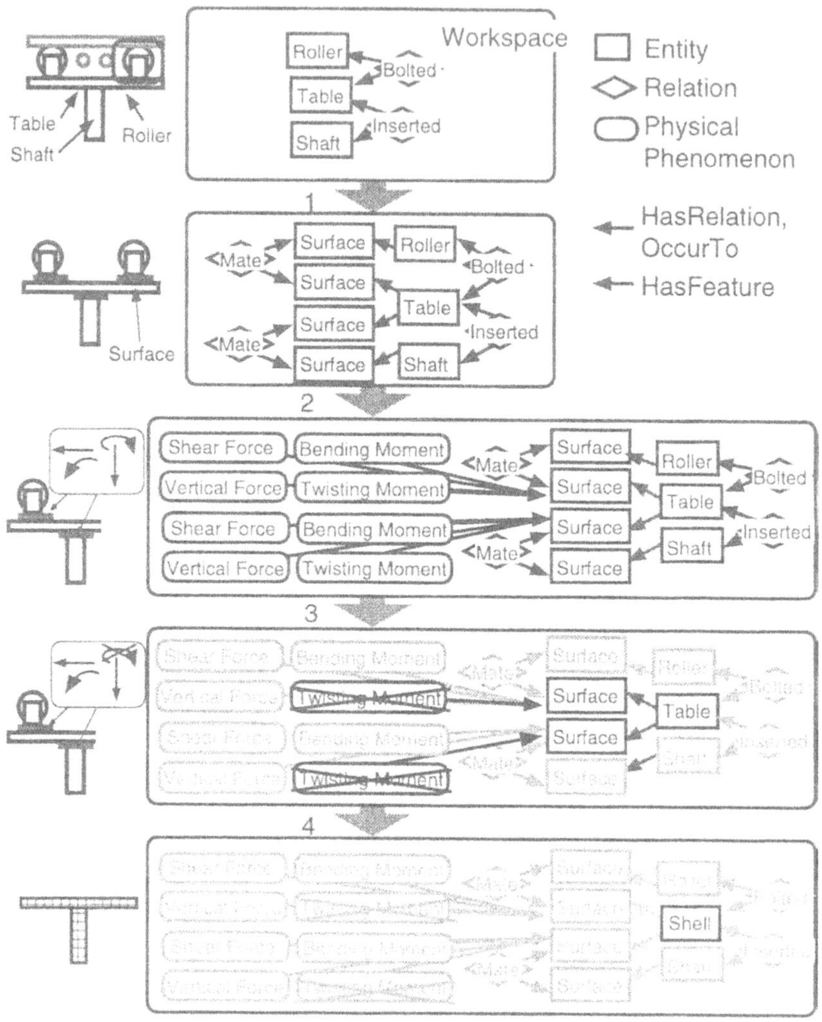

Figure 9: A Process of Finding Appropriate FEM Element for a Table

The designer selects one or a few parameters in the network. In this case, "Displacement of Table" and "Displacement of Axis" are considered. The value of "Displacement of Table" is expected small, because "Pallet" cannot be safely transferred to neighboring cells if "Displacement of Table" is large. Therefore, the designer tells the system to consider increasing of "Displacement of Table" to the model. According to Figure 7, the system proposes a possible way to increase "Force applied to the table" in order to increase "Displacement of Table," and advises the designer to consider the situation that the value of "Force" is large. In this case, the designer decides to analyze the turntable mechanism under the condition that the most load is applied to the table, and to simplify the structure of the turntable not to increase "Hardness of Table."

The designer also has to choose an appropriate tool for structural analysis. The current KIEF system offers FEM and BeamModeler (a simple tool we developed for analyzing strength of a beam based on strength of materials), and the designer can refer to the necessary information to use these specific tools. According to this information, the designer selects a tool.

In the modeling theory stage, the designer converts general concepts in the metamodel to the concepts specific to FEM. The ontology of FEM are defined in the model library for FEM. Figure 8(a) and 8(b) shows the hierarchical relationships among the ontology of FEM. Figure 8(d) is the definition of "Shell."

First, KIEF instantiates concepts about geometry in the workspace (Step 1 of Figure 9), because the ontology of FEM is related to that of geometry. These data can be instantiated by referring to the solid model.

Next, the system derives all forces and moments which will work on each surface by referring to the definition of constraints such as Figure 8(e) (Step 2 of Figure 9). In this case, these forces and moments are derived, because every part is bolted.

After that, the designer specifies some forces and moments that can be neglected. Then, the system proposes an appropriate finite element type for the given conditions with each definition of finite elements such as Figure 8(d) (Step 3 of Figure 9).

In this case, we assume the designer neglects twisting moment that works on the upper surface of the table. Then, the system proposes "Shell elements" for making mesh data of the turntable.

Finally, an aspect model of the FEM model can be built by repeating these steps (Step 4 of Figure 9).

In the tool stage, we build an FEM model on a specific FEM pre-processor (See Figure 10). The system also supports assigning data to the analysis model. For example, since we have to specify two surfaces of a part.

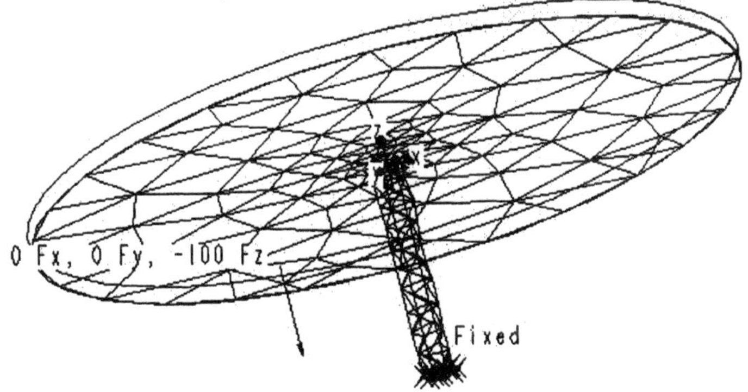

Figure 10: An FEM Model

in order to use "Shell Elements" on the FEM pre-processor we use, the system highlights the surfaces on which the designer neglects twisting moment.

6. DISCUSSION

In this research, we proposed formalized structure of knowledge about modeling processes, which was divided into four stages and also proposed how to support modeling on each stage.

In the design stage, the system detects problems to be considered, and the designer selects problems to be solved. Then, the system automatically extracts the reasoning rules relevant to the problems the designer selected.

Although one of the reasons to support the designer with KIEF is to tell what the designer cannot estimate, it takes considerable time to derive all possible phenomena if there are too many reasoning rules. There are some research reports that are categorized into the area called relevance reasoning in AI (e.g. Levy, 1997). Roughly speaking, it aims at deriving rules relevant only to the current focus for the efficiency of the reasoning. We implemented an algorithm to extract relevant rules according to the idea of relevance reasoning. In case of the turntable, the system works with only rules that have some connection to deformation.

In the analysis stage, to support the designer's decision making, we are interested in using a parameter network which represents qualitative relationships among parameters, and tried to use it to determine modeling assumptions such as neglecting detailed structure of the table and magnitude of load applied to the turntable. Although we believe there should be an algorithm that can make a better use of the network, the way we proposed in this research was simple. A modeling operation often influences a certain parameter both in the positive and negative directions. Therefore, we need a method to evaluate the extent of influences. We have a plan to implement Nayak's algorithm of order of magnitude reasoning (Nayak, 1992).

In the modeling theory stage, we considered that there existed ontology specific to each modeling theory. We studied reusability of universal ontology in our former research (Sekiya, 1996), and we believe the existence of such general ontology for the integration of various tools theoretically. Ontology that is dependent on a modeling theory, but independent of a modeling tool, supports integration of the same sort of tools for a certain modeling theory and representation of modeling knowledge specific to a certain modeling theory.

Choueiry proposes a framework for evaluating reformulation techniques for reasoning about physical systems (Choueiry, 1998). It is worth analyzing KIEF in their framework. Following the terminology they use, we do not have "Strategy" that is a sequence of constructing a specific model. Now we are planning that KIEF provides typical examples referred to when constructing a model. This idea can be categorized into "Strategy."

Ozawa also works on integrating engineering models similar to KIEF (Ozawa, 1998). The main difference between his work and ours is that he is trying to share models on the parameter level, whereas ours is on the conceptual level.

7. SUMMARY

In this paper we described knowledge used in a typical modeling process during engineering design, and we categorized it into four stages. We also described how to support each stage with KIEF. Particularly, in the first and second stages, we proposed methods for starting up the modeling process, and then building a model for analysis.

From a theoretical point of view, we still have to clarify mechanisms to determine a modeling goal. To support the designer to construct a model for the practical use, we have to develop a method to automate routine work of model building and to connect KIEF with other existing analysis tools for cooperative use.

ACKNOWLEDGMENT

This research was funded by the "Modeling of Synthesis" project of the Japan Society of for the Promotion of Science's Research for the Future Program under the contract number, JSPS-RFTF 96P00701.

REFERENCES

Addanki ,S., Cremonini, R., and Penberthy, J. (1991). Graphs of models, *Artificial Intelligence*, Vol. 51, No. 1-3, pp.145-177.

Choueiry, B. Y., McIlraith, S., Iwasaki, Y., Loeser, T., Neller, T., Engelmore, R. S., and Fikes, R. (1998). Thoughts Towards a Practical Theory of Reformulation for Reasoning About Physical Systems, *Working notes of the Symposium on Abstraction, Reformulation, and Approximation (SARA '98)*, Pacific Grove, CA, SA, pp.25-36.

Falkenhainer, B. and Forbus, K. (1991). Compositional modeling: finding the right model for the job, *Artificial Intelligence*, Vol. 51, No. 1-3, pp.95-143.

Fowler, J. (1995). *STEP for Data Management, Exchange and Sharing*, Technology Appraisals Ltd., First edition.

Ishii, M., Sekiya, T. and Tomiyama, T. (1995). A Very Large-scale Knowledge Base for the Knowledge Intensive Engineering Framework, In N.J.I. Mars (eds.): *KB & KS '95, the Second International Conference on Building and Sharing of Very Large-Scale Knowledge Bases*, IOS Press, Ohmsha, Amsterdam, Oxford, Tokyo, and Washington, DC, pp. 123-131.

Levy, A. Y., Iwasaki, Y., and Fikes, R. (1997). Automated Model Selection for Simulation Based on Relevance Reasoning, *Artificial Intelligence*, Vol. 96, No. 2, pp.351-394.

Nayak, P. (1992). Order of Magnitude Reasoning using Logarithms, In *The 3rd International Conference on Principles of Knowledge Representation and Artificial Intelligence*, pp.710-716, AAAI Press, San Jose.

Nayak, P. and Joskowicz, L. (1996). Efficient compositional modeling for generating causal explanations, *Artificial Intelligence*, Vol. 83, No. 1-3, pp.193-227.

Ozawa, M., Cutkosky, M. R., and Howley, B. J. (1998). Model Sharing among Agents in a Concurrent Product Development Team, In Finger, S., Tomiyama, T., and Mäntylä, M. (eds.): *Knowledge Intensive CAD Volume 3, Proceedings of the Third IFIP WG 5.2 Workshop on Knowledge Intensive CAD*, pp. 94-105.

Pos, A. (1997). *Automated Redesign of Engineering Models*, Ph.D. thesis, Twente University, The Netherlands.

Sakao, T., Kondoh, S., Umeda, Y., and Tomiyama, T. (1996). The Development of a Cellular Automatic Warehouse, In *IEEE/RSJ International Conference on Intelligent Robots and Systems '96 (IROS '96)*, pp. 324-331.

Sekiya, T. and Tomiyama, T. (1996). Case Studies of Ontology for the Knowledge Intensive Engineering Framework, In Finger, S., Mäntylä, M., and Tomiyama, T. (eds.): *Knowledge Intensive CAD Volume 2*, Chapman & Hall, pp. 139-156.

Tomiyama, T., Kiriyama, T., and Umeda, Y. (1994). Toward Knowledge Intensive Engineering, In Fuchi, K. and Yokoi, T. (eds.): *Knowledge Building and Knowledge Sharing*, Ohmsha, Tokyo, Osaka, and Kyoto.

Tomiyama, T., Umeda, Y., Ishii, M., and Yoshioka, M. (1996). Knowledge systematization for a knowledge intensive engineering framework, In Mäntylä, M., Tomiyama, T., and Finger, S. (eds.): *Knowledge Intensive CAD Volume 1*, Chapman & Hall, pp. 33-52.

Yoshioka, M., Nakamura, M., Tomiyama, T., and Yoshikawa, H. (1993). A design process model with multiple design object models, In *Design Theory and Methodology (DTM '93)*, ASME, New York, pp. 7-14.

5

Design History System: Data Models & Prototype Implementation

Jami J. Shah[1], S. Rangaswamy[1], Sohail Qureshi[1], Susan D. Urban[2]
[1]*Dept. of Mechanical & Aero. Engineering, Arizona State University, Tempe AZ85287, USA*
[2]*Dept. of Computer Science, Arizona State University, Tempe AZ85287, USA*

Key words: Design history, Product data management, Ontology

Abstract: This paper presents ISO/STEP compatible data models for digitally archiving the history of design projects. The two main components are a product core model and a process core model. The former relates product data to design process rationale and the latter encapsulates the design process itself. The process core model can represent process hierarchy, structure, logical and temporal relationships between processes and design steps. The core models are domain independent; specific schemas can be derived from the core models. A prototype Design History System has been implemented which can be accessed over the Internet with a web based user-interface. A relational-object database is used for design history archival. The system supports browsing, various types of queries, and dynamic schema evolution.

1. BACKGROUND

In today's large Corporations, product development teams are faced with many challenges. Under severe time and cost constraints, they must produce a design for a complex product that requires considerable resources to produce, often incorporates new technology and processes, and is expected to perform according to specifications with minimum cost and risk over its life cycle. George Santayana noted that "those who cannot remember the past are condemned to repeat it,"(Santayana 05). Thus, it makes sense for a design team to research similar past projects before and during product development. It is estimated that designers spend over 40% of their time looking for information. Some of the knowledge they require is archived in textbooks, journals, or company proprietary documents, etc. However, a large portion of it, comes from the company's past experience, and it is this knowledge that is often poorly documented..

Information that designers are interested in fall into three categories: physical attributes, performance characteristics, and design rationale. Since they are not trying to replicate the previous product, but to use it in designing a new one, they would like to understand not only the major hardware features, characteristics, and design parameters, but even more importantly, the rationale behind the choice of those features, characteristics, and parameters. In particular, they would like to see the analyses and design calculations that supported the choice of a particular set of characteristics.

In most large companies, product data is currently maintained in Product Data Management Systems (PDMs). Current PDMs are for the most part file-oriented and do not either store or reveal the semantics of the file contents. As a consequence, they provide a very meager means for relating product data with process or rationale. Also, PDMs do not capture much of the data they maintain. They obtain much of their data—e.g., manufacturing bills of materials (BOMs) and plans—by duplicating this data from other systems, where it is initially captured, and where it is also 'managed'. We need to go beyond PDM technology to create more comprehensive Design Information Systems (DIS) to support the work of design teams distributed in space and time. During the design process the DIS could provide support for better coordination of between team members. This would facilitate design change propagation throughout the project and provide an understanding in the future of the rationale used in design decisions. Before such information systems can be built we need to formulate data schemas that are rich, flexible, and extensible. This paper will discuss both the derivation of such a schema and the implementation of a prototype based on it.

2. LITERATURE REVIEW

Formal models for information representation have been developed in a fragmented manner. There is a set of ISO standards for representing (exchanging) detailed level geometric data and assembly structures (ISO 96). The standard is being extended gradually to include parametric geometry, constraints, construction history (Pratt 97) and some analysis data like FEA (ISO 96). There is no standard representation of performance parameters, function and behavior, or design process and rationale. Stanford's ontology editor uses KQML to specify domains of discourse among intelligent agents in terms of definitions of shared vocabulary (classes, relations, functions, and object constants) from a knowledge engineering point of view. Experiments at Stanford were conducted to determine what information should be captured on the basis of relative frequency of use (Baya92).

There are several computer-aided engineering design systems based on the hypertext paradigm (Brown89, Fu90, McCall89, Thompson90). Design rationale is built up by creating documents and links based upon hypertext. Other systems have tried to capture the "design trace", which is an execution trace of the CAD tools (Casotto94). DEDAL/Weblibrarian provides the means for a system model based indexing that is used in searching through hypermedia documents but it does not present the product or other types of data in a structured way (Baudin 93). *PartNet* uses the WWW for access to component catalog data; it assumes data retrieval and interpretation by human users and lacks structured representation of associated design procedures.

One argumentation model is the Issue Based Information System (IBIS) developed by Rittel for organizing the deliberation process that occurs during complex decision-making (Rittel 73). An IBIS model views the decision-making process in terms of issues (tasks, questions or problems), alternatives (proposals or concepts), arguments (evaluations) and decisions. It is possible to find whether an issue has been resolved or not, what decisions have been made, and the reasons for them (Chen 91, Conklin 88, Lubars 91). An extension of IBIS which would make it more applicable to the description of mechanical engineering design processes was proposed in (Ullman 95) and (Nagy 92). Lee (Lee 96) has provided a framework DRL (design representation language) that extends IBIS by adding more concepts such as goals, questions, procedures and viewpoints. Somewhat similar to IBIS is the QOC model proposed by MacLean (MacLean 96) in which, the logic that leads to each decision is modeled in terms of Questions (key issues), Options (possible answers) and Criteria (for comparing options).

A number of hypertext systems were developed to support frameworks for argumentation. Such systems included PHIDIAS (McCall et al. 94) and gIBIS (Conklin, 88) for the IBIS framework as well as EUCLID (Smolensky et. al. 87) and SIBYL (Lee 90) for other argumentative frameworks. PHIDIAS combines computer-aided design, argumentation, and multimedia capabilities (McCall 94). There have been attempts to combine argumentative approaches to capture design rationale and other design aids to improve the design process. Another system is the KBDS (King 95) system in which, a knowledge-based design system (KBDS) was used along with IBIS to develop a tool to support chemical plant design using design history. A system for conflict resolution in collaborative design called SHARED-DRIMS was proposed by (Pena-mora, 1996).

Case-based reasoning (CBR) is a general paradigm for problem solving based on the recall and reuse of specific past designs (cases). The three basic steps in a typical CBR cycle are: *find, retrieve, revise, and archive.* Many methods have been developed for each of these issues, such as *Archie* (Domeshek, 97), *Cadsyn* (Maher, 91), *Casecad* (Maher, 95), *Kritik* (Goel, 96), *Cadre* (Faltings, 97) and *Cadet* (Narasimhan, 97). *Casecad* and *Cadsyn* represent subcases with the Function Behavior Structure (FBS) framework which classifies the variables used to describe design cases into three semantically different categories. *Kritik*'s developers directly addressed the representation of causal behavior as sets of device states and transitions linking the states; these behaviors explain how the physical device's structural elements achieve its functions.

Commercial Product Data Management (PDM) systems do not support retrieval based on file contents and provide very limited support for design process representation. Current approaches for computer-based design retrieval fall well short of answering the types of questions that one human designer asks of another. The reason for this lack of sophistication is that design information is archived as either text/hypertext or data indexed in terms of a few pre-defined attributes.

Our previous ASU Design Information System (DIS) (Shah, 96) supported four information elements: product data, design steps, relationship of design steps to product data and rationale. The product data model is imported from STEP with modifications made to include design with features. The system was implemented on the World Wide Web and the data is stored in text files. This is a disadvantage because, complex data types cannot be handled and the system slows down as the text files get bigger. The work reported in this paper extends the ASU DIS system in several directions.

3. DIS CLASSIFICATION

In order to present the different research approaches to Design Information Systems under a common perspective, a taxonomy is presented here. The classification is based on six generic criteria:

1. Level of dynamic functionality: This criterion is a measure of both the extent of data processing and the control that the system has over the design process. At the lowest level is the archival retrieval of files like a PDM system which knows little about the contents. At the highest level is a pro-

active system that monitors conflicts, constrains violation, and automatically propagates design changes.

2. Level of abstraction: This criterion compares the levels of abstraction at which product data is captured. A system may support one or multiple levels. These levels may also be perceived as phases of the design process: the longer one gets into a project, the more information there is; for example, there is more detailed information available at the embodiment stage than at the early conceptual design stage.

3. Data organization: This criterion compares the level of formalization and structure of archived information. Unstructured text may require human interpretation while formal models may be thought of as computer understandable.

4. Granularity: Indication of the various levels of detail at which the design process information is captured, from microscopic actions, such as program log files to high level project planning information.

5. Data integration: This criterion refers to the data sharing architecture: centralized, distributed, or federated.

6. Schema flexibility: This categorizes information models according to the freedom they provide to the users to incorporate new applications via changes to the schema.

Table 1 is a comparison of five of the many design history systems described in the sections above: *PHIDIAS, DRIMS, C-DeSS, ASU-DHS* and *Cadre*. The Table shows that only passive design information systems have been built as prototypes. Most only capture a small fraction of design information and still lack formal structure. Also, systems either assume ownership of all data (centralize), or generate their own "overview" data, such as the IBIS approach. An integrated view of all design data in a distributed environment is done superficially today.

4. OVERVIEW OF RESEARCH

Except for highly routine designs, the product structure and design procedures are not known *a priori* ; this implies that the information schema evolves during the design process. Therefore, support for dynamic schema evolution and continual transformation of instance data between schema changes are fundamental requirements of any active or pro-active design archival system. A domain independent query language is another basic requirement for design retrieval. An indexing scheme is required to support user defined queries. Therefore, we need both topical models and integration infrastructure. Topical models are focused on specific aspects of design information (e.g., geometry, stress analysis, project management, etc.), while the integration model is needed to bring together product and process topical models without eliminating the flexibility to extend and develop models in localized domains. Various standard and pseudo standard topical models already exist but integration models for relating such information, at various levels of abstraction, to process information do not exist. The need for data organization, query language, and schema evolution all point to the use of database technology in the implementation of design archival systems.

Table 1 Comparison of Design Information Systems

Classification criteria	PHIDIAS	DRIMS	C-Dess	ASU-DIS	Cadre
Dynamic functionality					
Static file retrieval/ Browsing	•	•	•	•	•
Unstructured search	•	•	•	•	•
Structured queries	-	•	-	•	-
Reactive: Input checks	-	-	-	-	-
Proactice: Change propagation	-	-	-	-	-
Abstraction level					
Perceived need	•	•	•	•	•
Design specifications	•	•	•	•	-
Functional design	•	•	•	•	•
Embodiment design	•	•	•	•	•
Artifact type design.	•	•	•	•	•
Artifact instance design	•	•	•	•	•
Manufacturing process data	-	-	•	•	-
Production data	-	-	-	-	-
Data Organization					
Unstructured text	•	-	-	-	•
Partially structured	•	•	•	•	-
Fully Structured	-	-	-	-	-
Geometric rationale	•	-	•	-	-
Level of Granularity					
Commands/ actions log	-	-	•	•	-
Work session summaries	•	•	•	•	-
Design tasks	-	•	•	•	-
Design sub-project	-	•	•	•	-
Design project	-	•	•	•	-
Level of Integration					
Centralized (single source)	•	•	•	•	•
Distributed	-	-	•	•	-
Federated	-	-	-	-	-
Schema flexibility					
Pre-determined/ fixed schema	•	•	•	•	-
Branching in schema	-	-	•	•	-
Synthesis from a fixed set	-	-	-	-	-

Synthesis from an open set	-	-	-	-	-

The steps followed in the system development were as follows:

1. Study the morphology of design information and select topical models
2. Define domain independent integration model
3. Derive domain specific models for airframe design and analysis
4. Implement a Design History System (DHS) for archival and retrieval of design cases
5. Populate and test the DHS with specific cases

We examine the morphology of design information in Sec. 5 and then present an integration model in Sec. 6. Implementation issues are discussed in Sec. 7. Space does not permit us to discuss topical models; the reader is referred to (Qureshi 97a, 97b, Shyam 98).

5. MORPHOLOGICAL ANALYSIS

By morphology we mean the scope, content, internal structure, external relationships, temporal relations, role, usage and semantics of design knowledge, data, and information (information) needed to support the design process in a real-world corporate environment. We investigated the creation, organization, archival, communication, usage and management of product design data, information, and knowledge during the product development cycle in an industrial setting (an aircraft manufacturer). Both product and process knowledge were studied. To keep the project manageable, the emphasis was on the design phase; manufacturing and other downstream applications were out of scope, although any life cycle data used in design decisions (such as manufacturability) were within scope.

Basic information element-types include system constraints, product data elements, product data features, and design process steps. Also of interest are relationships among these elements—e.g., relationships between process steps and product data elements, relationships among system constraints, product data features, and rationale. We need to represent this information in a formal way. It is best to first consider one aspect or domain/task at a time (topical models), without worrying about the inter-relations (integration). Topical models will be discussed in this section, while the integration will be discussed in the next section.

Topical models for product data, design procedures, rationale, project management, and organizational data are needed for developing our system. Widely accepted topical models for product data already exist under the ISO/STEP standard for geometry, geometric tolerances, assembly structure, finite element analysis, manufacturing plans, and material specifications.

However, product models at higher abstraction levels, such function and behavior are either non-existent or not widely used. The same applies to design process and rationale, although IBIS may be considered a pseudo-standard. We needed to develop the process ontology further.

Since design processes can represent different types of activities, an ontology should be extensible in that the user can specialize the process class with user-defined processes. Subtype processes and supertype processes are specializations and generalizations of a process respectively; decomposition of a process is orthogonal to specialization or generalization of processes. The ontology framework must contain these capabilities. Process attributes can be categorized into: 1) attributes of processes, 2) process to information element relationships, and 3) and process-to-process relations. The class of attributes that describe a process represents important information about the process itself. Of interest is the status that a process is in. A process can be active, suspended, or resumed. In addition, a process can be tentative (the designer is exploring alternatives), committed (the process is chosen as part of the whole design process), or abandoned/failed (the process generated an unsatisfactory design). The input/output objects represent the objects that a process uses, creates or modifies. 'Uses-objects', 'creates-objects', 'modifies-objects', and 'deletes-objects' are the essential process-to-data relationships. For a particular process object and associated data objects (design specifications) there can be associated rationale and constraints. Sub-process and super-process attributes of a process represent the 'part-of' relationship between processes. A process is composed of a set of sub-processes. The sub-process and super-process attributes give information about the temporal relationship between processes (i.e., a sub-process will be performed within the time-frame of the parent process). But in general, additional temporal information is needed. Such information is provided by the dependency and temporal relationship attributes. Temporal relationships and dependencies among a related set of processes are: *depends-on, independent, parallel-with, mutually-exclusive-with,* and *synchronous*. Processes also require the definition of specific process operations. These operations model the various abstract and primitive activities that occur during design. An operation such as 'decompose' needs to be associated with the process meta-class object. The operation 'decompose' will take any process and relate the process to a set of new sub-processes or sub-tasks which is at a lower level of abstraction.

Two types of constraints must be supported for the description of design histories: Static constraints are those constraints that are typically associated with structural data (i.e., constraints expressible in a first-order logic constraint language, possibly supplemented with application-oriented functions). Dynamic constraints are important since they constrain relationships between processes or between processes and other information objects. Pre/post condition attributes of a process are one example of dynamic constraints.

A simplified form of IBIS is needed to capture rationale of a design and relationships of rationale to design processes, constraints, and data. A possible strategy is to scale down the IBIS structure to represent only issues, positions and arguments. In a simplified view, the justification may be considered to be the design rationale object. As an optional function, the post-condition attribute of a process may trigger a prompt to the designer for a rationale for the particular design action. Thus, rationale could be associated with design processes or objects at any level of abstraction and scope of the design. As with constraints and processes, rationale will be given object status to maintain uniformity of the information model and facilitate the definition, expression and manipulation of rationale.

The ontology given above for design process and rationale is domain independent. One may need to derive more specific models for domains of interest. We have derived ontologies for design and analysis of airframe structures, but this aspect of the research is not described in this paper; the reader is referred to (Qureshi 97b, Shyam 98) for more information.

6. INTEGRATION SCHEMA

The aim of the integration model is to provide a framework to relate topical models included in the design information capture system. The framework is developed by providing a basic skeleton called the "Integration Core Model" (ICM) which is a formal representation of the definition of a product in terms of one or more topical models. There are two major sub-divisions of the ICM: *Product Core* and *Process Core*. The Product Core Model provides the high level structure needed to associate process information to the product data and the Process Core Model provides the generic process information model that is needed to capture and organize process information. The ICM is developed to play the role of a generic resource similar to the integrated resources series of ISO 10303 standard.

6.1 Product Core Model

The Product Core Model defines the data-types necessary for establishing a framework for relating product data such as geometry, design procedures, function and behaviour attributes, and environmental information. The following is a description of selected Product Core Model entities. An EXPRESS-G representation of the Product Core Model is shown in Figure 1.

concept: Everything that is designed/developed is called a concept, meaning that each product would be a concept. By calling it a concept and not a product at this level, it becomes a generic representation without concern to the level of detail. Concepts have views, versions, context, relations, and description.

relations: This abstract entity represents the relations between concepts. The concepts may be related or relating to other concepts through explicit relationships in both sides. The relationships that a concept can bear with other concepts may be different each. For this reason, ***relations*** is an abstract class.

description: Such information includes, but is not limited to, properties associated with the product, their usage etc. This entity provides the attributes needed to uniquely identify a product. There is no commitment to any particular definition and the users of this model have the freedom to supply their own attributes that can uniquely identify a product in their environment.

product-process relations: link product models to process models.

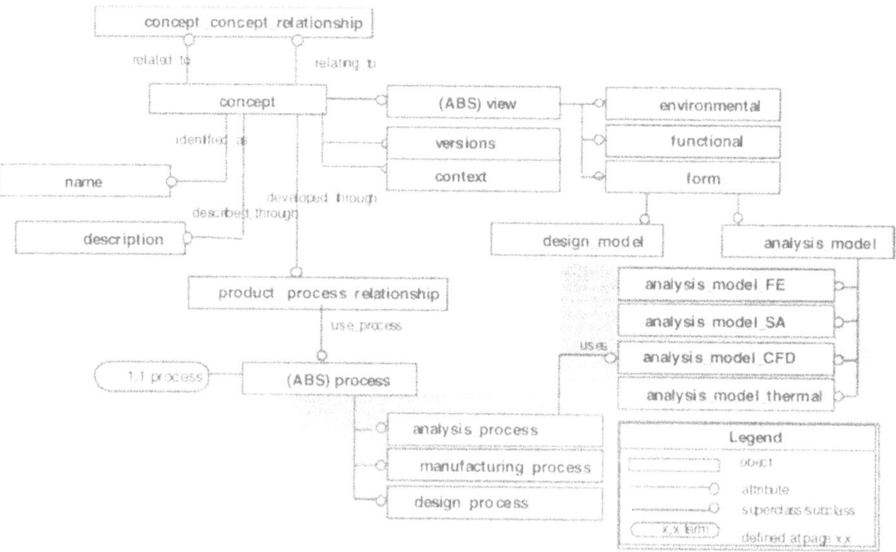

Figure 1 High Level Entities of the Product Core Model

(EXPRESS-G notation: boxes are entities; dark lines represent super-subclass relations; light lines represent attributes; little circles show direction of relation)

6.2 Process Core Model

A process can be described as it evolves and no *a priori* knowledge is necessary. Specialized processes are captured through survey studies along with the generic information that is common to all processes. The model also provides freedom for inclusion of specialized activities associated with the specialized processes. For example, a computational fluid dynamics (CFD) process would have specialized activities such as selection of flight parameters, evaluation of pressure distributions, specific to the CFD process. The EXPRESS-G representation of the model is shown in Figure 2.

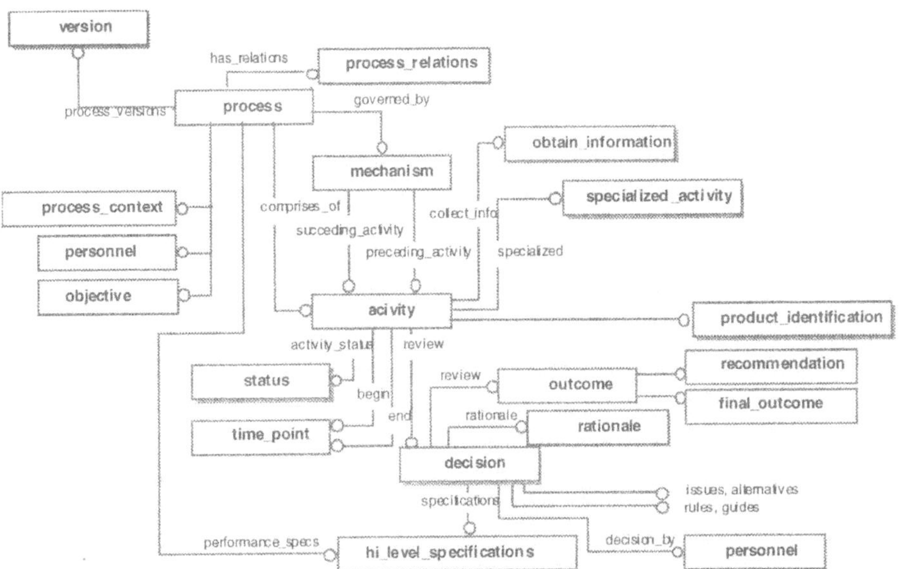

Figure 2 High Level Entities of the Process Core Model

The following information categories are used to describe the generic process information:

Mechanism: information about the sequence of *activities* that has to be maintained in order to run a process. The mechanism defines the relationship between various activities that constitute a process.

Personnel: information about the personnel involved in the process.

Decision Information: includes technical description of alternatives considered, outcome, personnel involved in decision making. The information is linked to rationale and outcome.

Rationale: Explanation of decisions made.

Time point: This information keeps track of what action was taken at what time so as to keep track of the process and plan for workflow.

Processes are associated with product data through relations defined in the product core model. The product data objects are used as inputs/outputs of a process activity. There is also a set of process attributes that define the relationships between various processes and these are expressed using mechanism information or process dependencies.

7. DESIGN HISTORY SYSTEM: IMPLEMENTATION

The following sub-sections describe the design and implementation of the second generation ASU design information capture system, DHS-2.

7.1 Database issues

Three requirements of the database management system are to faithfully represent the entities and complex relationships in the data model; to handle dynamic schema evolution; and to support user defined queries. Object oriented databases (OODB) can be used to support schema evolution, though they typically require recompilation to accommodate schema changes. In OODB all the data in a complex entity is stored in a single object. Therefore, the data in an entity is retrieved and modified as a single object. In a relational database, the same aggregate would be stored in multiple tuples scattered across multiple relations, requiring several operations to retrieve and modify it. It was thus decided to use an OODB.

The DBMS considered were ROSE, ITASCA and PSE-Pro. ROSE (Hardwick, 89) was selected because it was more stable, allows creation of objects in C++ or Java, and has a built-in connection to EXPRESS, the data modeling language of the ISO/STEP standard. ROSE also supports multiple versions of data and provides tools to aid the process of detecting differences between versions and merging versions of product data (Hardwick, 91). ROSE files can be converted to STEP Part21 format and vice-versa, a feature that can be very useful for a neutral storage in a central database.

7.2 DHS Architecture

Three types of interfaces need to be accommodated: schema definition/editing, populating the database with case histories, browsing/querying of design histories. All 3 functions could be carried out by the same user (designer), or by different people. Initially, a schema can be loaded from an EXPRESS file and subsequent changes made interactively. Also, the current system is based on interactive instantiation for archiving case histories using forms.

It was decided to build the DHS on top of the World Wide Web because it is a familiar interface to most people and designers feel comfortable working on it. The software for the client and the server is easily available for almost all platforms and is of a low cost or shareware. The web allows for remote access easily. Distance querying of the database information over the Internet does not require high bandwidth communication links. External security features can be easily implemented by using Javascript. There is also an option of building the system over an Intranet that is not accessible outside the organization. There is a possibility of referencing multimedia records such as graphics files, audio and video. Using the web for the UI, however, also has some disadvantages. There are only limited number of interaction techniques, such as "form input" and limited graphics input. Any higher level interactions have to be provided by external programs such as applets. Security is an important consideration in industrial applications. However, space does not permit us to describe this aspect of the implementation – see (Shyam 97) for details.

A high level architecture of DHS-2 is shown in Figure 3. The web server provides a link between the various clients accessing the system and the underlying application that connects to the DHS-2 database. The DHS-2 application contains a user interface engine to generate forms for user input based on the EXPRESS schema, and a backend to access the database for populating it and for queries. The following aspects of the DHS implementation are discussed below. form generation, the backend and web gateway to ROSE, history archival process, the designer's palette, dynamic schema evolution, and the query module.

7.3 Dynamic Form Generation

The UI, which is based on HTML forms is implemented over the World Wide Web. The UI is designed to perform the following functions:

1) Instantiate the Design History Database.
2) Delete an entity from the database.
3) Browse the instance data, the metadata and the EXPRESS schema.
4) Query the database.
5) Support dynamic schema evolution.

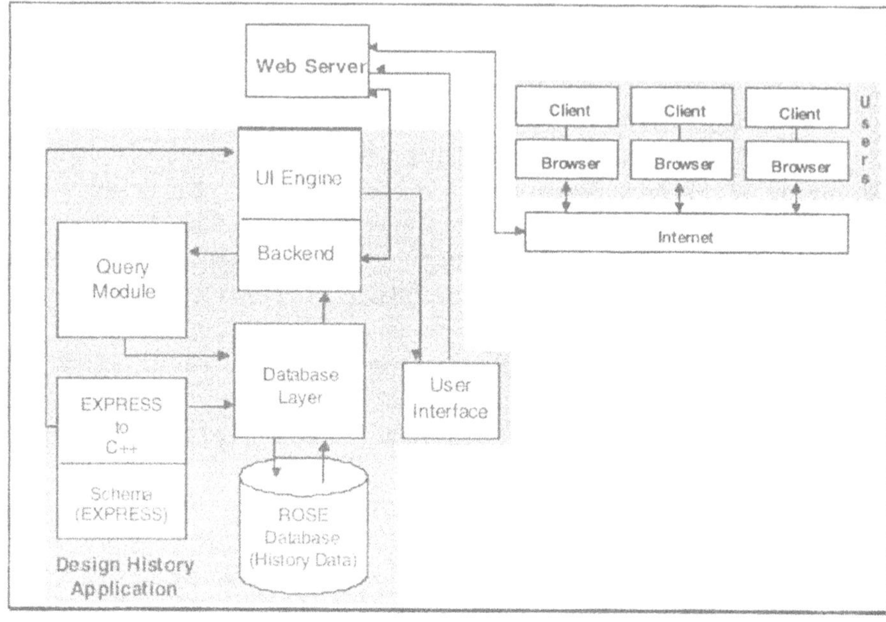

Figure 3 Conceptual Architecture of DHS-2

The forms that allow the user to populate design histories are generated automatically from the EXPRESS schema by the User Interface Engine. A typical instantiation form is shown in Figure 4. The UI Engine (Figure 5) contains an EXPRESS to HTML mapping tool. For every entity in the EXPRESS schema, HTML forms (like the one in Figure 4) are generated with input text fields, selection boxes etc. using the UI Engine. These HTML forms are used to populate the database based on the designers' input. The mapping has to proceed in a specific order because there may be complex entities that may reference other entities. First, all simple entities that have EXPRESS primitive types only as attributes are mapped. Next come all complex entities with references to other entities that have already been mapped. The third set is all supertypes with simple or complex entities or EXPRESS primitive types as attributes. The fourth set is all select types and enumeration types. The last to be mapped is the set of subtypes. A script has been implemented to create a list of entities in the order mentioned above. This list is the input for automating the entire process of form creation. This ordering is implemented in the Pre-Processor.

The output from the UI Engine consists of two files for each entity: one is a procedural file that contains the HTML definitions and the other is a script file that references the procedural file. When a form is requested by the client browser, the web server loads the script file to display the form.

ASU Design History System

phase_four:
review_results
input:
input_models
wind_tunnel_data:
identity
local_storage STR
sdm_location STR
cfd_results:
identity
local_storage STR
sdm_location STR
specification:
performance_specification
lift STR
drag STR
torque STR

evaluation_general:
e_general
standing
rating
good-0
comments:
rationale
comments STR
Edit image
test_hrs:
man_hours
design_hours STR
dhs_hours STR
evaluation_pressure_distribution
rating
good-0
evaluation_coefficient_of_lift
rating
good-0
evaluation_coefficient_of_drag
rating
good-0

7.4 Backend and Database Gateway

The backend is responsible for initial processing of the user input and depending on the user input, either more forms are displayed or a gateway is opened to the ROSE database. The backend is implemented as a CGI (Common Gateway Interface) program written in PERL (Practical Extraction and Report Language). The gateway to the ROSE database is implemented as a shell script for setting up environment and special ROSE variables, as well as, paths that have to be set before any ROSE operation can be performed.

For history archival (instantiation), which is described in detail in the next section, the backend program checks to see if all the information is received, then passes the data on to the database layer. For example, if the input form contains a select type and the selection made by the user is another EXPRESS entity, the backend has to display a new form for the selected entity. For deletion of an instance of an entity, a form is displayed that takes the name of the entity through a text box. Next, the form for that entity is displayed and the user has to put in one or more attribute values that uniquely identify that entity in the database. The particular instance is then removed from the database.

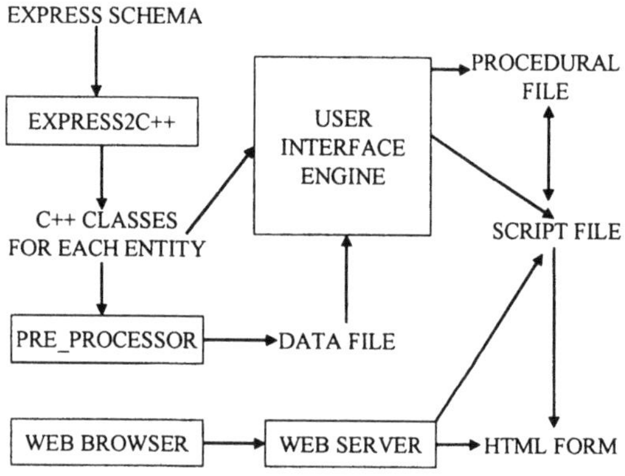

Figure 5 Generating html forms from schemas with the UI Engine

7.5 History Archival (Instantiation) Process

Histories can be archived based on the EXPRESS schema made current in the database. This does not mean that the schema itself cannot be changed; we will discuss dynamic schema evolution in a later section. For active projects, the company will need to determine the frequency of populating/updating the history. This could be at regular intervals, (e.g., once a week) or at the completion of significant sub-tasks, etc.

Archival requires interactive input via forms, such as the one in Figure 4. The EXPRESS schema is used as an input to the *express2c++* tool to generate the C++ class for each entity and a ROSE file that contains the EXPRESS Data Dictionary. After translation the C++ classes can be used in application programs that need to interact with the database, retrieving, manipulating and storing entities defined in the schema. Depending on the user input and the entity instantiated, the backend dynamically creates a C++ program, based on the constructor for that entity in the C++ program generated by the *express2c++* tool and the user input from the form. This is an important feature as it is required for the dynamic schema evolution also.

Figure 6 shows the process of design archival, i.e. database instantiation. When the user submits a data form, a gateway to the ROSE database is opened. The dynamic C++ program generator creates a new instantiation program based on the constructor and the user input. The program is run from within the web browser. The data goes into the ROSE database and the updated ROSE instance file is displayed on the web browser.

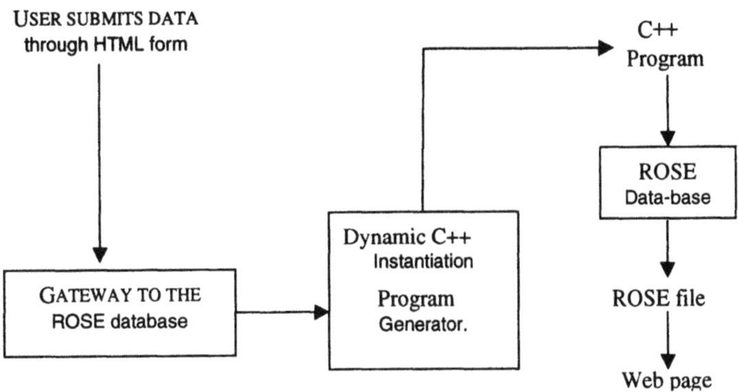

Figure 6 History archival (Instantiation) Process

During archival, the user also has the option of selecting entities for which earlier instances can be used. When this selection is made, the user can select the previous instance data and the UI is regenerated to include them as select types.

7.6 Database Layer

The database is stored as a ROSE file. There are two ROSE files for each EXPRESS schema definition. One stores the EXPRESS data dictionary and the other contains the instance data. Both ROSE files can be browsed from the user interface. New persistent objects are created in an application. ROSE applications read EXPRESS-defined objects into memory and write them to storage in clusters known as "design" objects. These RoseDesign objects hold the data objects and define operations that work on multiple objects. Objects are considered persistent if they are contained within a RoseDesign, because they can be written out to secondary storage. Objects that are not owned by a RoseDesign are considered non-persistent because they will be lost when the program has finished running. An object may belong to only one RoseDesign at any given time. In addition to belonging to a design, a persistent object has an EXPRESS data-dictionary definition, called its domain, and a unique 160-bit object identifier, called an OID. This extra information, along with a reference to the owning design, is stored in a helper object called a manager. Instances of the RoseManager class are associated with each persistent object. Within a schema design, EXPRESS definitions are stored as instances of the RoseDomain and RoseAttribute classes. Each RoseAttribute object describes a storage slot. Depending on the EXPRESS definition, this storage slot could be an entity attribute, one component of a select, or the elements of an aggregate. The EXPRESS Data Dictionary is a compiled description of the data structures defined by an EXPRESS schema. The description is stored as a RoseDesign containing RoseDomain and RoseAttribute objects.

7.7 Designer's Palette

Non-geometric rationale is entered through the text boxes provided by the user interface. Geometric data, which is defined via CAD systems, is translated into 2D (GIF) or 3D (VRML) formats. These images can be annotated and comments can be added to express rationale, by using the "Designer's Palette". The "Designer's Palette" is a Java applet that can be viewed from within the web browser. The modified images, once entered into the Design History database, can be viewed over the Web and provide a visual browsing of geometry rationale. An advantage of using image files is that it conveys the message more clearly than simple text. The image shown in Figure 7 was annotated using this functionality.

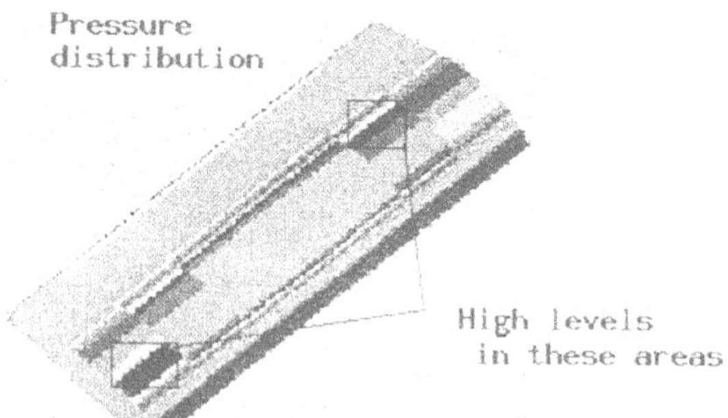

Figure 7 Archiving and annotating graphical data

With every occurrence of rationale in the schema, the UI Engine puts a hyperlink to the Java applet, along with the regular text-box for input of rationale as text. The applet allows the user to load any image file in *gif* or *jpeg* format. Portions of the image can be highlighted and comments can be added or fresh drawings can be created. Once the comments and alterations have been made, the new modified image file is stored and its location is put into the text area for rationale in the original form from which the link was made. The modified image file is displayed when the ROSE file is loaded by the browser.

7.8 Query module

The querying facilities provided in DHS-2 to extract useful information from the ROSE database are based on the various functions provided by the ROSE library to traverse, search and locate objects in memory. As in the case of instantiation, C++ programs are generated based on the type of query and the backend runs these programs to give an output. Since a RoseDesign object is the basic unit of I/O for STEP data, most of these services operate within the scope of a single design.

When the user submits a query through the web browser, it goes to the server. The server runs the backend, which does the initial processing and selects the appropriate query handler from the query module. Then, the database layer runs the query using the form input, the query handler and the relevant C++ classes. It fetches the data from the database and displays it back to the user.

Queries in DHS-2 are divided into three categories: Standard database queries, pre-defined queries, and user-defined queries.

<u>Standard database queries (domain independent)</u>

1. Generate a list of all instances of an entity along with its attributes.
2. Objects that match certain constraints: Operators <, >, ≥, =, ≠, have been implemented. These are particularly useful to locate values of numerical attributes.
3. AND/OR constraints: Queries such as "display a list of Points where x=0 AND/OR y>0" have been implemented.

<u>Pre-defined queries (specific to design rationale)</u>

1. What was the objective of design task "x"?
2. Why was/was not alternative "x" approved?
3. What were the results of the evaluation "type y" of design "x"?
4. What were the recommendations to solve problem " y" in "x"?
5. What were the alternatives generated for design "x"?
6. What kind of analysis was performed on design "x"?
7. What was the overall rating for design "x" and why was it rated so?
8. What were the performance specs. and how did design "x" perform?
9. What were the rules that governed design "x"?
10. What were the design constraints?

An example of results of query type #4 is shown in Figure 8. In this example, "y" is aerodynamics and "x" is a specific wing design.

User defined (Dynamic) Query generation

There is an option available under 'DHS specific queries' that can be used for dynamically generating new queries that could help other designers. The user can formulate a query question that would be visible to other designers accessing the query page. Then, the user enters the entity and attribute information for the query. When the user hits the submit button, the new query is generated, and when the query page is reloaded, this new query becomes visible. The person setting up the query drafts the text in which entity and attribute names are embedded.

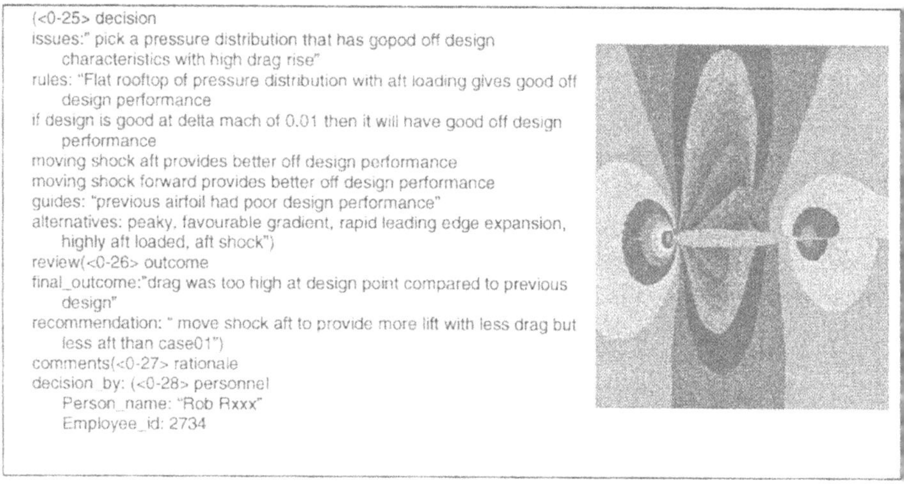

```
(<0-25> decision
issues:" pick a pressure distribution that has gopod off design
    characteristics with high drag rise"
rules: "Flat rooftop of pressure distribution with aft loading gives good off
    design performance
if design is good at delta mach of 0.01 then it will have good off design
    performance
moving shock aft provides better off design performance
moving shock forward provides better off design performance
guides: "previous airfoil had poor design performance"
alternatives: peaky, favourable gradient, rapid leading edge expansion,
    highly aft loaded, aft shock")
review(<0-26> outcome
final_outcome:"drag was too high at design point compared to previous
    design"
recommendation: " move shock aft to provide more lift with less drag but
    less aft than case01")
comments(<0-27> rationale
decision_by: (<0-28> personnel
    Person_name: "Rob Rxxx"
    Employee_id: 2734
```

Figure 8 Results of query #4 on design 1

7.9 Dynamic Schema Evolution

The designer can modify the schema or add new entities by using the *text editor* or the *expgedit* tool provided by *Steptools*. Dynamic schema evolution provides the following three options:

1) *Attribute changes only:* Addition or deletion of attributes.

2) *Entity changes*: Addition or deletion of entities; also attribute changes.

3) *New schema*: For an entirely new schema or major schema changes.

The "attribute changes" option recompiles the new schema and generates a new set of procedural files and script files that reflect the changes made. (The operations are shown in Figure 9) It also generates a new backend for processing. If the new schema is instantiated with data, the new data goes into the same database file as the earlier data. If attributes are added, the new instance data for the new attributes is copied over to the older instances.

The "entity changes" option proceeds in the same manner as before, except that the preprocessor file is changed to include the new entities. Here again, if instances are created, the new entity instances are copied over to the previous instances.

In the "new schema" option, the database is created at a new directory location and a new set of user interfaces and backends are created at that location. The user interface then performs the same actions as before at the new location and will initialize the database and make necessary changes to the user interface. The process is shown in Figure 9. All actions can be performed from the web browser itself. Another useful feature is that the system can display the difference between two schemas. The interface takes in the names of two schemas and gives a ROSE difference file as an output which shows the difference between the two schemas.

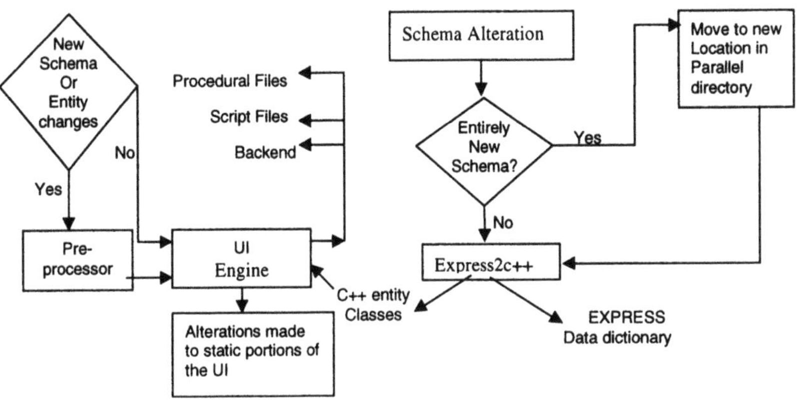

Figure 9 Dynamic Schema Evolution

8. DISCUSSION

We implemented the DHS as part of a larger project to create an Integrated Product Design Environment (IPDE) in which several design and analysis applications interact with a common data repository through Design Access Interfaces (DAI). All product data is based on STEP Application protocols AP203, AP224, and AP209. The Product and Process Core Models were domain independent and designed to be compatible with STEP. Domain specific schema for airframe design and analysis was the derived from the core model. The prototypes DHS uses this derived model and interacts with the IPDE in the same way as other applications used in the pilot project, such as CATIA for geometric design and PATRAN for FEA.

Thus, apart from having its own private database, DHS gets and puts data in the shared database at the start and end of each session, respectively. The role of DHS in the IPDE is to explain what each of the design iterations achieved and how. Two design case histories were then documented in DHS and Company personnel were able to access the system remotely via the Internet. Even this limited experiment revealed the problems of design information availability. Also, the instantiation process was quite labor intensive.

There are three areas in particular that industry may find appealing: (1) use of STEP standards in data modeling, (2) application of commercial database technology in data archival and retrieval, and (3) use of the WWW in generating the user interface. Despite these features, we are a long way from getting industry to shift from passive file management to active information integration. Barriers preventing this from happening include the following: large volumes of data produced by diverse application programs used by different groups of engineers and other involved in product development; lack of time and/or motivation on the part of designers to document design rationale; lack of commercial systems taking this approach; and heavy investment needed to set up and maintain design information systems.

One solution for reducing the volume of data to archive is to be selective, i.e., we could store only the most critical data based on frequency of re-use or the relative importance for cost or performance. Studies are needed to determine what data should be archived for most benefit.

REFERENCES

Baudin, C.; Underwood, Jody G.; Baya, Vinod, (1993),"Question –based Acquisition of Conceptual Indices for Mutlimedia Design Documentation", In proceedings of the 11th National Conference on Artificial Intelligence AAAI-93, Washington, D. C., pp. 454-458, July.

Baya, Vinod and Leifer, Larry, (1995), "Understanding Design Information Handling Behavior Using Time and Information Measure". *ASME Design Engineering Technical Conference*, Volume 2.

Brown D. C.; (1989), "Using Design History System for Technology Transfer", Proceedings of the MIT JSME Workshop on Cooperative Product Development, November 1989, pp. 545-559.

Casotto A.; Newton A. R.; Sangiovanni-Vincenetelli A.; (1994), "Argumentation-Based Rationale: What Use at What Cost?", *International Journal of Human-Computer Studies*, v40, n4, pp. 603-652.

Chen A., (1991), "A computer-Based Design History Tool", Thesis for the Department of Mechanical Engineering, Oregon State University.

Conklin, J., M. Begeman, (1988), "Gibis: a Hypertext Tool for Exploratory Policy Discussion", *Proceedings of the Conference on Computer Supported Cooperative Work*, September 1988, pp 140-152.

Conklin, Jeffrey E. & Burgess-Yakemovic, KC. (1996) "A Process-Oriented Approach to Design Rationale". Thomas Moran & John Carrol eds. Design Rationale: Concepts, Techniques, and Use. Lawrence Erlbaum Associates: New Jersey.

Domeshek E. and Kolodner J., (1997), "The Designer's Muse," in Issues and Applications of Case-Based Reasoning in Design, M.L. Maher and P. Pu, eds., Lawrence Erlbaum Associates, Hillsdale, N.J., pp. 11-38.

Faltings, Boi, (1997), "Case Reuse by Model-based Interpretation." In: Issues and Applications of Case Based Reasoning in Design, Maher M. L., Pu P., eds. Lawrence-Earlbaum Publishers.

Fu H.; Bansal, R.; Haggerty C. M.; Posco P.; (1990), "Hyperinformation Systems and Technology Transfer", Proceedings of the 1990 ASME International Computers in Engineering Conference and Exposition.

Goel, Ashok. et al. (1996), "Explanatory Interface in Interactive Design Environments". Artificial Intelligence and Design Conference. Stanford, July.

Hardwick M. and Spooner D., (1989), "The ROSE Data Manager: Using Object Technology to Support Interactive Engineering Applications", *IEEE Transactions on Knowledge and Data Engineering*, Vol. 1, No.2, pp. 285-289.

Hardwick, M.; Spooner, D.; (1989)," The ROSE Data Manager: Using Object Technology to Support Interactive Engineering Applications", *IEEE Transactions on Knowledge and Data Engineering*, Vol. 1, No. 2, pp. 285-289.

ISO Ind. Automation Systems, (1996), "Part 209 Application Protocol: composite and metallic structural analysis and related design", IDO/CD 10303-209.

ISO. (1996) "Guidelines for the Development and Approval of STEP Application Protocols. Volume 1.2,ISO TC 184/SC4 N433. Pages 4-5.

King, J.M.P., René Bañares-Alcántara, Ballinger and Lakshmanan R., (1995), "Using Design History to Support Chemical Plant Design", *The 1995 IChemE Research Event, First European Conference*.

Lee, J., (1990), "SIBYL: A Qualitative Decision Management System." In Artificial Intelligence at MIT: Expanding Frontiers, P. Winston, S. Shellard, Eds. The MIT Press, Cambridge, Mass., 1990, pp. 104-133.

Lee, J., Lai, K., (1996), "What's in Design Rationale". Thomas Moran & John Carrol Eds. "Design Rationale: Concepts, Techniques, and Use". Lawrence Erlbaum Associates: New Jersey.

Lubars, M D., (1991), "Representing Design Dependencies in an Issue-Based Style". *IEEE Software*. Pages 81-89.

MacLean, et al. (1996), "Questions, Options, and Criteria: Elements of Design Space Analysis". Thomas Moran & John Carrol Eds. Design Rationale: Concepts, Techniques, and Use. Lawrence Erlbaum Associates: New Jersey.

Maher M.L., Balachandran B., and Zhang D.M., (1995), Applications of Case-Based Reasoning in Design, M.L. Maher and P. Pu, eds., Lawrence Erlbaum Associates, Hillsdale, N.J.

Maher, M.L., and Zhang, D.M., (1991), "CADSYN: Using Case and Decomposition Knowledge for Design Synthesis". In Gero, J.S. (ed.). Artificial Intelligence in Design.

McCall, R. J.; (1989), "MIKROPOLIS: A Hypertext System for Design", Design Studies, V10(4), October 1989, pp. 228-238.

McCall, R., Bennett, P., and Johnson, E., (1994), "An Overview of the PHIDIAS II HyperCAD System." In Reconnecting: ACADIA '94, A. Harfmann and M. Fraser (eds.) *Association for Computer Aided Design in Architecture*, pp. 63-74.

Nagy, R.L., et al., (1992), "A Data Representation for Collaborative Mechanical Design". *Research in Engineering Design*, Volume 3, pp. 233-242.

Narashiman S., Sycara K., and Navin-Chandra D., (1997), "Representation and Synthesis of Non-Monotonic Mechanical Devices," Issues and Applications of Case-Based Reasoning in Design, pp. 187-220.

Ng, Jason L., (1993), "GSQL: A mosaic gateway to SQL", http://www.ncsa.uiuc.edu/SDG/People/jason/pub/gsql

Pena-Mora, F. & Vadhavkar, S., (1996), "Design Rationale and Design Patterns in Reusable Software Design". *Artificial Intelligence and Design Conference.* Stanford.

Pratt, M.; (1997), "Parametric Representation and Exchange (PAREX), Part 1: Overview and General Principles", ISO 14959-1: Draft.

Qureshi, S., (1997), "Integration Framework for Electromechanical Design Information", PhD Thesis, Arizona State University.

Qureshi, Sohail M., Shah, Jami J. et al. (1997), "Process Modeling to Support Design Process History Databases". *ASME Design Engineering Technical Conference.*

Rittel, H.W.J. and Weber, M.M., (1973), "Dilemmas in General Theory of Planning", *Policy Sciences*, pp. 155-169.

Santayana G.; (1905), "The Life of Reason".

Schenck, Douglas & Wilson, Peter., (1995), "Information Modeling the EXPRESS Way", Oxford University Press: New York.

Shah, J., Urban S., Bliznakov., (1996), "Database Infrastructure for Supporting Engineering Design Histories", *Computer Aided Design,* Volume 28, pp. 347-360.

Shah, J.J. et al. (1993), "Development of Machine Understandable Language for Design Process Representation". ASME, Design Theory and Methodology Conference. Albuquerque, NM.

Shyam R., (1998), "System for archival & retrieval of design history", MS thesis, Mech. Eng., Arizona State University.

STEP, (1996), http://www/scra.org/uspro//projects//std00026.html, 1996.

Thompson J. B.; Lu S. C.; (1990), "Design Evolution Management: A Methodology for Representing Design Rationale", 1990 ASME Design Technical Conference, Chicago, IL, Sept. 1990, pp. 185-191.

Ullman, David G., Paasch, Robert, (1995), "Design History, Design Rationale and Design Intent System development issues", *Design Engineering Technical Conference.*

PART FOUR

KNOWLEDGE INTENSIVE CAD (KIC)

6

Modeling of Product Life-cycle Knowledge and Data for an Intelligent Concurrent Design System

Deyi Xue
Department of Mechanical and Manufacturing Engineering, The University of Calgary, Calgary, Alberta, Canada T2N 1N4

Key words: Product life-cycle, Concurrent design, Artificial intelligence, Optimization, Object-oriented modeling

Abstract: This paper discusses the issues in modeling product life-cycle knowledge and data for an intelligent concurrent design system. Requirements for intelligent concurrent design are first outlined. Mathematical formulation for intelligent concurrent design is then introduced. Development and implementation of an intelligent concurrent design system and its applications are subsequently presented based upon the theoretical research results. A case study example is given at last to demonstrate the effectiveness of the introduced methods. This research focuses on the following four issues: (1) representation of various product life-cycle aspects, (2) automated generation of product life-cycle aspects, (3) maintenance of relations among product life-cycle aspects, and (4) identification of the optimal design considering relevant product life-cycle aspects.

1. INTRODUCTION

1.1 Product life-cycle and concurrent design

A product changes from its birth to its death through a sequence of life-cycle phases, including design, production process planning, manufacturing, inspection, distribution, operation/maintenance, and disposal/recycle. With the advances in computer technologies, many of the product development activities have been automated by introducing computer-based systems, such as Computer-Aided Design (CAD), Computer-Aided Process Planning

(CAPP), Computer-Aided Manufacturing (CAM), and so on (Chang, Wysk, and Wang, 1991; Singh, 1996). Many intelligent systems have also been developed for further improving the computer-based product development systems (Kusiak, 1992; Dong, 1994). Despite of the progress, information in most of these automated and intelligent systems still flows only in one direction – from design to other downstream product development phases. Since many re-designs have to be conducted to achieve good evaluation in these downstream product life-cycle aspects, the sequential product development process requires long product development lead time.

Concurrent design is an approach to incorporate considerations in different downstream product development life-cycle aspects, including manufacturing, assembly, maintenance, disposal/recycle, etc., into design phase, thus generating the design with the best overall life-cycle performance (Kusiak, 1993; Prasad, 1996). Because evaluations to these downstream product development aspects are carried out simultaneously during the design phase, concurrent design approach can reduce the number of costly re-designs and shorten product development lead time. Many industrial companies have employed this approach for improving the competitiveness of their products (Kusiak, 1993; Prasad, 1996).

The research on computer-aided concurrent design was initiated by the early work on *feature recognition* (Choi, Barash, and Anderson, 1984; Henderson, 1984). Feature recognition is an approach to automatically extract the geometric features, such as holes and slots, to be produced by certain manufacturing operations from the CAD database for planning production process and evaluating the design from manufacturing point of view. Due to the difficulty in feature extraction, another approach, called *feature-based design* that defines features as a library and uses the features to model a design, has been employed by many researchers (Pratt, 1984; Luby, Dixon, and Simmons, 1986; Shah and Rogers, 1988). Detailed review on feature recognition and feature-based design can be found in Reference (Shah and Mantyla, 1995).

To improve design with good evaluation in downstream product development life-cycle aspects, research on *design-for-X* was started by incorporating considerations in these life-cycle aspects into the early design phase. Typical downstream life-cycle aspects considered in design-for-X methods include manufacturing (Bralla, 1986; Dong, 1993), assembly (Boothroyd and Dewhurst, 1983), maintenance (Makino, Barkan, and Pfaff, 1989; Gershenson and Ishii, 1993), disposal/recycle (Zhang *et al.,* 1997), etc. Many advanced computational techniques, including constraint-network (Young, Greef, and O'Grady, 1992), optimization (Dowlatshahi, 1992), etc., have been employed for automating concurrent design processes.

1.2 Knowledge intensive engineering

As the result of market competition and technology advances, more products are manufactured nowadays to satisfy the increasing demand from customers. The current mass production paradigm brings tremendous advantages to us such as to improve the quality of living. Despite of these advantages, problems arose due to the mass production. These problems, called modern evils by Yoshikawa (Yoshikawa, 1993), are caused by natural constraints (e.g., materials, energy, and environmental capacity), social constraints (e.g., market and transportation), and human constraints (e.g., acceptance of high technology) (Tomiyama, 1997).

To solve these problems in the current mass production paradigm, a new manufacturing paradigm, namely Post Mass Production Paradigm (PMPP), was proposed (Tomiyama, 1997). PMPP aims at reducing the volume of production and consumption to an adequate and manageable size considering the limitations of natural, social, and human resources, while improving our living quality. In PMPP, the economical growth is decoupled from the resource/energy consumption and waste creation.

To reach the goal of PMPP, the past evaluation of living quality in terms of quantitative sufficiency must be replaced by the future evaluation in terms of qualitative satisfaction. The economic development therefore relies on the creation of high value products using intellectual resources rather than natural resources. Knowledge plays a crucial role in developing the value-added products.

Since the development of a product involves a sequence of life-cycle phases, the concept of *knowledge-intensive engineering*, which aims at organizing the knowledge at different life-cycle stages in a flexible manner to generate more added-value to products, was proposed (Tomiyama, 1994).

This research focuses on improving the current data-centered CAD systems into the next generation CAD systems – the knowledge intensive CAD systems. In knowledge intensive CAD systems, different product life-cycle knowledge is described in different modules. The relevant life-cycle knowledge is used when required to evaluate the design from a certain product life-cycle aspect. Since both the knowledge and data play important roles in the knowledge intensive CAD systems, modeling of product life-cycle knowledge and data is addressed in this paper.

1.3 Previous research on intelligent concurrent design

During the past years, the author has devoted the efforts on the development of an intelligent concurrent design system that supports the activities in all product development life-cycle aspects (Xue and Dong,

1993; Dong, Hu, and Xue, 1994; Xue and Dong, 1994; Xue, Rousseau, and Dong, 1996; Xue, 1997; Xue and Dong, 1997).

In this research, first modeling of product life-cycle aspects was studied (Xue and Dong, 1993). The three major life-cycle aspects, design, geometry, and manufacturing, are modeled by aspect primitives called features, including design features (mechanisms and components such as a gear and a shaft), geometry features (geometric primitives such as a box and a cylinder), and manufacturing features (geometric elements to be produced such as a hole and a slot). Representation of features follows the scheme of a product modeling language – Integrated Data Description Language (IDDL) (Tomiyama and ten Hagen, 1987; Xue *et al.,* 1992), which was originally developed at University of Tokyo. A system combining knowledge-based reasoning and optimization was developed for generating aspect models automatically and identifying the optimal design (Xue and Dong, 1994). Due to the large size of feature library, a design-function based design feature coding system and a manufacturing-function based manufacturing feature coding system were introduced for organizing feature library and for automatically generating design candidates and planning production process (Xue and Dong, 1997). Since production cost is a key measure for evaluating design from manufacturing point of view, the cost models considering different production processes and tolerance requirements were then developed (Dong, Hu, and Xue, 1994). An optimization model was developed for achieving the design with the best tradeoff between functional performance and production cost (Xue, Rousseau, and Dong, 1996). A number of global optimization models were also introduced to identify the optimal design (Xue, 1997).

The goal of the research presented in this paper is to further develop the intelligent concurrent design system and its applications with focus on modeling product life-cycle knowledge and data. The requirements for intelligent concurrent design are discussed first. The mathematical formulation for intelligent concurrent design is then introduced. The development and implementation of the intelligent concurrent design system and its applications are subsequently presented based upon the theoretical research results. Effectiveness of the introduced methods is illustrated using a case study example at the end of this paper.

2. REQUIREMENTS FOR INTELLIGENT CONCURRENT DESIGN

The requirements for intelligent concurrent design were achieved based upon an extensive study on the activities in concurrent design. These requirements are summarized as follows:

1. *An efficient method for modeling product life-cycle aspects should be introduced.*
   The different product life-cycle aspects, including design, manufacturing, assembly, and so on, should be described as aspect models. Each aspect model is composed of aspect descriptions for representing and evaluating the product from that life-cycle perspective. To improve the modeling efficiency, aspect models should be constructed using aspect building primitives. A building primitive is represented by a group of relevant descriptions for a particular purpose in the product development process. For instance, descriptions of a gear can be grouped as a building primitive for modeling a design candidate, and a hole can be described by a collection of geometric elements to be produced by a certain manufacturing operation. These building primitives also serve as the elements for evaluating the product aspect models. Descriptions in aspect models, including data and their relations, are classified into two categories: qualitative descriptions and quantitative descriptions. Different aspect models are associated by their relations.
2. *An automated product life-cycle aspect model generation mechanism should be achieved.*
   This mechanism aims at further improving the efficiency of constructing product life-cycle aspect models and their relations. Since the aspect models and their relations are built based upon relevant knowledge in product development process, a knowledge-based system is required to generate these aspect models and their relations automatically. In addition, because the development of a product undergoes a sequence of processes, including design candidate generation, design geometry modeling, manufacturing operation identification, and so on, this evolutionary nature of product realization process should also be represented.
3. *An integrated environment to maintain the relations among aspect models should be developed.*
   The aspect models are used for representing the same product from different life-cycle perspectives. Aspect models are associated by their relations. Because a concurrent design is carried out by considering these different life-cycle aspects simultaneously, a mechanism to maintain the relations among aspect models in an integrated environment is required.

The relations include qualitative relations and quantitative relations. Any change in one aspect model should be propagated to other aspect models automatically using these relations.

4. *An optimal design model considering all relevant product life-cycle aspects should be identified.*
   Because the same design requirement can be reached by alternative design candidates and different design parameter values, a mechanism to identify the optimal design alternative and its parameter values considering relevant life-cycle aspects should be developed. The product life-cycle aspect performance measures, including manufacturability, assemblability, serviceability, disposalability/recyclability, etc., should be employed for evaluating the product from the different product life-cycle aspects. Optimization approach can be used to achieve this objective.

The mathematical models and the intelligent concurrent design system were developed based upon the requirements summarized above. Details of these mathematical models and system implementation are presented in the following sections.

3. MATHEMATICAL FORMULATION FOR INTELLIGENT CONCURRENT DESIGN

A number of mathematical models have been developed for modeling intelligent concurrent design. The intelligent concurrent design system and its applications were implemented based on these mathematical models.

3.1 A feature-based product life-cycle aspect representation model

Models of different product life-cycle aspects are called aspect models, including design aspect model, $\boldsymbol{M}^{(D)}$, manufacturing aspect model, $\boldsymbol{M}^{(M)}$, and so on. These aspect models are built using aspect primitives, namely aspect features (Xue and Dong, 1993). An aspect feature, $F_i^{(P)}$ $(i=1,2,\ldots,n_F^{(P)})$, is represented by a group of relevant descriptions in the aspect model for a particular product development purpose. The superscript *(P)* of $F_i^{(P)}$ denotes the life-cycle aspect of the feature, such as design aspect, *(D)*, manufacturing aspect, *(M)*, and so on. For instance, a motor is a design feature for creating rotational motion, and a pocket is a manufacturing feature to be produced by a milling machining operation. A feature usually consists of quantitative descriptions called attributes. An attribute, $A_{ij}^{(P)}$, of the feature, $F_i^{(P)}$, is described by

$$A_{ij}^{(P)} = A_{ij}^{(P)}(F_i^{(P)}), \quad i = 1,2,\cdots,n_F^{(P)}; j = 1,2,\cdots,n_{A_i}^{(P)} \tag{1}$$

For instance, rotational speed and output power are two attributes of a motor.

Features and attributes are associated by their qualitative relations, $R_{Fl}^{(P)}$, and quantitative relations, $R_{Am}^{(P)}$, respectively. These relations are defined as

$$R_{F_l}^{(P)} = R_{F_l}^{(P)}(F_1^{(P)}, F_2^{(P)}, \cdots, F_{n_F^{(P)}}^{(P)}), \; l = 1,2,\cdots,n_{R_F}^{(P)} \tag{2}$$

$$R_{A_m}^{(P)} = R_{A_m}^{(P)}(A_1^{(P)}, A_2^{(P)}, \cdots, A_{n_A^{(P)}}^{(P)}), \; m = 1,2,\cdots,n_{R_A}^{(P)} \tag{3}$$

For example, the connection relation between a gear and its shaft is a qualitative relation, while the relation between the speeds of the gear and the shaft is a quantitative one.

An aspect model, $\boldsymbol{M}^{(P)}$, consists of aspect features, $\boldsymbol{F}^{(P)}$, attributes of these features, $\boldsymbol{A}^{(P)}$, qualitative relations among features, $\boldsymbol{R}_F^{(P)}$, and quantitative relations among attributes, $\boldsymbol{R}_A^{(P)}$, as defined by

$$\boldsymbol{M}^{(P)} = \{\boldsymbol{F}^{(P)}, \boldsymbol{A}^{(P)}, \boldsymbol{R}_F^{(P)}, \boldsymbol{R}_A^{(P)}\} \tag{4}$$

where,

$$\boldsymbol{F}^{(P)} = \{F_1^{(P)}, F_2^{(P)}, \cdots, F_{n_F^{(P)}}^{(P)}\} \tag{5}$$

$$\boldsymbol{A}^{(P)} = \{A_1^{(P)}, A_2^{(P)}, \cdots, A_{n_A^{(P)}}^{(P)}\} \tag{6}$$

$$\boldsymbol{R}_F^{(P)} = \{R_{F_1}^{(P)}, R_{F_2}^{(P)}, \cdots, R_{F_{n_{R_F}^{(P)}}}^{(P)}\} \tag{7}$$

$$\boldsymbol{R}_A^{(P)} = \{R_{A_1}^{(P)}, R_{A_2}^{(P)}, \cdots, R_{A_{n_{R_A}^{(P)}}}^{(P)}\} \tag{8}$$

A product, $\boldsymbol{P}$, is defined by all its life-cycle aspect models, $\boldsymbol{M}$, and their relations, $\boldsymbol{R}_F$ and $\boldsymbol{R}_A$, using

$$\boldsymbol{P} = \{\boldsymbol{M}, \boldsymbol{R}_F, \boldsymbol{R}_A\} \tag{9}$$

where, $\boldsymbol{M}$ is a collection of aspect models described by

$$\boldsymbol{M} = \{\boldsymbol{M}^{(D)}, \boldsymbol{M}^{(M)}, \cdots\} \tag{10}$$

3.2 A product realization process model

The product aspect models are built gradually from design to other downstream life-cycle aspects. Usually design candidates are first created based upon design requirements. Product geometry is then achieved to model design details. Manufacturing descriptions are subsequently obtained from the product geometry. In this research, a product realization process model was introduced for representing this progressive nature of product development activities. This model is an extension of the General Design Theory (GDT), in which a design is considered as a process of mapping from function space to attribute space (Yoshikawa, 1981; Tomiyama and Yoshikawa, 1987).

In the product realization process model, new product descriptions, M', at a certain product development stage are derived from the product descriptions, M, at an earlier product development stage using relevant knowledge, K, as described by

$$M \cap K \Rightarrow M' \tag{11}$$

In this equation, $\cap$ and $\Rightarrow$ are logical symbols representing AND relation and description derivation relation respectively. The relations among the derived data are of two types: AND relations and OR relations. For instance, the two machining operation descriptions derived by

$$\textit{internal thread} \cap K_1 \Rightarrow \textit{drilling} \cap \textit{threading} \tag{12}$$

have an AND relation, while the two design candidate descriptions generated by the following two equations

$$\textit{rotational motion} \cap K_2 \Rightarrow \textit{electrical motor} \tag{13}$$

$$\textit{rotation motion} \cap K_3 \Rightarrow \textit{gasoline engine} \tag{14}$$

have an OR relation.

3.3 A data relation maintenance model

Since different product life-cycle aspect models are used for representing different aspects of the same product, any change in one aspect model should be propagated to other aspect models to keep the consistency of the product database. In this research, the consistency of aspect models is maintained using the relations among these aspect models including qualitative relations among features and quantitative relations among attributes.

In the process of product development, since a piece of product description is usually derived from other descriptions using relevant knowledge, change of an earlier created description should have influence on the derived descriptions. For instance, the two machining operation descriptions in Eq. (12) are derived from the internal-thread manufacturing feature. If the internal-thread manufacturing feature is removed from the database, the two derived machining operation descriptions should also be deleted. This dependency relation is described by

$$d_j \leftarrow d_1, d_2, \cdots, d_n \tag{15}$$

where, d_i could be a feature, an attribute, a qualitative relation among features, or a quantitative relation among attributes.

A quantitative relation among attributes can be further described by

$$A_j = A_j(A_1, A_2, \cdots, A_n) \tag{16}$$

where, A_j is calculated using A_1, A_2, ..., A_n as input attributes.

3.4 An optimal concurrent design model

Since design requirements can be satisfied by alternative design candidates, each of these candidates is further described by attributes with different values, in this research an optimal concurrent design model was introduced to identify the optimal design alternative and its attribute values considering relevant life-cycle aspects. The optimization is conducted at two different levels: alternative optimization level and attribute optimization level.

A feasible design alternative is modeled by a number of features and their attributes. Since the qualitative descriptions of features remain the same for a design alternative, a feasible alternative, $\boldsymbol{P}_i$, can therefore be described by a collection of attributes:

$$P_i = \{A_{i1}, A_{i2}, \cdots, A_{in_i}\} \tag{17}$$

The optimal attribute values regarding one design alternative are obtained using constrained optimization approach:

$$\underset{w.r.t.\ A_{i1}, A_{i2}, \cdots A_{in_i}}{Min} \quad f_i(A_{i1}, A_{i2}, \cdots, A_{in_i})$$

subject to:

$$h_{ij}(A_{i1}, A_{i2}, \cdots, A_{in_i}) = 0, \ j = 1,2,\cdots,k_i$$

$$g_{ij}(A_{i1}, A_{i2}, \cdots, A_{in_i}) \le 0, \ j = k_i + 1, k_i + 2, \cdots, m_i \tag{18}$$

The objective function, $f_i(A_{i1}, A_{i2}, \ldots, A_{in_i})$, is an evaluation measure of the design from a certain product life-cycle perspective, such as manufacturing.

The optimal objective function evaluation measure is described as $f_i(P_i^*)$. The optimal alternative is identified from all possible alternatives using

$$\underset{w.r.t.\ P_i^*}{Min} f_i(P_i^*) \tag{19}$$

where P_i^* is iterated among the feasible alternatives with the optimal attribute values.

4. DEVELOPMENT OF AN INTELLIGENT CONCURRENT DESIGN SYSTEM AND ITS APPLICATIONS

Based upon the mathematical formulation introduced in the previous section, an intelligent concurrent design system was developed for automating concurrent design activities. In this system, product life-cycle aspects are described by aspect models, as shown in Figure 1. The mathematical models introduced in the previous section were implemented as follows: (1) The product life-cycle aspects are modeled using a feature representation language. (2) The product realization process model is automated through knowledge-based inference. (3) The data relations among aspect models are maintained through data relation networks. (4) The optimal concurrent design is identified using a multi-level optimization approach. The system was implemented using Smalltalk, an object oriented programming language (Goldberg and Robson, 1983).

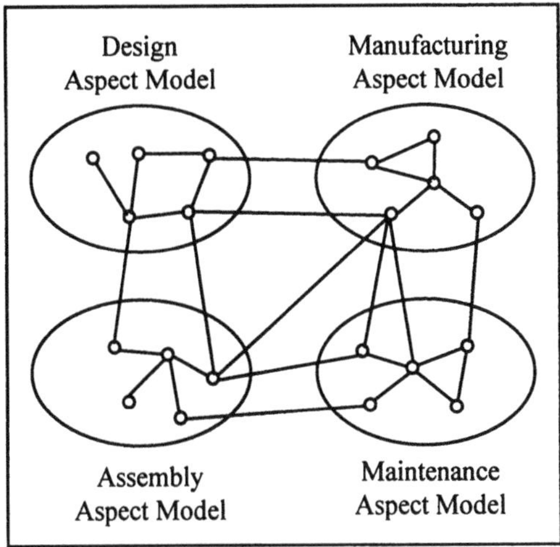

Figure 1. Aspect models of a product

Many industrial applications were also developed using the intelligent concurrent design system. One of these applications is used for designing building products for a local manufacturing company – Gienow Building Products Ltd. Many examples used in this paper were implemented for this application.

4.1 Modeling product life-cycle aspects using a feature representation language

In the feature-based product life-cycle aspect representation model introduced in Section 3.1, features are primitives for modeling product life-cycle aspects including design, manufacturing, and so on. In the intelligent concurrent design system, a feature representation language was introduced for modeling these aspect features.

In the feature representation language, features are described at two different levels, class level and instance level, corresponding to generic feature libraries and specific data for modeling particular products, respectively. Class features are used as templates for creating instance features. Object-oriented programming approach is employed for implementing class features and instance features.

Class features are used for modeling product libraries. All class features are organized in a hierarchical data structure. A new class feature is defined as a sub-class of an existing class feature. All the descriptions in a super-class feature are inherited by its sub-class features automatically. The top level class feature is a built-in class feature called Feature. Examples of class feature definitions used for the building product design application are shown in Figure 2. A class feature has 4 types of major components: (1) element-features, (2) attributes, (3) qualitative relations among features, and (4) quantitative relations among attributes.

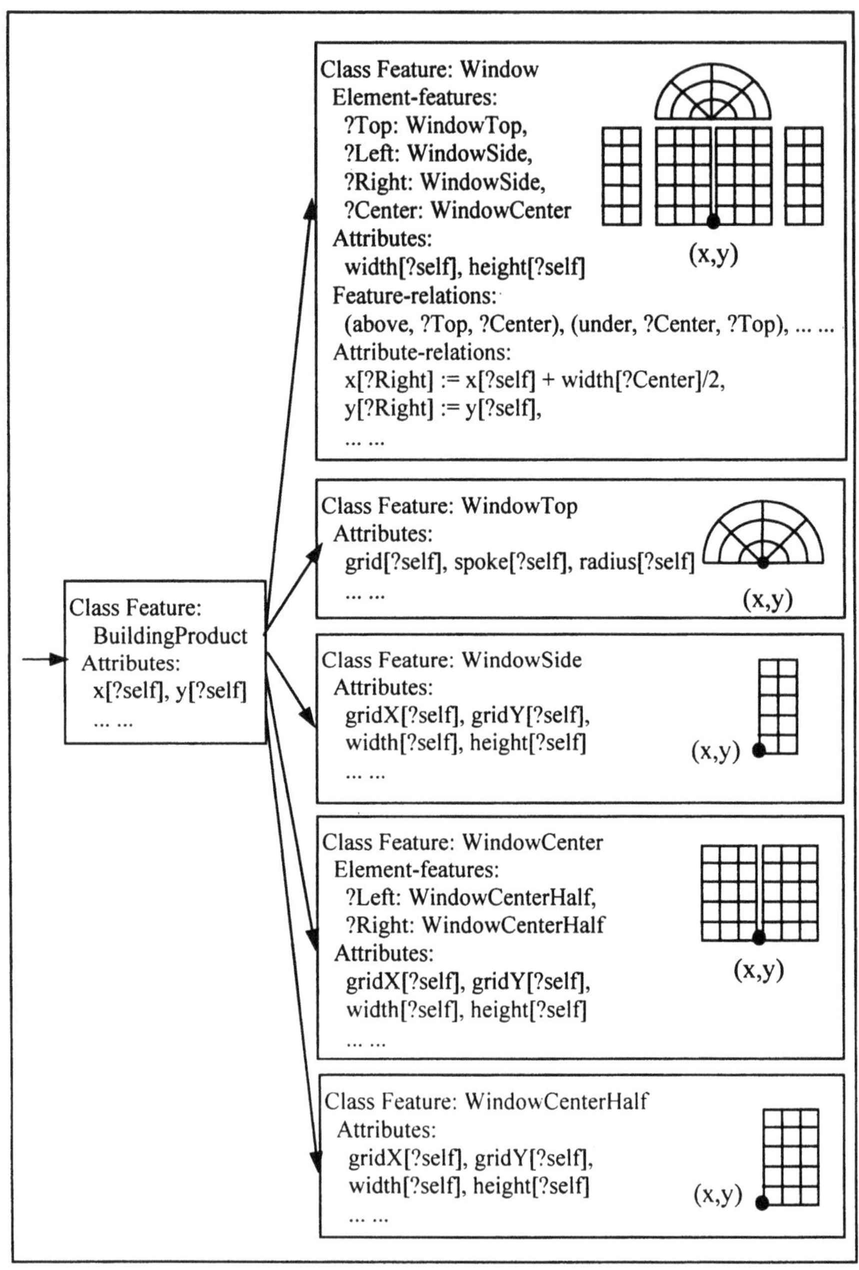

Figure 2. Class feature definitions

An element feature is a component that composes the feature being defined. For instance, the Window class feature, shown in Figure 2, is composed of four element features. An element feature is defined by a variable and its class feature type. A variable is described by a string starting with "?". In the class feature Window, the four element features are associated with four variables: ?Top, ?Left, ?Right, and ?Center. When an instance feature is generated using this class feature as the template, the element features should also be created according to their class feature types defined in the class feature. The variables that are associated with element features can be used in other parts of the class feature definition. For instance, the four variables in class feature Window are used for defining feature relations and attribute relations of this class feature. The feature itself is associate with a built-in variable ?self. When a class feature is used for generating an instance feature, all the variables, representing element features, should be replaced by the actual element instance feature names in the created instance feature.

An attribute is a piece of quantitative description of a feature. An attribute is described by an attribute name and an attribute value. In a class feature definition, an attribute can be associated with a default value. Attributes are used in the form of attribute[feature] in other parts of the feature definition. For instance, width[?Center] in Figure 2 represents the attribute width of the feature ?Center.

A qualitative relation among features is described by a predicate, in the form of $(x_1, x_2, ..., x_n)$, where $x_1, x_2, ..., x_n$ are terms of this predicate represented by strings (e.g., above, under), integers (e.g., 25, −14), floats (e.g., 2.5, 1.2e–25), variables (e.g., ?Left, ?Center), and attributes (e.g., width[?self], height[?self]). A predicate without variable terms is called a fact.

A quantitative relation among attributes is defined by a function with a number of input attributes and one output attribute, as shown in Figure 2. Syntax of functions follows the syntax of Smalltalk. Element feature variables and attributes are also allowed in function definitions.

Instance features are generated from class features and used for modeling actual products. When a class feature is selected as the template for generating an instance feature, the element features defined in this class feature should also be created as instance features. All the descriptions defined in the class feature and its super-class features are inherited by the generated instance feature automatically. Figure 3 shows the instance features that are generated from the class features given in Figure 2 for representing a window product. In an instance feature, the variables in its class feature definition, representing element features, are replaced by the names of the actually created element instance features. Descriptions of instance features can be modified, added, and deleted.

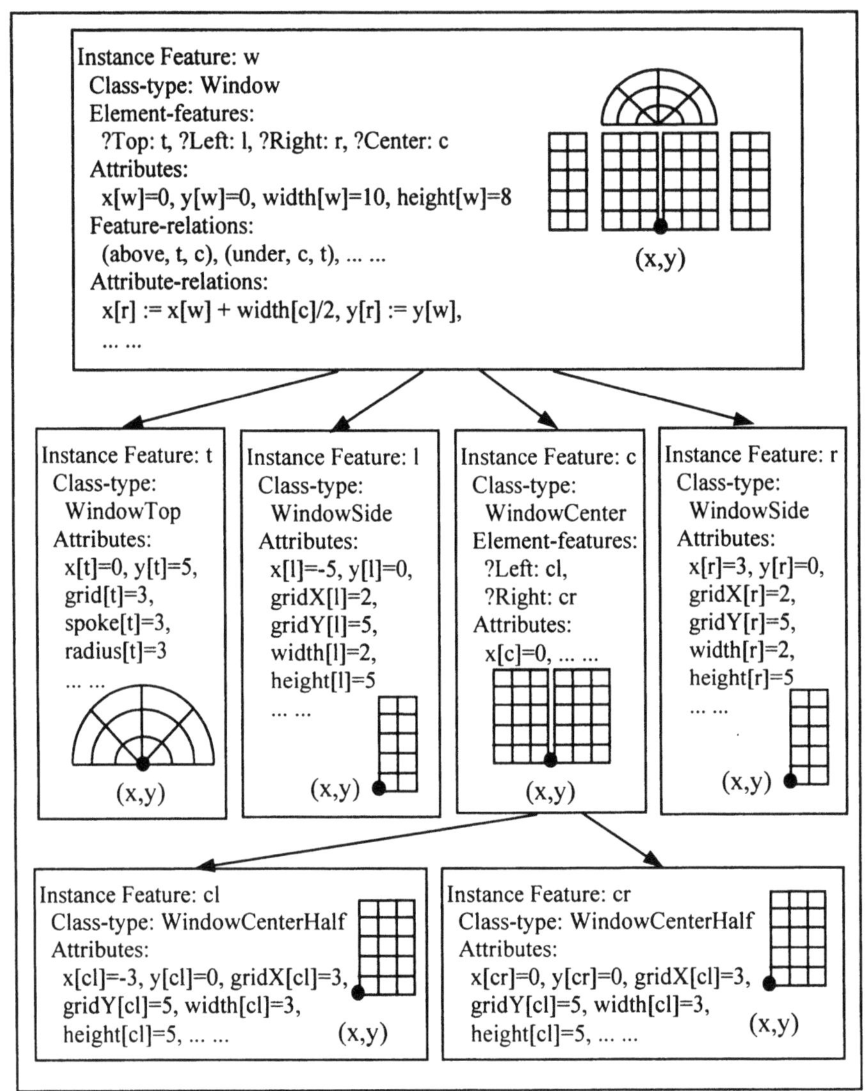

Figure 3. Instance feature definitions

4.2 Automating product realization process through knowledge-based inference

In Section 3.2, product realization process is modeled by mapping among different product development life-cycle aspects. In the intelligent concurrent design system, the mapping process is described by an AND/OR graph, as shown in Figure 4. In this graph, product descriptions, including features, attributes, qualitative relations among features, and quantitative relations among attributes, are described by nodes. The AND and OR relations among sub-nodes are achieved using the knowledge as described in Eqs. (12), (13) and (14).

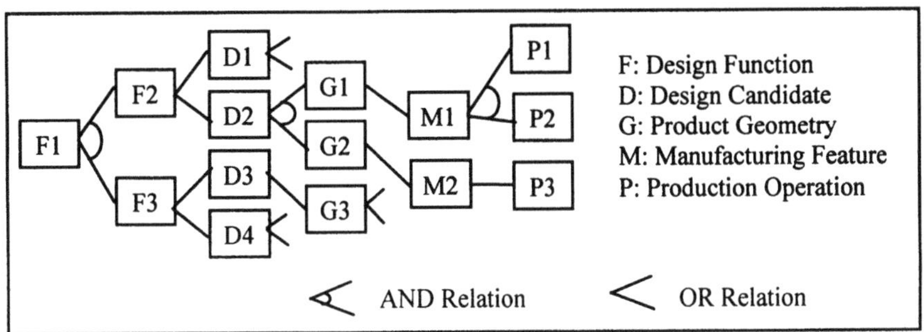

Figure 4. An AND/OR graph of product realization process

To automate the product realization process, a knowledge base system has been developed for generating the AND/OR graph through knowledge-based reasoning. In this system, product development knowledge is described by rules. Rules are grouped as rule-bases. The idea for organizing rules in groups follows the concept introduced for the Intelligent Integrated Interactive CAD (IIICAD) system (Tomiyama and ten Hagen, 1987; *Xue et al.*, 1992).

A rule-base is defined by a rule-base name and a collection of rules, as shown in Figure 5. Each rule description consists of a rule name and the rule itself in the form of IF-THEN data structure representing a piece of cause-result knowledge. Both the IF part and the THEN part of a rule are described by a number of patterns linked with logical-and (&). A pattern is described by a predicate in the form of $(x_1, x_2, ..., x_n)$, where $x_1, x_2, ..., x_n$ are terms described by strings, numbers, variables, and attributes. The condition part and result part of a rule are used for matching, creating, deleting, and modifying the data in product models, including features, attributes, qualitative relations among features, and quantitative relations among attributes, through knowledge-based inference.

To improve the efficiency of reasoning, only partial database and partial knowledge base are considered during product development process. Since an instance feature is composed of element features, attributes, qualitative relations among features, and quantitative relations among attributes, an instance feature is such a database unit selected for inference. The partial knowledge base used in inference is a collection of selected rule-bases.

Therefore, each instance feature is associated with a number of rule-bases. This idea is illustrated in Figure 6.

```
Rule-base: WindowDesign

Rule: changeLeftGridY
IF (left, ?L) & (center, ?C) & (<>, gridY[?L], gridY[?C]) &
   (message, 'gridY values of left and center are not equal!') &
   (confirm, 'Do you want to change gridY of left?')
THEN (=, gridY[?L], gridY[?C])

Rule: changeCenterGridY
IF (left, ?L) & (center, ?C) & (<>, gridY[?L], gridY[?C]) &
   (message, 'gridY values of left and center are not equal!') &
   (confirm, 'Do you want to change gridY of center?')
THEN (=, gridY[?C], gridY[?L])
... ...
```

Figure 5. A rule-base definition

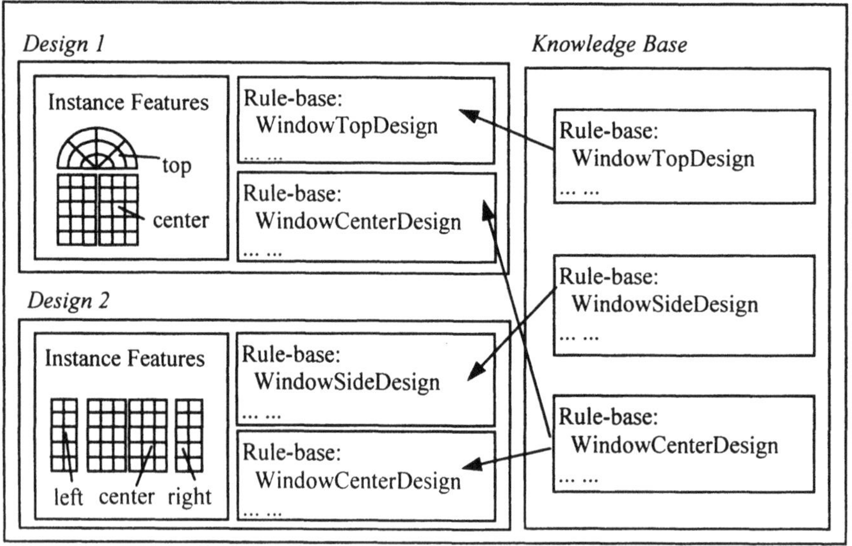

Figure 6. Selection of partial knowledge base and database in product design

During the process of knowledge-based product modeling, first an instance feature is selected as the partial database to be considered in inference. A number of rule-bases are then selected as the partial knowledge for this instance feature. All the rules in these rule-bases should be registered in this instance feature. The inference is conducted first by matching the condition parts of all the registered rules with the instance feature database. If multiple rules are matched, the best rule is then selected and the result part of this rule is executed. In this research, the first matched rule is considered as the best rule to be fired.

The AND/OR graph of product realization process is also generated by rule-based reasoning. When condition part of a rule matches with the database, the data created by executing the result part of this rule should have an AND relation. If several rules match with the same data, the data generated by executing these rules have an OR relation. Figure 7 shows the AND/OR graphs generated through rule-based reasoning.

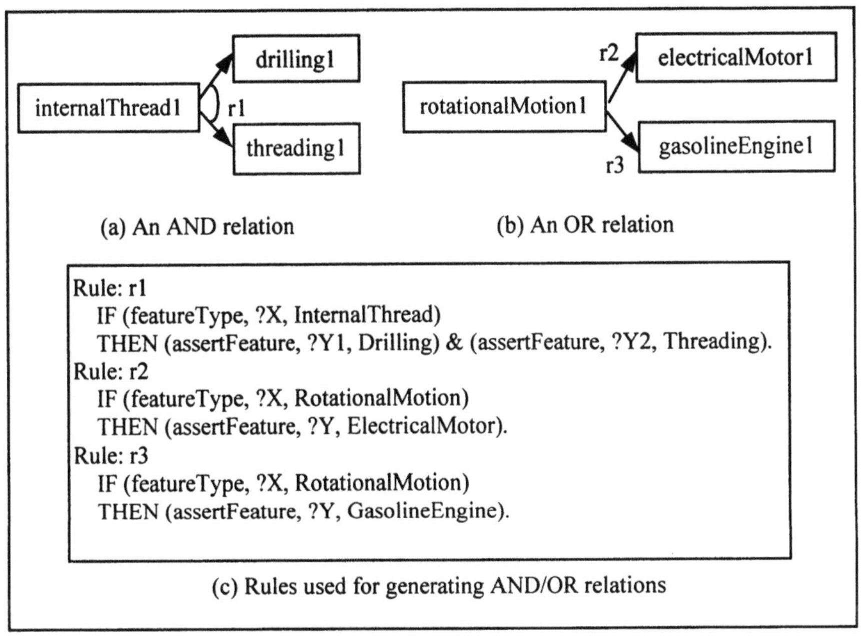

Figure 7. Generation of AND/OR graphs through rule-based reasoning

4.3 Maintaining data relations among aspect models through data relation networks

In Section 3.3, a data relation maintenance model was introduced for keeping the consistency of the product database using qualitative dependency relations among features and quantitative relations among attributes. In the intelligent concurrent design system, these two types of relations among product data are described by two associated networks, *feature relation network* and *attribute relation network*. The consistency of the product life-cycle aspect models is maintained using these two data relation networks. Any change in one life-cycle aspect is propagated automatically to other aspects through the data relation networks.

The feature relation network is described by an AND/OR tree of the product realization process. This network is composed of instance features and their dependency relations, which are generated either manually or through knowledge-based system. Other feature descriptions, including element features, attributes, qualitative relations among element features, and quantitative relations among attributes, are associated with these instance features. A feature relation network, representing two design alternatives shown in Figure 8 (a), is given in Figure 8 (b).

Product realization process alternatives, such as design alternatives or production process alternatives, can be achieved from the AND/OR tree of a feature relation network. An alternative is described by a collection of instance features. The process to identify product realization process alternatives is formulated in the following steps:

1. From the AND/OR tree, select the instance feature that needs alternative subsequent product realization processes.
2. If a selected instance feature has descendant instance features with an AND relation, all these descendant instance features should be selected.
3. If a selected instance feature has descendant instance features with an OR relation, only one of these descendant instance feature should be selected.

Steps 2 and 3 are conducted continuously until no selection is required.

In the example shown in Figure 8, two alternatives, described by instance features of (1) doorWindow1, door1, window1, win2Frame1, dl1, dc1, dr1, s1, wl1, and wr1, and (2) doorWindow1, door1, window1, win3Frame1, dl1, dc1, dr1, s1, wl2, wc2, and wr2, are obtained from the AND/OR tree.

For each product realization process alternative, the quantitative relations among attributes then form another network, called attribute relation network. An attribute relation network is composed of two types of nodes: attribute nodes and function nodes. A function node is linked with a number of input attribute nodes and one output attribute node. The attribute relation network for the first design alternative is shown in Figure 8 (c).

4.4 Identifying the optimal concurrent design using a multi-level optimization approach

In Section 3.4, an optimal concurrent design model was introduced to identify the optimal design considering relevant product life-cycle aspects. In the intelligent concurrent design system, this optimal concurrent design model was implemented using a multi-level optimization approach, based upon the optimization algorithms introduced in (Xue, 1997).

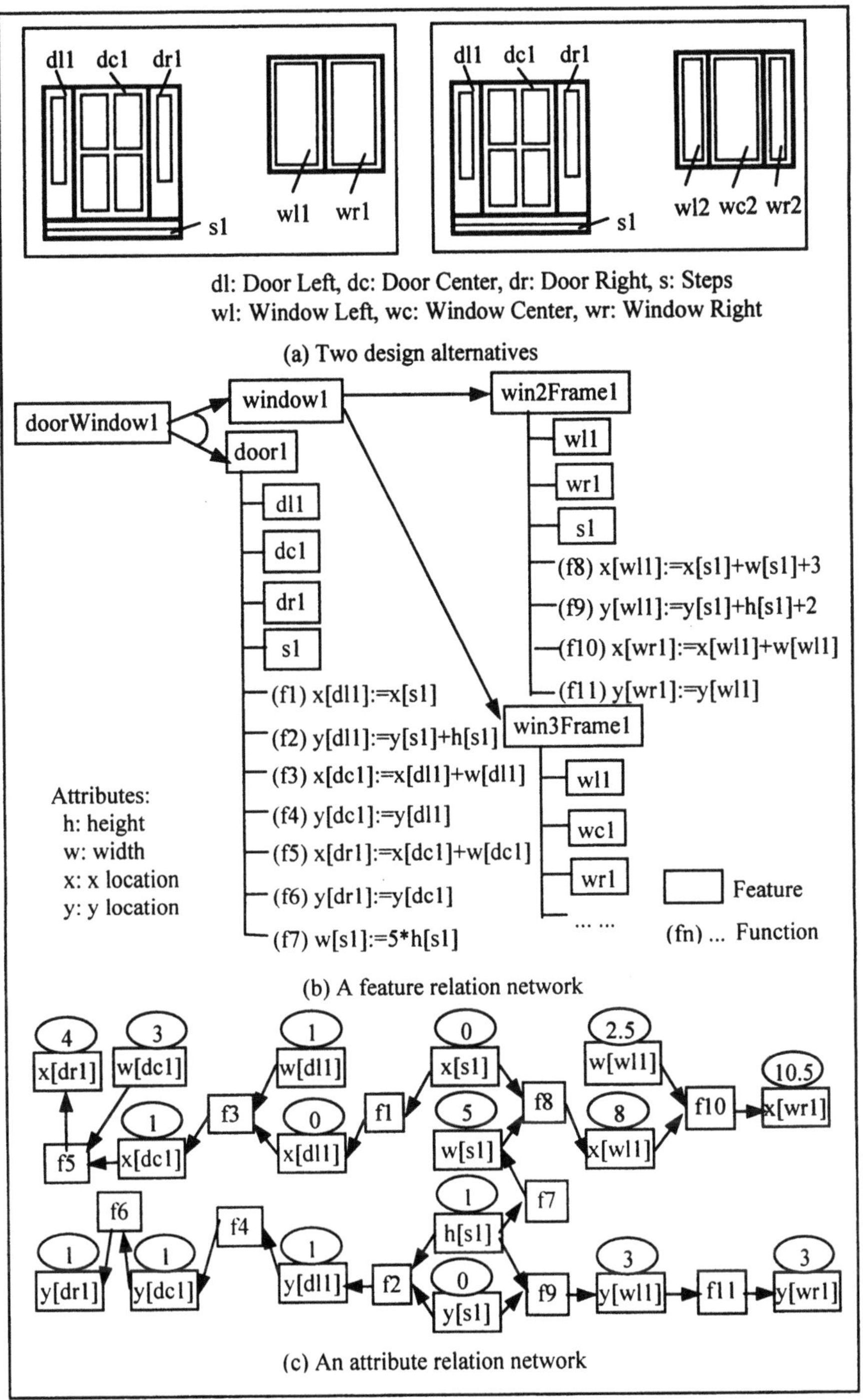

Figure 8. Maintenance of data relations

Since product realization process can be described by many alternatives, and each of these alternatives can be further described by attributes, the optimization is conducted at two different levels: attribute optimization level and alternative optimization level. First feasible design alternatives, which are described by instance features and relevant descriptions, are obtained from the AND/OR graph using the method introduced in Section 4.3. For each alternative, attribute optimization is carried out to identify the optimal attribute values using constrained optimization search. The optimal alternative is achieved from all the feasible alternatives at alternative optimization level. Many advanced optimization methods, including genetic algorithm and simulated annealing, were employed for improving the search efficiency and quality (Xue, 1997).

The objective function selected for optimization is based upon the concurrent design requirements. In the previous research for improving manufacturability, three types of objective functions have been introduced (Xue, Rousseau, and Dong, 1996). They are: (1) production cost function, (2) production time function, and, (3) combined cost and time function. Suppose production cost and time regarding *i*-th alternative are represented by $C_i(A_{i1}, A_{i2}, \ldots, A_{in_i})$ and $T_i(A_{i1}, A_{i2}, \ldots, A_{in_i})$ respectively, the objective function $f_i(A_{i1}, A_{i2}, \ldots, A_{in_i})$ in Eq. (18) can be represented by one of the three functions shown in Table 1. The α and β in this table are weighting factors between 0 and 1 for representing the importance of production cost and time in manufacturability evaluation.

Table 1. Objective functions considering manufacturability

Manufacturability Considerations	Objective Functions
Production cost only	$C_i(A_{i1}, A_{i2}, \ldots, A_{in_i})$
Production time only	$T_i(A_{i1}, A_{i2}, \ldots, A_{in_i})$
Both production cost and production time	$\alpha_i\, C_i(A_{i1}, A_{i2}, \ldots, A_{in_i}) + \beta_i\, T_i(A_{i1}, A_{i2}, \ldots, A_{in_i})$

5. IMPLEMENTATION OF THE INTELLIGENT CONCURRENT DESIGN SYSTEM

The intelligent concurrent design system was implemented using Smalltalk, an object oriented programming language (Goldberg and Robson, 1983), based upon the methods introduced in Section 4. Figure 9 shows the architecture of this implemented system. Users of this system are classified into two types: knowledge modeling users and product modeling users. The knowledge modeling users use two interface windows, *Class Feature Browser* and *Rule-Base Browser,* to model knowledge libraries including class features and rule-bases. The product modeling users use *Instance*

Feature Browser to model product database by generating instance features. Instance features are created from class features either manually or through rule-based inference. The consistency of the database is maintained by the data relation maintenance module using qualitative relations among features and quantitative relations among attributes. The optimal design and its attribute values considering relevant life-cycle aspects are identified through optimization using the optimal design identification module. A snapshot of the implemented system is shown in Figure 10.

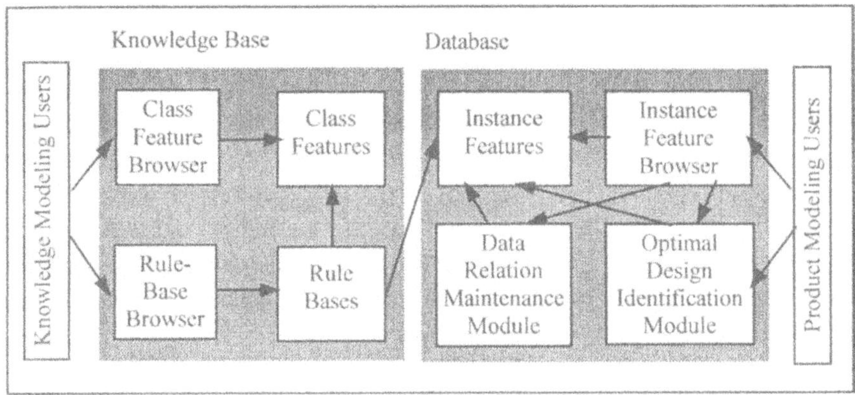

Figure 9. Architecture of the intelligent concurrent design system

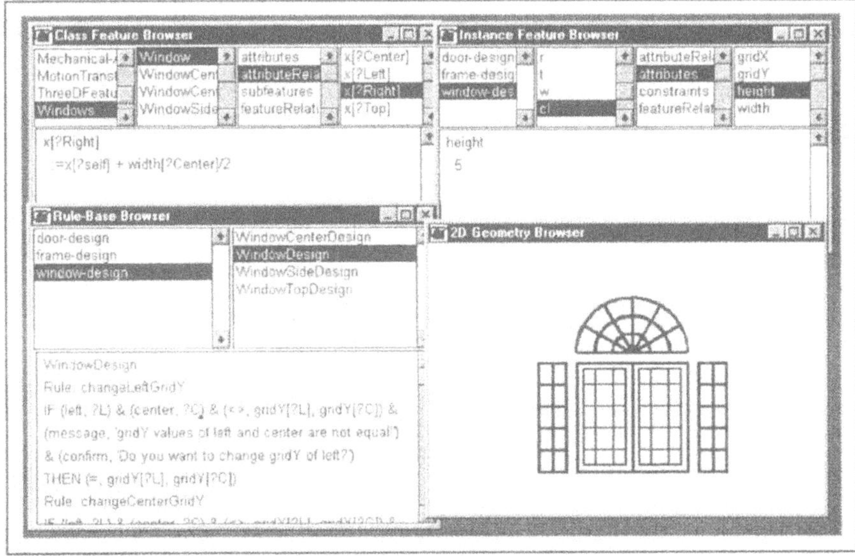

Figure 10. A snapshot of the implemented system

An industrial application for designing building products has also been developed for a local industrial company – Gienow Building Products Ltd., using the implemented system.

6. A CASE STUDY EXAMPLE

In this section, a case study example is given to show how a concurrent design is conducted to achieve the optimal design alternative and its attribute values using the introduced method.

The problem is to design a window frame with 2 glass panels. The required dimensions for this window are 150 cm by 100 cm. Two design candidates, *c1* and *c2* as shown in Figure 11 (a) and (b), are created from the design requirements. The width of the frame material is 5 cm. Through strength analysis, the length x must be long enough to support the whole window frame based upon the following two constraints: (1) x must be at least 20 cm, and (2) x must be greater than $0.035L$, where L is the total frame length in the 150 cm by 100 cm window area.

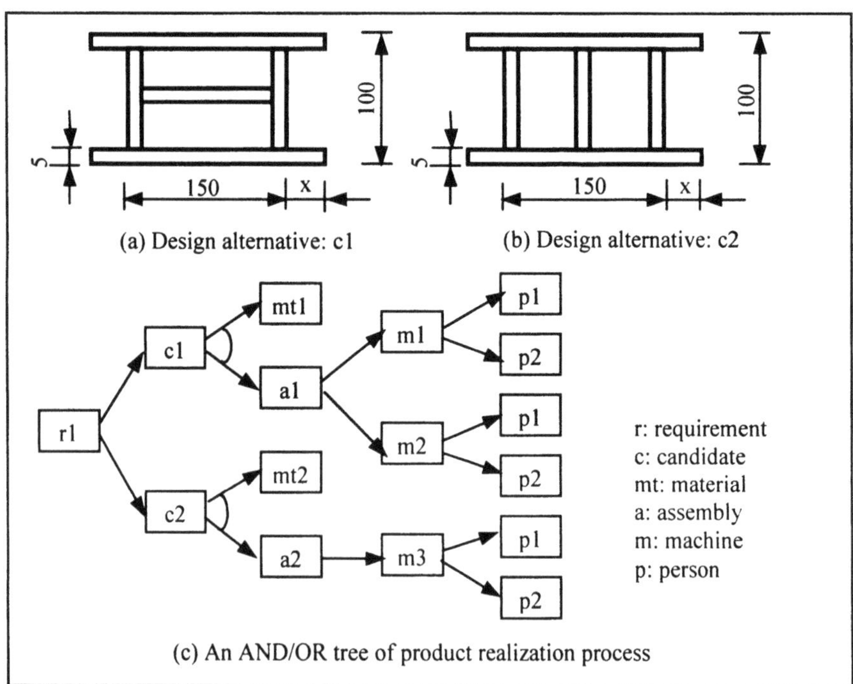

Figure 11. A case study example

Each of these design candidates is produced by processes of material ordering and assembly. The assembly process for candidate *c1* can be conducted using machine *m1* or *m2*. Each of these machines can be operated by person *p1* or *p2*. The assembly process for candidate *c2* can be conducted by machine *m3*, which is also operated by *p1* or *p2*. The AND/OR graph of the product realization process, which is generated through knowledge-based reasoning, is illustrated in Figure 11 (c). The nodes in the AND/OR graph are described by instance features, which are generated from class features. It requires 6 minutes for machine *m1*, or 3 minutes for machine *m2* to produce the candidate *c1*. It requires 6 minutes for machine *m3* to produce candidate *c2*. The unit machine costs and labor costs are given in Table 2. The unit cost of material is *$0.05/cm*.

Table 2. Unit costs for different machines and persons

Machines and Persons	Unit Costs ($/hour)
m1	10
m2	30
m3	15
p1	25
p2	30

From the AND/OR tree, six manufacturing alternatives are generated, as shown in Table 3. For each alternative, the length attribute *x* of the frame is selected as the variable at the attribute optimization level. The total production cost is selected as the objective function to be minimized for this problem. Using the cost models introduced in Table 2, the total cost is a function of the selected variable attribute for each alternative.

Table 3. Feasible alternatives and their optimal attribute values

Alternatives	Optimal Attribute Values (cm)	Costs ($)
1. r1, c1, mt1, a1, m1, p1	$x[c1]^*=21.7$	38.84
2. r1, c1, mt1, a1, m1, p2	$x[c1]^*=21.7$	39.34
3. r1, c1, mt1, a1, m2, p1	$x[c1]^*=21.7$	38.09
4. r1, c1, mt1, a1, m2, p2	$x[c1]^*=21.7$	38.34
5. r1, c2, mt2, a2, m3, p1	**$x[c2]^*=20.0$**	**36.5**
6. r1, c2, mt2, a2, m3, p2	$x[c2]^*=20.0$	37.0

The optimal attribute value regarding one alternative is identified using constrained optimization. For instance, attribute optimization for the first alternative is formulated as:

$$\underset{w.r.t.\ x[c1]}{Min}\ cost[mt1] + cost[m1] + cost[p1]$$

$$= 0.05(620 + x[c1] * 4) + 6 \times 10/60 + 6 \times 25/60$$

subject to:

$$x[c1] \geq 20$$

$$x[c1] \geq 0.035 \times 620$$

The optimal attribute value is achieved as:

$$x^{*}[c1] = 21.7\ (cm)$$

and the total cost is calculated as *\$38.84*. In the same way, the minimum costs for other alternatives are calculated as shown in Table 3. The optimal alternative is then identified from all the feasible alternatives.

7. CONCLUSIONS

In this research, modeling of knowledge and data for an intelligent concurrent design system is discussed.

The different product life-cycle aspects, including design, manufacturing, etc., are modeled by aspect primitives called features. A feature is a collection of qualitative and quantitative descriptions and their relations. Features are described at two levels, class level and instance level, representing product modeling libraries and actual product data, respectively. Instance features are generated using class features as their templates. The product realization process is modeled by an AND/OR tree. Generation of product models is carried out either manually or through knowledge-based inference. Rules are used for representing the product modeling knowledge and are organized in rule-bases. The qualitative and quantitative relations among product life-cycle aspects are maintained by two associated networks, the feature relation network and the attribute relation network. Any change can be propagated to other parts through these two associated networks. The optimal design alternative and its attribute values are identified by a multi-level optimization approach.

The introduced method has greatly improved the product modeling efficiency. This approach also provides a platform for developing the next generation CAD systems with intelligent concurrent design capabilities.

ACKNOWLEDGEMENTS

I would like to give my thanks to my graduate student, S. Yadav, at University of Calgary for his work on improving and implementing the intelligent concurrent design system, and Prof. D. H. Norrie at University of Calgary for his collaboration on developing the industrial application. I would also like to thank Prof. H. Yoshikawa and Prof. T. Tomiyama at University of Tokyo, and Prof. Z. Dong at University of Victoria for their support in developing the product description language and the early version of the intelligent concurrent design system. Financial support from the grant of Natural Sciences and Engineering Research Council (NSERC) of Canada and Gienow Building Products Ltd. is also acknowledged.

REFERENCES

Boothroyd, G. and Dewhurst, P. (1983) *Design for Assembly: A Designer's Handbook*, Boothroyd Dewhurst Inc., Wakerfield, RI.

Bralla, J. G. (ed.) (1986) *Handbook of Product Design for Manufacturing*, McGraw-Hill.

Chang, T. C., Wysk, R. A., and Wang, H. P. (1991) *Computer-Aided Manufacturing*, Prentice Hall.

Choi, K., Barash, M., and Anderson, D. (1984) "Automatic Recognition of Machined Surfaces from a 3-D Solid Model," *Computer-Aided Design*, Vol. 16, No. 2, pp. 81-86.

Dong, Z. (1993) "Design for Automated Manufacturing," *Concurrent Engineering: Automation, Tools, and Techniques*, Kusiak, A. (ed.), John Wiley & Sons, pp. 207-234.

Dong, Z. (ed.) (1994) *Artificial Intelligence in Optimal Design and Manufacturing*, Prentice Hall.

Dong, Z., Hu, W., and Xue, D. (1994) "New Production Cost-tolerance Models for Tolerance Synthesis," *Journal of Engineering for Industry, Transaction of ASME*, Vol. 116, pp 199-206.

Dowlatshahi, S. (1992) "Product Design in a Concurrent Engineering Environment: An Optimization Approach," *International Journal of Production Research*, Vol. 30, No. 8, pp. 1803-1818.

Gershenson, J. and Ishii, K. (1993) "Life-cycle Serviceability Design," *Concurrent Engineering: Automation, Tools, and Techniques*, Kusiak, A. (ed.), John Wiley & Sons, pp. 363-384.

Goldberg, A. and Robson, D. (1983) *Smalltalk-80: The Language and Its Implementation*, Addison-Wesley.

Henderson, M. R. (1984) "Extraction of Feature Information from Three Dimensional CAD Data," Ph.D. Dissertation, Purdue University.

Kusiak, A. (ed.) (1992) *Intelligent Design and Manufacturing*, John Wiley & Sons.

Kusiak, A. (ed.) (1993) *Concurrent Engineering: Automation, Tools, and Techniques*, John Wiley & Sons.

Luby, S. C., Dixon, J. R., and Simmons, M. K. (1986) "Creating and Using a Feature Databases," *Computers in Mechanical Engineering*, Vol. 5, No. 3, pp. 25-33.

Makino, A., Barkan, P., and Pfaff, R. (1989) "Design for Serviceability," *Proceedings of the 1989 ASME Winter Annual Meeting*, San Francisco, CA.

Prasad, B. (1996) *Concurrent Engineering Fundamentals: Volume I*, Prentice Hall.

Pratt, M. J. (1984) "Solid Modeling and the Interface between Design and Manufacturing," *IEEE Computer Graphics and Application Magazine*, pp. 52-59.

Shah, J. J. and Mantyla, M. (1995) *Parametric and Feature-Based CAD/CAM*, John Wiley & Sons.

Shah, J. J. and Rogers, M. T. (1988) "Functional Requirements and Conceptual Design of the Feature-based Modeling System," *Computer-Aided Engineering Journal*, Vol. 5, No. 1, pp. 9-15.

Singh, N. (1996) *Systems Approach to Computer-Integrated Design and Manufacturing*, John Wiley & Sons.

Tomiyama, T. (1994) "From General Design Theory to Knowledge-Intensive Engineering," *Artificial Intelligence for Engineering Design, Analysis, and Manufacturing*, Vol. 8, No. 4, pp. 319-333.

Tomiyama, T. (1997) "A Manufacturing Paradigm towards the 21st Century," *Integrated Computer Aided Engineering*, Vol. 4, pp. 159-178.

Tomiyama, T. and ten Hagen, P. J. W. (1987) "The Concept of Intelligent Integrated Interactive CAD Systems," CWI Report No. CS-R8717, Centre for Mathematics and Computer Science, Amsterdam, The Netherlands.

Tomiyama, T. and Yoshikawa, H. (1987) "Extended General Design Theory," *Design Theory for CAD, Proceedings of the IFIP Working Group 5.2 Working Conference 1985 (Tokyo)*, Yoshikawa, H. and Warman, E. A. (eds.), North-Holland, Amsterdam, pp. 95-130.

Xue, D. (1997) "A Multilevel Optimization Approach Considering Product Realization Process Alternatives and Parameters for Improving Manufacturability," *Journal of Manufacturing Systems*, Vol. 16, No. 5, pp. 337-351.

Xue, D. and Dong, Z. (1993) "Feature Modeling Incorporating Tolerance and Production Process for Concurrent Design," *Concurrent Engineering: Research and Applications*, Vol. 1, pp. 107-116.

Xue, D. and Dong, Z. (1994) "Developing a Quantitative Intelligent System for Implementing Concurrent Engineering Design," *Journal of Intelligent Manufacturing*, Vol. 5, pp. 251-267.

Xue, D. and Dong, Z. (1997) "Coding and Clustering of Design and Manufacturing Features for Concurrent Design," *Computers in Industry*, Vol. 34, pp. 139-153.

Xue, D., Rousseau, J. H., and Dong, Z. (1996) "Joint Optimization of Performance and Costs in Integrated Concurrent Design: Tolerance Synthesis Part," *Engineering Design and Automation*, Vol. 2, No. 1, pp. 73-89.

Xue, D., Takeda, H., Kiriyama, T., Tomiyama, T., and Yoshikawa, H. (1992) "An Intelligent Integrated Interactive CAD – A Preliminary Report," *Intelligent Computer Aided Design*, Waldron M. B., Brown, D., and Yoshikawa, H. (eds.), North-Holland, Amsterdam, pp. 163-192.

Yoshikawa, H. (1981) "General Design Theory and CAD Systems," *Man-machine Communication in CAD/CAM*, Sata, T. and Warman, E. (eds.), North-Holland, Amsterdam, pp. 35-58.

Yoshikawa, H. (1993) *Techno-Globe*, Sangyo Chosa-kai, Tokyo.

Young, R. E., Greef, A., and O'Grady, P. (1992) "An Artificial Intelligence-based Constraint Network System for Concurrent Engineering," *International Journal of Production Research*, Vol. 30, No. 7, pp. 1715-1735.

Zhang, H. C., Kuo, T. C., Lu, H., and Huang, S. H. (1997) "Environmentally Conscious Design and Manufacturing: A State-of-the-Art Survey," *Journal of Manufacturing Systems*, Vol. 16, No. 5, pp. 352-371.

7

Model Sharing among Agents in a Concurrent Product Development Team

Masanori Ozawa[1], Mark R. Cutkosky[2] & Brian J. Howley[2]

[1] *Visiting scholar, Center for Design Research, Stanford University from Corporate Research and Development Center, Toshiba Corporation*

[2] *Center for Design Research, Stanford University*

Key words: Performance Sizing, Lumped Parameter Model, Compositional Modeling Language (CML), Ontology, Java Agent Template (JAT), DVD, Pick Up Head, Concurrent Engineering, Open Knowledge Base Connectivity (OKBC), Open I-DEAS™, Matlab™.

Abstract: We describe a project involving the use of software agents for concurrent engineering of electromechanical products. The agents are a mix of autonomous programs and software interfaces for human specialists in an engineering team. Our goal is to accelerate the design process by reducing delays associated with the exchange of design information, including models, constraints, objectives, and dependencies associated with each agent. Part of this effort involves methods for representing and exchanging design information in a human/machine-readable form. In this paper we focus on the sharing of information in models, such as the lumped-parameter models of electromechanical systems that engineers often use in the early stages of design. We first review the design information-sharing problem and examine the different levels of abstraction and detail at which such information is represented and shared. We then introduce a representation language and information-sharing infrastructure that we have employed for an agent-based concurrent engineering system. We illustrate some of the issues involved in our approach with a short scenario involving the redesign of an optical pick-up head for DVD (digital versatile disc) players. We then discuss our plans for extending the system to allow more general exchanges of engineering models among agents.

1. INTRODUCTION

One of the major challenges associated with the design of modern consumer products is the need to integrate mechanical, electrical, optical and software components in a compact, low-cost system. The design of such devices as DVD and CDROM players typically involves a team of specialists who exchange models, preferences, decisions and constraints as the design progresses. Delays are introduced when such information is not transferred efficiently among human specialists and among the engineering programs they use.

A way to address this problem is to represent the engineering team as a set of agents that adhere to a common communication language and protocol. The agents can be autonomous programs that perform a specific function or software interfaces through which human specialists exchange information between their own engineering tools and those of the rest of the team. Our work on agent-based engineering teams has involved two efforts: the development of software for coordinating the actions of agents by dynamically tracking the dependencies among their decisions, tasks and goals, and the development of methods for capturing and exchanging the information that agents need to share in a machine-readable form. The focus of this paper is the second effort; the agent coordination problem is discussed in other publications [Petrie, Webster and Cutkosky, 1995].

Our approach to representing and sharing design information among agents is a specialized subset of the Knowledge Sharing effort in the Artificial Intelligence community [Olsen et al, 1995, Iwasaki et al 1997, Falkenhainer et al, 1994]. The sharing of information among agents is supported by a common ontology [Gruber, T. R., 1993] (a set of terms and definitions in the product domain) and a compositional modeling language (CML) in which models can be created such that conventions, constraints, applicability conditions and assumptions are defined formally and ultimately grounded in logic.

1.1 Levels of information sharing in design

The sharing of design information can take place at a variety of levels, ranging from detailed numerical representations, such as FEM mesh for a component, to abstract principles (e.g., of energy conservation in a circuit). Choueiry et al [1998] have proposed a "theory of model reformation for reasoning about physical systems" which provides a useful framework for examining the different levels at which engineering information is used and exchanged. They describe the process of composing and analyzing models as a sequence of steps, as shown in Figure 1.1. The process begins with a task description, including an underlying domain theory (representation of the relevant physical laws, properties of components, etc.), modeling assumptions (for example, that the temperature will remain within some range) and a scenario that captures the particular conditions that hold during the task.

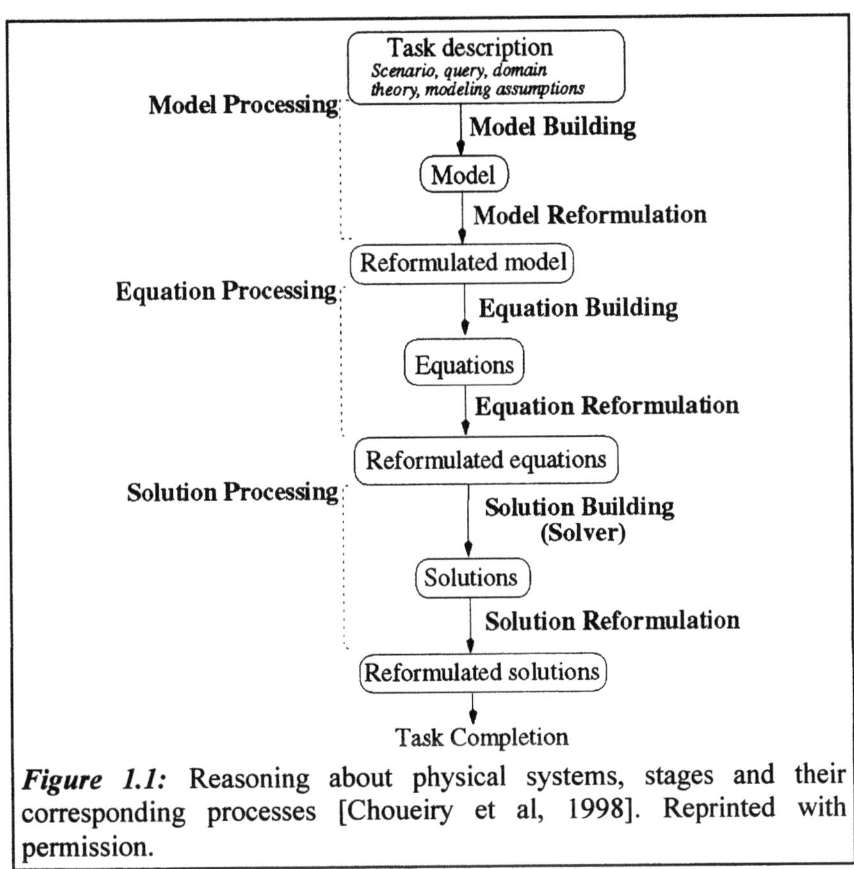

Figure 1.1: Reasoning about physical systems, stages and their corresponding processes [Choueiry et al, 1998]. Reprinted with permission.

The steps shown in Figure 1 can also be applied to engineering analyses. Given a task description, the first step is to compose models appropriate for the task. A model at this point often consists of knowledge of the physical structure (components and their topology, for example) as well as knowledge of the relevant physical phenomena, including the conditions under which they are active. The models may also be transformed, or reformulated, to improve their suitability for addressing the task. For example, a continuous model may be discretized. The next step is to generate equations from the models. The equations may also be reformulated or transformed for ease of analysis and solution. For example, the equations may be transformed from cartesian to polar coordinates or from time domain to frequency domain. The final step is solution processing, which may involve analytic or numerical solution. The solution may also be reformulated the better to answer particular questions.

In an engineering team, there will be multiple specialists or agents going through steps like those in Figure 1.1, and each stage will typically involve sharing information. Table 1 is an attempt to distinguish among the main levels of detail and their associated uses. At the highest level are representations used primarily in the conceptual design stages for communication among human experts. These models are often difficult to encode in a machine-understandable form. At the next level are ontologies and information such as assumptions and constraints associated with the model-building and model-reformation stages of analysis. Generation of machine-interpretable models and ontologies is challenging and time consuming, but can be accomplished using research tools like CML [Falkenhainer et al, 1994, Bobrow et al, 1996], to be discussed in the next section. The next level in the table involves equations. Automatic generation and manipulation of equations is possible with commercial tools like Mathematica™[i], which is used as the "equation processor" and "equation solver" in the CML environment. The most common levels of information sharing for integrated engineering tools are levels (d) and (e), exchanging model parameters and numerical data sets.

Table 1: Knowledge representation levels in different design stages

Knowledge representation level	Tool, Mean (examples)	Processing stage
a: Conceptual Model-Market needs, Specifications	Methodologies: QFD, TRIZ, Morphological Chart Method Tools: Rapid, 3D-Live	Task Description
b: Ontologies, Model Fragments, Constraint set	Languages: Ontolingua, CML, etc.	Task Description, Model Processing
c: Mathematical Equations	Tools: Mathematica, Maple, Design Sheet, CDME	Equation Processing, Solution Processing
d: Design Parameters	Tools: MATLAB, 3D-CAD (I-DEAS etc.), CDME	Task Description, Solution Processing
e: Product Model- 2D/3D models, FEM models	Tools: I-DEAS, Pro-E, Rapid, 3D-Live Standards: IGES, STEP, VRML etc.	Model Processing, Solution Processing

In level (e), models can involve detailed information e.g., not only part geometry, but also physical properties, geometric constraints, and even the history of modeling operations on each part. However, such data intensive models do not translate well between different applications despite progress on standardized product formats such as STEP[ii] .

Although levels (d), (c) and (b) are increasingly abstract and difficult to exchange among automated agents, they are also increasingly flexible and

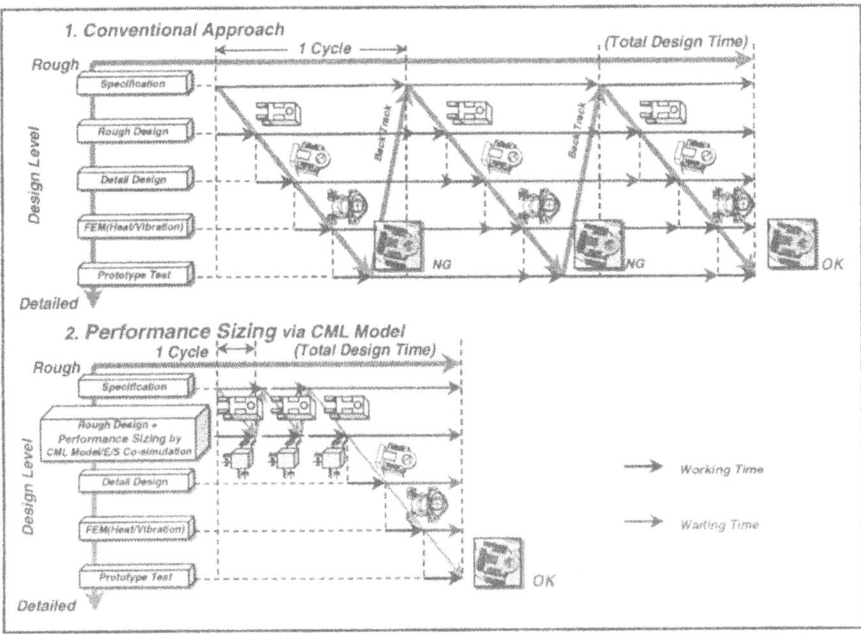

Figure 1.2: Reducing delays in the early ("Performance Sizing") stages of design through better sharing of information among agents [Ozawa, Iwasaki and Cutkosky 1998].

adaptable for early design stages when the form of a design may be changing dramatically. The hypothesis guiding our work is that by exchanging models at the earliest design stages it is possible to execute more design tasks in parallel and evaluate design trade-offs before the detailed design phase. We call this early stage evaluation "**Performance Sizing**" [Ozawa, Iwasaki, and Cutkosky 1998]. Performance Sizing, as shown in Figure 1.2, can lead to a significant reduction in the amount of backtracking and delays caused by conflicts and misunderstandings that is otherwise commonplace in designing complex electromechanical systems.

In the next sections we describe briefly the approach we have taken for sharing such information among agents in a concurrent engineering system. We start with a brief description of CML and how it is used.

2. COMPOSITIONAL MODELING LANGUAGE

In this section we briefly describe CML and its characteristics that make it suitable for developing engineering models for early-stage design. For a more detailed discussion see [Ozawa, Iwasaki and Cutkosky 1998].

Compositional modeling is a paradigm for formulating a behavior model of a physical system by composing descriptions of symbolic and mathematical properties of individual system components. CML is a general-purpose declarative modeling language for representing physical knowledge required for compositional modeling. CML is intended to facilitate model sharing between research groups, many of which have long been using similar languages. These languages are based primarily on the language originally defined by Qualitative Process Theory [Forbus 1984] and include the languages used for the Qualitative Physics Compiler [Farquhar 1994], compositional model formulation [Falkenhainer 1991], and the Device Modeling Environment [Low and Iwasaki 1993]. CML is fully translatable to the knowledge interchange format (KIF)[Genesereth and Fikes 1992].

A domain theory in CML is a finite set of the following top-level forms:

- **defEntity** for defining properties of persistent objects (e.g., resistors, containers).
- **defModelFragment** for describing the behavior of modeled entities under explicitly specified conditions. Model fragments are used to describe phenomena that arise out of the interactions of a composite set of objects (e.g., collisions or flows), or the behavior of a single object (e.g., a resistor, pump, or valve).
- **defScenario** for defining initial value problems consisting of a set of objects, their configuration, and initial values for the quantities that describe them.

To predict the behavior of a physical system in some domain, knowledge about the physics of the domain is captured in a general purpose *domain theory* that describes classes of relevant objects, phenomena and systems. A domain theory in CML consists of a set of definitions, called *model fragments* and *entities*, each of which describes a piece of the domain's physics or objects. Once the domain theory has been constructed, it can be used to model different physical devices under a variety of conditions. The description of a specific system or situation being modeled is called a *scenario*. The scenario includes an initial configuration of the device, the initial values of some of the parameters that are relevant to modeling it, and perhaps conditions that further characterize the system. The CML implementation automatically identifies those model fragments that are applicable to the scenario. These model fragments are composed into a single model that comprises both a symbolic description and a set of governing equations. The equations may be solved or simulated to produce a behavioral description. Because the conditions under which the model fragments hold are stated explicitly in the domain theory, the system is able to assemble new models that describe the device as it moves into new operating regions. The full specification of the languages can be found in [Falkenhainer et al. 1994].

CDME is a web-based interface through which users can compose and interact with models in CML [Iwasaki et al, 1997]. If users define the domain theory in CML, and initial conditions or simulation conditions, etc. in a scenario, CDME will automatically interpret those definitions, convert them into an internal logical model, and prepare a procedure for numerical calculation. Currently, "Mathematica™" is the solver used in CDME. In addition, CDME can extract and generate equations from the CML model for use with an external solver or simulator.

Interaction between CML models and scenarios and external agents is accomplished using the Open Knowledge Base Connectivity (OKBC) protocol from the Stanford Knowledge Systems Laboratory [Chaudhri et al, 1997]. OKBC provides access to the classes, individuals, slots, facets, etc., of the CML library. OKBC is based on the Generic Frame Protocol (GFP) [Karp, Myers, Gruber, 1995].

3. LOGICAL DESCRIPTION OF VIRTUAL PUH MODEL IN CML

To investigate the sharing of models among engineering agents, we used CML to build models of the pick-up head (PUH) of a DVD optical disk device. The models capture several different domains of physical behavior, and the interactions between them. A CAD drawing of the PUH and its major components is shown in Figure 3.1. Figure 3.2 shows some of the CML models for the PUH, including rigid body and heat transfer dynamics.

The dynamics include nonlinear changes in magnetic field strength as a function of actuator displacement and changes in ambient temperature.

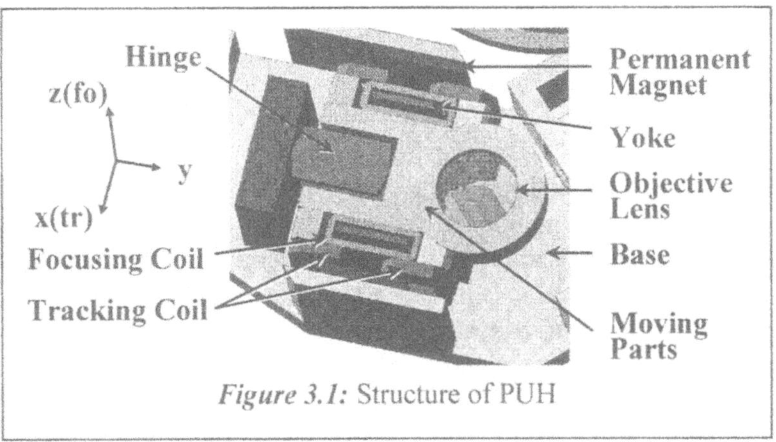

Figure 3.1: Structure of PUH

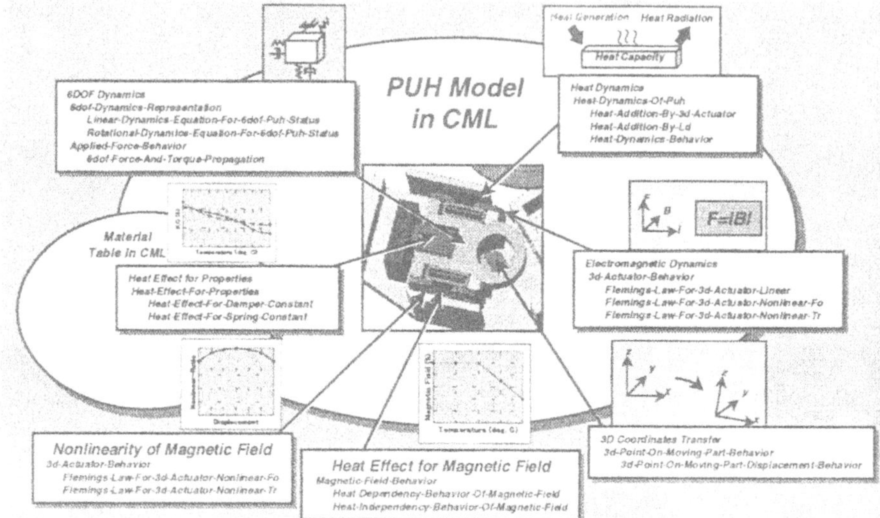

Figure 3.2: PUH Model in CML

3.1 6-DOF Rigid Body Dynamics

The moving part of the PUH can be approximated as a rigid body with six degrees of freedom (6-DOF), suspended by a combination of linear and rotational stiffness and damping elements. Voice coil motors actuate the body in two directions to achieve focus and maintain tracking. In Figure 3.1, the focus direction is along the z axis and the tracking direction is along the x axis.

The actuation force, F, is governed by Fleming's law ($F=iB_o r_{mt}\ r_{md}\ l$), where l is the effective length of the coil in the magnetic field. The strength of the magnetic field varies as a function temperature and actuator displacement. These dependencies are captured by the parameters r_{mt} and r_{md}, which are further described in Sections 3.3 and 3.4. A detailed description of the CML model fragments is given in [Ozawa, Iwasaki and Cutkosky 1998].

3.2 Temperature Dependency of Material

High-polymer materials are often used in the flexure (hinges) of the PUH to provide controlled motion of the lens with respect to the base. The stiffness and damping parameters of these materials are often temperature-dependent. The changes in stiffness and damping must be accounted for when designing the servo system. The heat dependent stiffness (k) and damping (c) are expressed by equations (3.2.1 - 3.2.3).

$$k(t_{PUH}) = k_{20} \cdot e^{\{-c_k \cdot (t_{PUH} - 20)\}} \qquad (3.2.1)$$

$$c(t_{PUH}) \propto \frac{\sqrt{m \cdot k(t_{PUH})} \cdot \tan\delta}{\sqrt{1 + \tan^2\delta}} \qquad (3.2.2)$$

$$\tan\delta = c_{c1} \cdot e^{(c_{c2} \cdot t_{PUH})} \qquad (3.2.3)$$

K_{20} ≡ spring constant at 20 (c°)
c_k, c_{c1}, c_{c2} ≡ constants that are peculiar to each high-polymer material

3.3 Temperature Dependency of Magnetic Field

Magnetic fields of permanent magnets are also affected by temperature. Although the sensitivity is not high at normal room temperatures, it may be a concern in automotive applications where the ambient temperatures around the PUH exceed 80° C and the surface temperatures of actuator coils can exceed 120° C.

An approximate expression of the temperature dependency is given by equation (3.3.1).

$$\begin{cases} r_{mt} = 1.0 & (t_{PUH} \le t_{cr}) \\ r_{mt} = 1.0 - c_{mt} \cdot (t_{PUH} - t_{cr}) & (t_{PUH} > t_{cr}) \end{cases} \qquad (3.3.1)$$

In this equation, c_{mt} and t_{cr} are constants that are peculiar to each magnetic material, c_{mt} is the slope of the curve shown in Figure 3.2 and t_{cr} is the critical temperature at which the magnetic field starts to be weakened by heat.

For certain materials, a more accurate model may be available in the form of a look-up table or a function. Such models can be incorporated using the "Blackbox Function" of CML. Explicit conditions can be imposed on the applicability of such blackbox models.

3.4 Non-Linearity of Magnetic Field

Ideally, the field produced by the permanent magnet should be uniform over the range of motion of the actuator coils to obtain maximum servoing accuracy. However, the field usually weakens somewhat near the edges. This effect is captured by the ratio, r_{md},, where the full strength of the field corresponds to a value of rmd,=1.0 at the center of the field.

A typical curve of r_{md}, is illustrated in the lower left corner of Figure 3.2. This information is entered into CML in the form of a table.

3.5 Simulation Results

Co-simulation results of PUH heat and rigid body dynamics are shown in Figures 3.3 and 3.4. The results were obtained using CDME. Figure 3.3 shows the change in material and magnetic properties over a change in PUH temperature. Figure 3.4 compares PUH dynamic response at two different temperatures. The simulation captures physical interactions that are normally characterized by separate design disciplines.

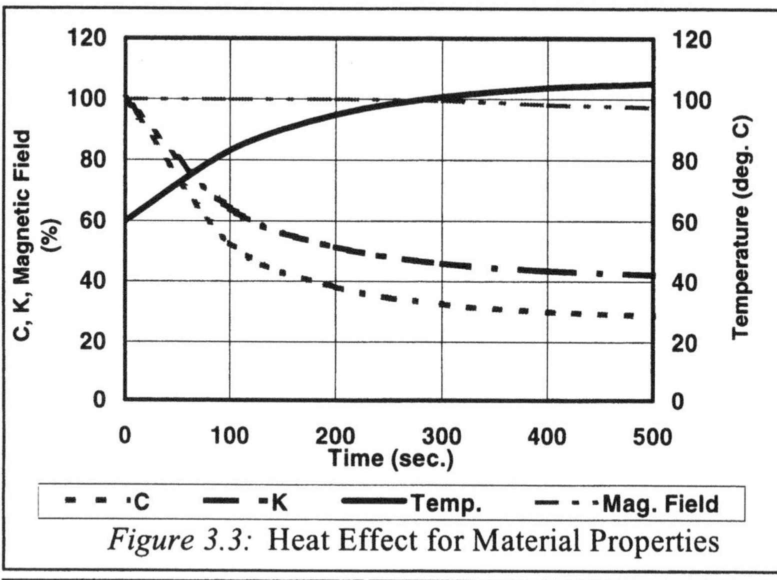

Figure 3.3: Heat Effect for Material Properties

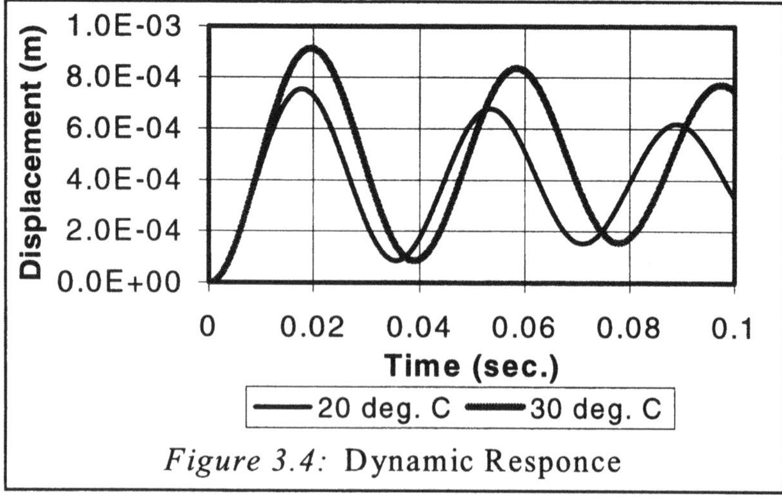

Figure 3.4: Dynamic Responce

4. CML/MATLAB/I-DEAS INTEGRATION

Although cross-disciplinary simulations can be performed entirely within CML/CDME, we do not anticipate that this will be the usual approach. As discussed in Section 2, CML is an object-oriented, declarative language that emphasizes expressiveness and re-use of models and model fragments. It is not optimized for numerical efficiency. Moreover, we believe that most engineers will prefer to use their own specialized tools for computationally intensive analyses and simulations. The role of CML/CDME is to provide models that these engineers can interact with (publish, view, query, and refine).

4.1 Agent Infrastructure

To support interaction with CML, we have developed an agent-based framework as shown in Figure 4.1. This approach is based on the agent-interaction technology described in Cutkosky *et al* [1993]. The engineers and their tools interact through agents using the emerging standard communications language, KQML (see http://www.cs.umbc.edu/kqml/ for the current KQML standard). The communications are built on open Internet standards, TCP/IP, SMTP, and FTP.

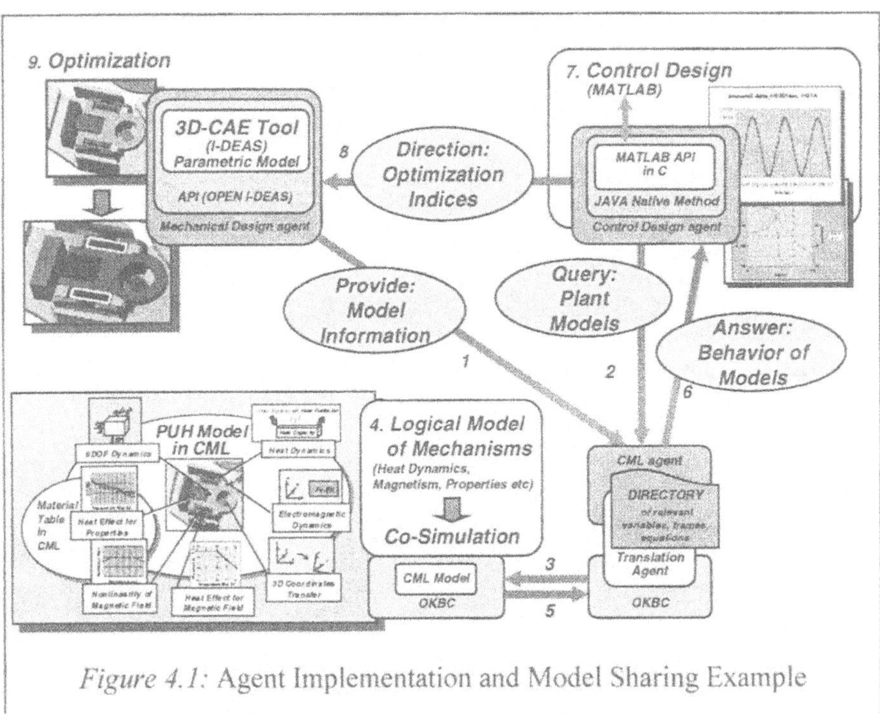

Figure 4.1: Agent Implementation and Model Sharing Example

To facilitate the wrapping of commercial engineering tools we have developed the Java Agent Template (JAT). A description of JAT is beyond the scope of this paper, but details on the beta-release of JAT can be found at http://java.stanford.edu. Briefly, JAT is a package of programs written in the Java language that allow users to quickly create new software "agents" that communicate over the Internet. JAT facilitates especially construction of agents that send and receive messages in KQML and provides services including name registration, queuing and buffering of messages, connect/disconnect and security. Agents can be stand-alone programs or applets, downloaded through a standard web browser. Interfaces have been created for programs written in C++ and Lisp as well as Java.

4.2 Agent Interaction Example

Figure 4.1 shows an example exchange that we have implemented with three agents:

- a Mechanical Design agent, which is an interface for a human designer using the I-DEAS™[iii] CAD package and responsible not only the geometric optimization but miscellaneous design trade-offs on physical performances described in Section 3.1 –3.4
- a Control Design agent, which is an interface to a servo designer using the Matlab™[iv] controls toolbox
- a CML agent, which maintains the CML models of the PUH domain and design scenario. The CML agent uses OKBC and a Java

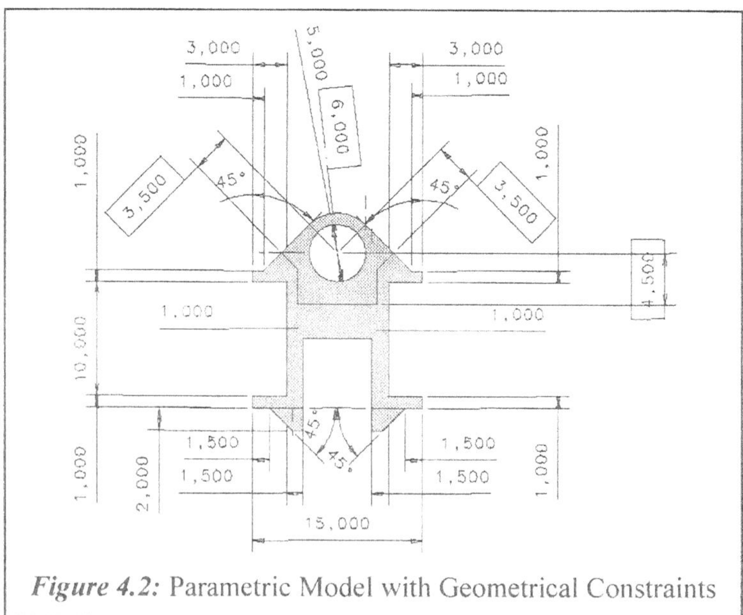

Figure 4.2: Parametric Model with Geometrical Constraints

translation agent to communicate with other agents. The Translation Agent converts between the (verbose) internal CML variable names and shorter task-specific names used by the other agents in the scenario.

Table 2 is a partial listing of these terms.

The interaction illustrated in Figure 4.1 has the following sequence:

1) The Mechanical Design agent uses the CAD tool to create an initial PUH design as a collection of parametric models. (Figure 4.2 shows a parametric model of the PUH "bobbin" in more detail). Parameter values describing the properties of the PUH (e.g., overall mass, moments of inertia, stiffness) are transmitted to the CML model via the Translation Agent.

2) The Control Design queries the CML model to obtain values for PUH mass, spring constant and other model parameters. A sample request is shown in Figure 4.3.

3) The requests are translated and submitted as a set of queries to CML.

4) CML composes a model of the PUH dynamics and computes changes to the spring constant, damping, and magnetic field strength parameters as a function of temperature.

5) CML returns the parameters.

6) Parameter values are translated and passed back to the Control Design agent as KQML messages.

7) The servo designer analyzes the plant response and determines the need to reduce PUH mass.

8) The Control Design agent sends a message to the Mechanical Design agent requesting a reduction in the moving mass.

```
Control Design Agent query to CML Agent:
 (ask-one
  :sender   Control Design Agent
  :receiver   CML Agent
  :language   KIF
  :content    (get-initial-values :values Mx))

 CML Agent response:
 (reply
  :sender   CML Agent
  :receiver   Control Design Agent
  :language   KIF
  :content    (initial-values Mx 0.002))
```

Figure 4.3: Example message exchange between the Control Design agent and the CML agent.

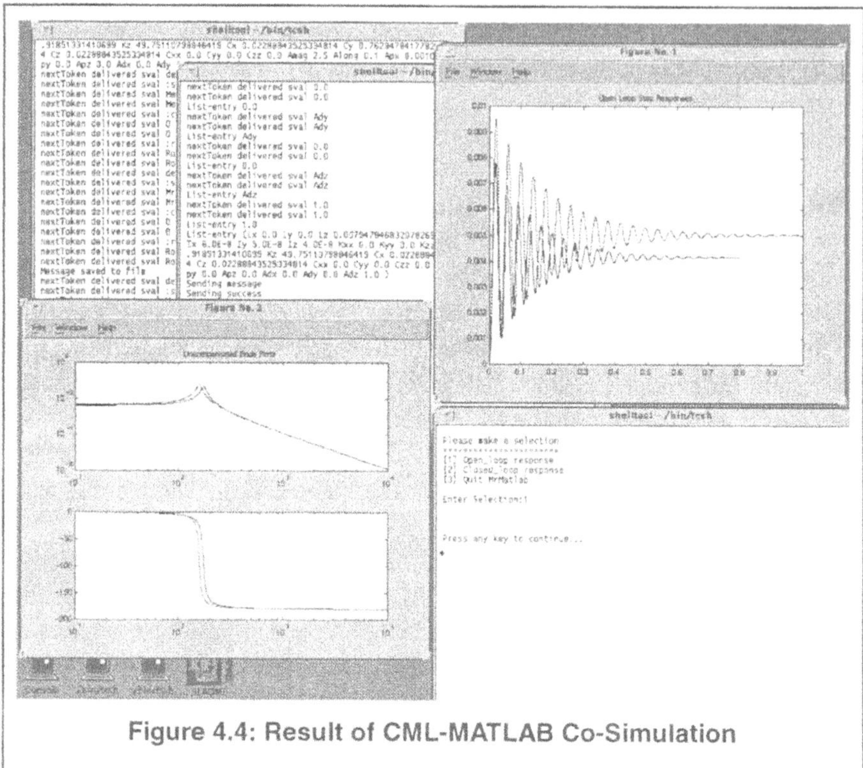

Figure 4.4: Result of CML-MATLAB Co-Simulation

A sample KQML message exchange between Control Design agent and the CML agent is shown in Figure 4.3. The query contains the performative “ask one” and specifies the intended recipient, and the contents of the question.

The “get-initial-values” and the model parameter “Mx” are part of a shared ontology between the Control Design agent and the CML agent. The content expression is written in Knowledge Interchange Format, (KIF). The translation agent, shown towards the bottom of Figure 4.1, converts the expression “Mx” to the internal CML label “M-X”, “The-3D-Mass,” using Table 2.

Figure 4.4 is the screen shot of the Control Design agent’s desktop and includes information on the message exchange, parameter values, and results of the agent’s analysis. Figures 4.5 and 4.6 show the analysis results in more detail. Figure 4.5 shows the open loop response at different temperatures (20 C and 30 C respectively), and Figure 4.6 shows the closed loop system is temperature insensitive (the two curves are indistinguishable).

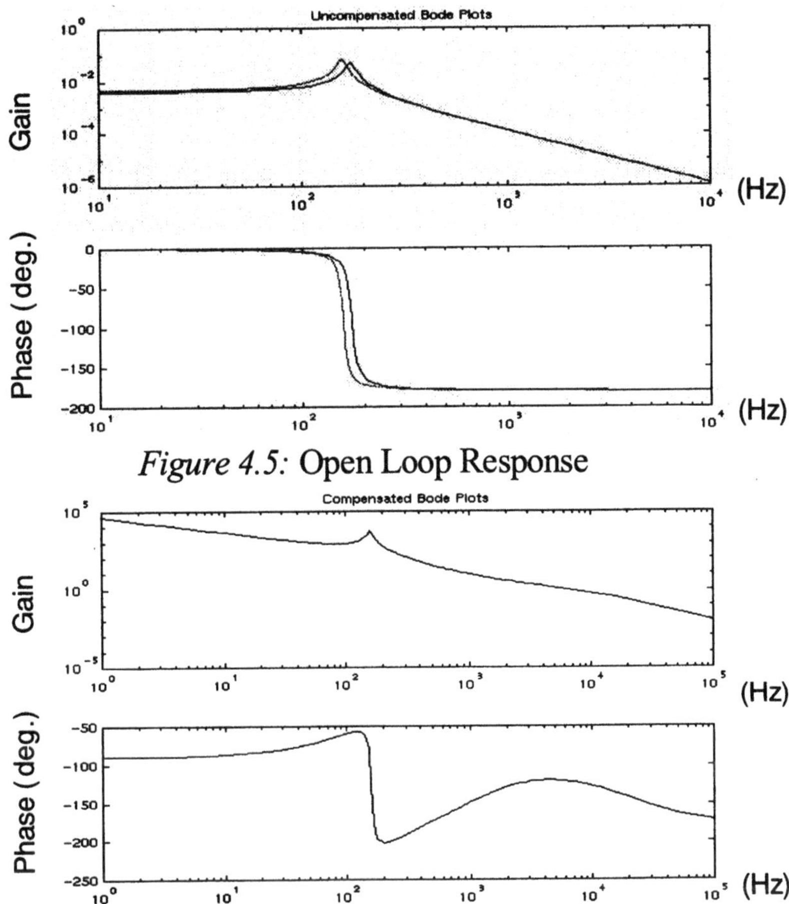

Figure 4.5: Open Loop Response

Figure 4.6: Closed Loop Response with Servo Agent

Table 2: Partial Listing of Terminology Translation Table

Matlab Agent name	MechaAgent name (CML cross reference)	Description
Mx	"M-X", "The-3D-Mass"	Effective PUH mass in X direction
Kx	"K-X", "The-K-Matrix"	Linear spring constant along the X direction
Cx	"C-X", "The-C-Matrix"	Linear damping coefficient along the X direction
Ix	"I-Xx", "The-3d-Inertia-Tensor"	PUH X axis inertia through mass center
Krx	"Kr-X", "The-K-Matrix"	Torsional spring constant about the X axis
Crx	"Cr-X", "The-C-Matrix"	Torsional damping coefficient about the X axis
l_track	"Effective-Length", "The-3d-Actuator-Tr"	Tracking actuator coil length
b_track	"Magnetic-Induction", "The-3d-Actuator-Tr	Tracking actuator air gap flux density
s_track	"Directional-Sine-Against-Magnetic-Field", "The-3d-Actuator-Tr"	Tracking actuator coil winding perpendicularity
dx_track	"Direction-Cosine-For-X", "(Direction-Vector-For-3d-Applied-Force(Generated-Force The-3d-Actuator-Tr))"	X axis component of tracking actuator's direction of applied force
ax_track	"X-Coordinate", "(Location-For-3d-Applied-Force(Generated-Force The-3d-Actuator-Tr))"	X component of the tracking actuator's point of application
cgx	"X-Coordinate", "The-Center-Of-Gravity"	X component of the PUH center of mass
Lx	"X-Coordinate", "The-Focal-Point"	X component of the PUH center of focus

5. DISCUSSION

In this section we discuss some of the issues that arose during our development of the system used for the example exchange in Figure 4.1.

5.1 Levels of the Information Sharing

It is useful to reconsider Table 1 in light of the simple example described in the last section. The example involved sharing of information at the parameter level (d) in the table. The sharing just of parameters could have been accomplished with agents that did not use CML models but instead used a common domain model and table of terms, such as in Table 2. In addition, sharing of models at the level of numerical data could be accomplished using commercial technology. Indeed, it is common to exchange 3D geometry models between CAD systems such as I-DEAS™ and FEM solvers such as Nastran™ and Abacus™.

In fact, our view is that the main point of creating models in CML is to publish them so that others, outside of one's own area of expertise, can assimilate them. As an example, consider what it takes for a control engineer to incorporate models of laser optics and actuators into the controller of a DVD device. Before she can use the models, she needs to understand the terminology associated with models (what parameters, physical units, reference frames, etc. are involved) and what underlying domain theory the models are built upon. In addition, there may be limits to the applicability of the models, or additional constraints affecting some of the model parameters, which must be understood before the models can be used correctly. The more explicitly and formally these terms, conventions and limitations are defined, the more likely that non-experts will be able to use the models and the less chance there is for accidental misuse.

The extreme case of writing models for non-experts is to develop models that can be assimilated by software agents, defined in this context as programs that automate some elements of an engineering task. An example might be a controller design agent that specifies the parameters of a linear controller in response to stated objectives and a description of the system to be controlled. In this case it is necessary to develop machine-interpretable representations of the following:

- Definitions of all terms used in the model, especially those related to inputs and outputs - for example, whether the torque output of a motor is in Newton meters or gram centimeters and whether the position of a servomechanism is assumed to be a continuous function or discretized.

- The underlying knowledge in which a model is grounded - for example, how a model of robot dynamics is grounded in rigid body dynamics, kinematics, coordinate frames, vectors, etc.
- Conditions under which the model(s) are valid and conditions under which to change from one model to another - for example, that the field strength of a pair of magnets is constant below 100°C, but varies as an inverse function of temperature above 100°C.

The design exchange in Section 4 is an example of information exchange at the parameter level. As information is exchanged, each agent must reformulate parameter values into a model suitable for the agent's design specific task. The results of the agent's design or analysis generally affect the value of other design parameters which in turn are communicated to other agents. This process leads to an iterated approach to system design as illustrated in Figure 5.1. A disadvantage to this approach is that the information exchange is constrained to a set of mutually agreed upon (hence predetermined) parameters. More powerful representations will allow information exchange at the equation level, as shown in Figure 5.2. Equation level information is not constrained to a set of predefined parameters and allows a high level of design optimization.

5.2 Models for sharing versus models for internal use

The Mechanical Design agent has the task of modifying the geometry of the parts to meet functional and physical requirements. The modification of part geometry requires expertise and is best done by a human engineer using a parametric CAD system. The parametric CAD model (see Figure 4.2) involves constraint equations that relate the various geometric parameters. While it would certainly be possible to express these constraints in CML, and accomplish parametric model updating via communication between the CAD agent and CML, this would be a cumbersome approach. The point here is that since geometry modification requires human expertise, and since the model used for accomplishing the modifications is encoded efficiently within the 3D CAD system, we should not treat it as a model to be published and possibly assimilated by other agents. On the other hand, complicated dependencies or trade-off problems involving multiple agents should probably be modeled in CML and solved either using the CDME environment, or exported as equations to be used with a solver such as Design Sheet [Rebby, Fertig and Smith, 1998] that is specialized for trade-off studies.

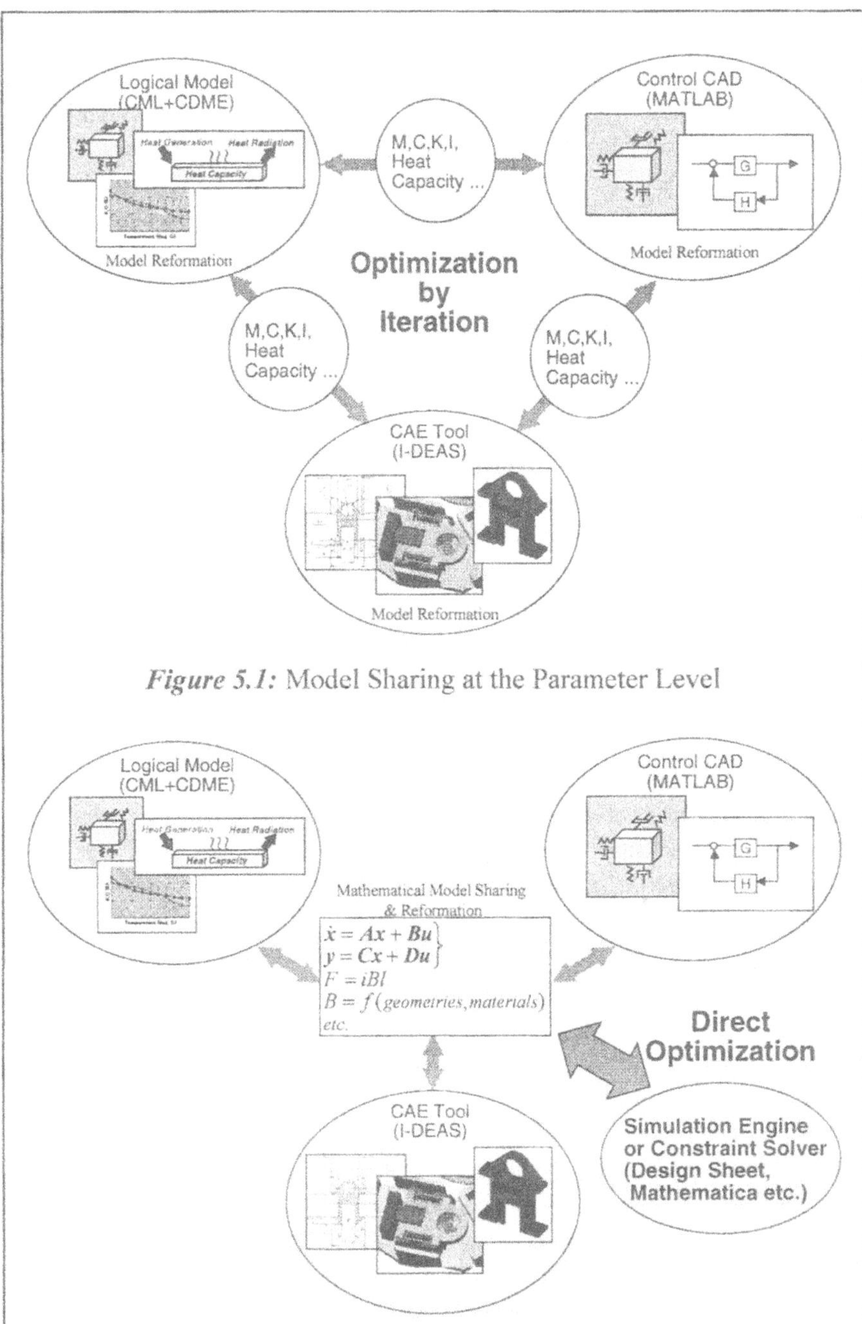

Figure 5.1: Model Sharing at the Parameter Level

Figure 5.2: Model Sharing at the Mathematical Model Level

6. CONCLUSIONS AND FUTURE WORK

In our current implementation, parameters are shared among CML, MATLAB, and I-DEAS (level d in Table 1: see Figure 5.1). Model parameters are partially listed in Table 2. Under the model assumptions shared by these agents the parameters in Table 2 provide a complete description of the PUH dynamics. But without a set of shared assumptions, parametric information is not sufficient. For example parametric values alone do not guarantee a consistent set of units, nor do they define a reference coordinate system. Without making model assumptions explicit, values for inertia moments could be reasonably interpreted to be either about the PUH mass center or flexure.

In future work, we intend to support information sharing at the mathematical model level (see Figure 5.2). Information sharing at the mathematical model level reduces the model reformulation task, and increases flexibility because models are no longer constrained to a pre-defined format. For instance, the temperature dependency of the damping coefficient can be readily expressed at the equation level. Additionally, model information will be augmented with applicability conditions to make modeling assumptions explicit. For example, the spring-mass-damper model of the PUH dynamics is only valid over a range of frequencies, beyond which PUH flexible modes become significant. Applicability conditions will help ensure models are used correctly and reduce design errors.

We are also eager to extend our concurrent system to address other engineering functions. Namely, we are trying to integrate the control logic model for the tracking, focusing and seeking controllers with our PUH model in the example. In this phase, we expect hybrid (continuous/discrete) modeling and simulation [Carlson and Gupta, 1997 and Mosterman, Zhao and Biswas, 1998] to be an important key technology to overcome the differences of granularity and behaviors of each simulation model.

ACKNOWLEDGMENTS

The authors would like to thank the past and the present members of the Super Design Technology: Toshiba-Stanford project, Gautam Biswas and Sheila McIlraith for their advice and assistance in this work. We gratefully acknowledge the contributions of Yumi Iwasaki, Tony Looser, James Rice, Robert Engelmore, and Richard Fikes from the Stanford Knowledge Systems Lab for their help with CML, CDME and OKBC. We also acknowledge the help of HeeCheol Jeon, Neeraj Shodhan and Liang Zhu with Java Agent Template/OKBC interface, Matlab API and Open I-DEAS integration.

The work at CDR has been supported by Toshiba Corporation and DARPA under Navy contract N00014096-1-0679.

REFERENCES

Bliznakov, Plamen I., Shah, Jami J., and Urban Susan D., "Integration Infrastructure to Support Concurrence and Collaboration in Engineering Design" Proc. of ASME Design Engineering Technical Conference and Computers in Engineering Conference, 1996, Irvine CA.

Bobrow, D., Falkenhainer, B., Farquhar, A., Fikes, R., Forbus, K., Gruber, T., Iwasaki, Y., Kuipers, B., "A Compositional Modeling Language", 96 AAAI Technical Report WS-96-01, 1996, Fallen Leaf Lake, CA.

Carlson, Bjorn and Gupta, Vineet, "The hcc Programmers Manual", (http://ic-www.arc.nasa.gov/people/vgupta).

Chaudhri, V. K., Farquhar, A., Fikes, R., Karp, P. D., and Rice, J. P., "Open Knowledge Base Connectivity 2.0", Artificial Intelligence Center, SRI International, 21 July 1997.

Choueiry, Berthe Y., McIlraith, Sheila, Iwasaki, Yumi, Loeser, Tony, Neller, Todd, Engelmore, Robert S., and Fikes, Richard, "Thoughts Towards a Practical Theory of Reformulation for Reasoning About Physical Systems", Working notes of the Symposium on Abstraction, Reformulation, and Approximation (SARA'98), 1998, Pacific Grove, CA, USA, pp. 25-36.

Cutkosky, M. R., Engelmore, R. S., Fikes, R. E., Genesereth, M. R., Gruber, T. R., Mark, W. S., Tenenbaum, J. M. and Weber, J. C. "PACT: An Experiment in Integrating Concurrent Engineering Systems" IEEE Computer, 1993, Vol. January pp. 28-38.

Diaz-Calderon, Antonio, Paredis, Christiaan J. J., Khosla, Pradeep, "A Modular Composable Software Architecture for the Simulation of the Mechatoronic Systems", Proc. of ASME Design Engineering Technical Conference and Computers in Engineering Conference, 1998, Atlanta, GA.

Falkenhainer, B., Farquhar, A., Bobrow, D., Fikes, R., Forbus, K., Gruber, T., Iwasaki, Y., Kuipers, B., "CML: A Compositional Modeling Language", Technical report KSL-94-16, 1994, Knowledge Systems Laboratory, Stanford University.

Farquhar, A., "A Qualitative Physics Compiler", Proc., Twelfth National Conference on Artificial Intelligence, 1994, Seattle, Washington, The AAAI Press/The MIT Press.

Forbus, K. D., (1984). "Qualitative Process Theory." Artificial Intelligence, 1984, vol. 24, pp. 85-168.

Genesereth, M. R. and Fikes, R. E., "Knowledge Interchange Format, Version 3.0 Reference Manual", Technical report Logic-92-1, Stanford University Logic Group, 1992.

Gruber, T. R. (1993). "Toward principles for the design of ontologies used for knowledge sharing", International Journal of Human-Computer Studies, special issue on Formal Ontology in Conceptual Analysis and Knowledge Representation, August 1993 (Available as technical report KSL-93-04, Knowledge Systems Laboratory, Stanford University.

Gruber, Tom R. and Gautier, Pierre O., Machinegenerated Explanations of Engineering Models: a Compositional Modeling Approach. In Proc. of the 13th IJCAI, pages 1502-1508, Chamb'ery, France, 1993.

Iwasaki, Y., Farquhar, A., Fikes, R., and Rice, J., "A web-based compositional modeling systems for sharing of physical knowledge", Proc. of the 15th International Joint Conference on Artificial Intelligence, AAAI Press/The MIT Press, August 1997.

Karp, P. D., Myers, K. L., Gruber, T., "The Generic Frame Protocol", Proc. of the Fourteenth International Joint Conference on Artificial Intelligence, 1995, Montreal, pp768-774.

Kiriyama, T., Tomiyama, T., and Yoshikawa, H., "Building a physical feature database for integrated modeling in design" In The Sixth International Workshop on Qualitative Reasoning about Physical Systems, 1992, pp. 124-138.

Mosterman Pieter J., Zhao, Feng, and Biswas, Gautum, "Sliding Mode Model Semantics and Simulation for Hybrid System", Lecture Notes in Computer Science: Hybrid Systems V, Springer Verlag, Berlin-Heidelburg, 1998.

Olsen, G., R., Cutkosky, M., Tenenbaum, J., M., and Gruber, T., R., "Collaborative Engineering Based on Knowledge Sharing Agreement", CONCURRENT ENGINEERING, June 1995, Vol. 3, No. 2, pp. 145 – 159.

Ozawa, M., Iwasaki, Y., Cutkosky, M., R., "Multi Disciplinary Early Performance Evaluation via Logical Description of Mechanisms: DVD Pick Up Head Example" Proc. of ASME Design Engineering Technical Conference and Computers in Engineering Conference, 1998, Atlanta, GA.

Petrie, C. J., Webster, T. and Cutkosky, M.R., "Using Pareto Optimality to Coordinate Distributed Agents," AIEDAM Vol. 9, 1995, pp. 269-281.

Phang, Francis, Bae, Seokhoon, and Wallace, David, "A Web-based Collaborative Design Modeling Environment", IEEE 7th Intl. Workshops on Enabling Technologies; Infrastructure for Collaborative Enterprise, 1998 (WET ICE '98: http://www.cerc.wvu.edu/WETICE/), Stanford, CA.

Reddy, S. Y., Fertig, K. W., and Smith, D. E. "Constraint Management Methodology for Conceptual Design Tradeoff Studies" Proc. of ASME Design Engineering Technical Conference and Computers in Engineering Conference, 1998, Sacramento, CA.

---

[i] http://www.wri.com

[ii] http://www.iso.ch/, http://www.scra.org/pdesinc.html, http://www.steptools.com/library/standard/

[iii] I-DEAS™, Open I-DEAS™ : http://www.sdrc.com

[iv] http://www.mathworks.com

8

Design-to-Manufacture Information Transfer in the Context of Solid Freeform Fabrication Technologies

David W. Rosen
Georgia Institute of Technology, United States of America

Key words: Solid Freeform Fabrication, Distributed Product Realization, Process Planning, Engineering Design, Decision-Based Design, Rapid Tooling Testbed

Abstract: With Solid Freeform Fabrication (SFF) technologies, the possibility of implementing a VLSI-like metaphor for design-manufacturing information transfer is enabled. That is, it has been hypothesized that a standard interchange format for SFF can be developed that enables design activity to be separated from manufacturing activity and that little additional communication between design and manufacturing organizations is necessary. In this paper, this hypothesis is explored for various points along the product design time-line. At earlier times in the design process, the requirements for a standard interchange format change as do requirements on SFF process planning. Advantages and disadvantages of early transfer of design information are presented. A system architecture and information models are discussed for enabling design-manufacturing transfers at various points in the design timeline. Examples are presented that illustrate progress toward this architecture and demonstrate the capabilities and limitations of our progress.

1. INTRODUCTION

Increased competition is forcing product realization to change: to become faster and to leverage facilities and expertise, wherever they may be. Imagine a product realization environment in which engineers collaboratively develop, build, and test solutions to design-manufacture problems encountered in product realization processes. In this paper, I present progress toward this vision, highlighting information requirements at the design-manufacture interface. This work is in the context of the Rapid Tooling TestBed (RTTB), a distributed computing environment and design methodology that incorporates rapid prototyping and rapid tooling technologies (Allen & Rosen, 1997). The RTTB is intended to support the design of parts and molds, the selection of prototyping technologies and vendors, and the fabrication of those parts and molds. The RTTB integrates design process and fabrication process models with product models to enable a designer to instantiate an approved design process with the appropriate tasks, personnel, vendors, software, and equipment.

The purpose of this paper is to present conditions under which design representations can be transferred to a manufacturing organization. The research question that is addressed here is:

How early, and under what conditions, can design representations be transferred to manufacturing?

This problem is explored in the context of the RTTB and SFF technologies. By "transferred to manufacturing," I mean that the manufacturing organization assumes responsibility for delivering parts or product with little additional input from the designer(s). A design representation that can be transferred to manufacturing meets the objectives of a VLSI-like interface between design and manufacturing. This representation must be process independent, but must contain enough information to enable the manufacturing organization to fabricate the artifact. Since SFF technologies build parts using a large number of simple, well understood operations, it is hypothesized that process planning can be based on powerful geometric decomposition algorithms, enabling the automation of process planning and the prediction of part properties. Such a situation achieves the desired VLSI-like interface.

The problem defined by the research question can be restated more informally as "who is responsible for design-for-manufacturing (DFM)?" DFM is often difficult for mechanical parts since significant manufacturing knowledge is required to adjust part designs to aid manufacturability by a specific process. Small design changes can cause large changes in the manufacturing process or may render that process infeasible. However, if the manufacturer understands the purpose of a design and its functional requirements, then the manufacturer may be in a better position to adjust the design to facilitate manufacturing without compromising functionality. Thus, the research question asks if design representations can be developed that enable the manufacturer to perform DFM.

The baseline case is the usage of service bureaus by engineering organization for prototype parts, generally fabricated by SFF technologies. Typically, an engineer will send a STL file electronically to a service bureau, the part will be fabricated, then shipped overnight so the engineer receives it in 2-3 days. The STL file is a well-known standard interchange format, but it has significant disadvantages (Kumar & Dutta, 1997).

In Figure 1, three candidate points are shown where this design-to-manufacture transfer could occur, indicated by the numbered circles (D-M Interfaces in the Figure key). The Geometric Tailoring activity indicates any design operations required to ensure manufacturability, such as adding rounds and draft to an injection molded part. Should the design or manufacturing organization be responsible for geometric tailoring? Referring back to Figure 1, it is clear that a manufacturing process and a part material must be selected prior to fabrication. Again, which organization should be responsible for doing so?

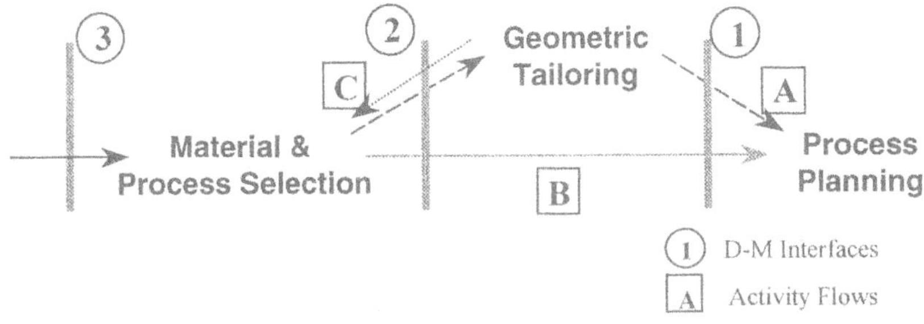

Figure 1. Design-Manufacture Interfaces and Activity Flows.

Figure 1 shows three different sequences of activities, labeled by the letters in squares. In some cases, no geometric tailoring may be necessary, indicated by flow B. For example, when a company orders a stereolithography part from a service bureau, they probably did not change the part design to facilitate the SLA process. Sometimes a geometric tailoring event is required, such as in injection molding; this is flow A. Flow C indicates iteration between material & process selection and geometric tailoring. Such an iterative flow is necessary if the selection depends upon the extent or nature of part redesigns to facilitate fabrication. In the STL baseline case, transfer point 1 is used, no geometric tailoring would be performed, and the designer may or may not have specified the material or process to be used, but would have likely described his requirements verbally to the service bureau.

Three questions follow from the main research question above:

1. If the manufacturing organization selects the material and process, what information must be in the design representation to facilitate this selection?

2. To what extent can design activity be manufacturing process independent (i.e., no DFM)?
3. Conversely, can design requirements be communicated to the manufacturing organization such that adjustments to the part to facilitate manufacture result in parts that satisfy the design requirements?

Questions 1 and 3 will be directly addressed in this paper.

Investigating design representations further, Figure 2 shows a set of design and manufacturing hierarchies along with potential places where design-manufacturing transfer occur. At present, solid and other geometric models without tolerances and surface finish specifications can be transferred, assuming that the parts are to be manufactured using SFF technologies (STL file format). We are currently researching the transfer of design representations with tolerance and surface finish specifications, along with additional requirements for SFF technologies. At higher levels of information content, it is unclear if general purpose design-manufacture transfers can be achieved, in part because there are no widely accepted languages for specifying engineering requirements.

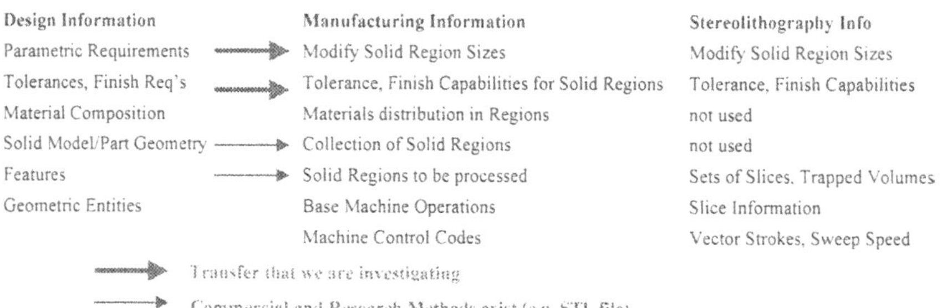

Figure 2. Information Hierarchies for Transferring Product Representations from Design to Manufacturing.

In Section 2 of this paper, the approach to the research is covered with an emphasis on the major bodies of literature underlying the research. In Section 3, the RTTB architecture is briefly described, outlining the major software modules and the distributed computing environment being constructed. Given the desired software architecture, information modeling requirements are discussed in Section 4 to support this architecture. In Section 5, three examples are presented that illustrate different design-manufacture transfer situations. These examples demonstrate one approach at achieving design-manufacture transfer at earlier points in the design process and highlight the challenges in doing so. The paper concludes with summary observations and directions of future work.

2. RESEARCH APPROACH

There is a tremendous amount of literature that could be referenced in support of this paper. In the interests of brevity and focus, two areas will be emphasized, that of decision making in design and process planning for SFF technologies. Both the selections (materials and processes) in Figure 1 and the geometric tailoring activity can be modeled as decisions. Clearly material selection is a selection decision. Geometric tailoring is a multiobjective decision with dimensions as variables; this can be formulated as a multiobjective optimization problem.

2.1 Decision-Based Design

We use the framework of *Decision-Based Design,* DBD, for describing a typical product realization process. In Decision-Based Design, decisions serve as markers to identify the progression of a design from initiation to implementation to termination. The implementation of Decision-Based Design can take different forms. In mechanical engineering there is an increasing awareness that decisions made by designers could be the key element in the development of design methods that facilitate design for the life cycle and foster concurrency in the process, for example, Hazelrigg (1996), Suh, (1990), and Whitney, et al. (1988) support this notion as well. Our approach is called the **D**ecision **S**upport **P**roblem (DSP) Technique (Mistree et al., 1990). It has been developed and implemented to provide support for human judgment in designing systems that can be manufactured and maintained.

The DSP Technique consists of three principal components: a design philosophy rooted in systems thinking, an approach for identifying and formulating Decision Support Problems (DSPs), and software, the DSIDES, package (Mistree et al., 1993). The DSP Technique requires that a designer implement two phases, namely, a meta-design phase and a computer-based design phase. Meta-design is accomplished through *partitioning* a problem into its elemental DSPs and then devising a *plan* of action.

Decision Support Problems provide a means for modeling decisions encountered in design and the domain specific mathematical models so built are called *templates*. Multiple objectives, quantified using analysis-based "hard" and insight-based "soft" information, can be modeled in the DSPs. For real-world, practical systems, all of the information for modeling systems comprehensively and accurately in the early stages of the project may not be available. However, solutions to DSP's can be used to support a designer's quest for a superior solution. Formulation and solution of DSPs provide a means for making the following types of decisions:

- *Selection* - the indication of a preference, based on multiple attributes, for one among several alternatives (Mistree et al., 1989).
- *Compromise* - the improvement of an alternative through modification (Mistree et al., 1990 and Mistree, et al., 1993).

Word formulations of the Decision Support Problems are shown in Table 1. Note that each is described by a set of keywords (Given, Find, Identify, etc.) and descriptors (alternatives, attributes, importances, etc.) which form a language for describing decision problems. The math form of the compromise DSP is shown in Figure 3. There is a 1-to-1 correspondence between word and math forms of this DSP; furthermore, specific forms of bounds, constraints, and goals and deviation functions ensure that all compromise DSP's are structured in the same manner, essentially defining a mathematical language for specifying such problems. It is important to note that the compromise DSP is an extensive of goal programming methods, where the purpose is to satisfy "rigid" objectives, called constraints, and to meet "soft" objectives, called goals, as well as possible, provided significant flexibility in solving problems. Hence, the compromise DSP is not a traditional multiobjective optimization formulation.

In addition to selection and compromise decisions, combinations of decisions in coupled, hierarchical or non-hierarchical forms are possible; selection/selection, compromise/compromise and selection/compromise decisions may be coupled (Bascaran et al., 1989; Herrmann & Allen, 1999).

Table 1. Word Formulations for Selection and Compromise Decision Support Problems

Selection DSP	Compromise DSP
Given: Alternatives from which to select.	**Given**: Alternative to be improved through modification.
Identify: Key attributes that influence the selection of alternatives. Relative importances of attributes.	**Find**: Values of System Variables. Values of Deviation Variables.
Rate: Alternatives with respect to each attribute.	**Satisfy**: Goals, Constraints, Bounds
Rank: Order the alternatives in terms of preference.	***Minimize**: Deviation of solution from goals.*

2.2 SFF Process Planning

Currently there is a great deal of literature available for process planning of SFF technologies such as stereolithography. This literature spans from topics such as build process optimization, to inaccuracy prediction and correction, and support structure generation. The work presented in this paper relates to process planning issues.

Given:

An alternative to be improved through modification.

Assumptions used to model the domain of interest.

Find:

System variables values:	X_i	$i = 1, \ldots, n$
Deviation variables values:	d_i^-, d_i^+	$i = 1, \ldots, m$

Satisfy:

Bounds: $X_i^{min} \leq X_i \leq X_i^{max}$		$i = 1, \ldots, n$
System constraints:	$g_i(\mathbf{X}) \leq 0$	$i = 1, \ldots, p$
System goals:	$A_i(\mathbf{X}) + d_i^- - d_i^+ = G_i$	$i = 1, \ldots, m$
Deviation variables:	$d_i^-, d_i^+ \geq 0, d_i^- \cdot d_i^+ = 0$	$i = 1, \ldots, m$

Minimize:

Archimedean deviation function: $Z = \Sigma W_i (d_i^- + d_i^+)$, where $\Sigma W_i = 1$, W_i □ 0

Figure 3. Mathematical Formulation of the Compromise Decision Support Problem

Many researchers have investigated adaptive slicing of parts for layer based fabrication. The objective of adaptive slicing is to develop a slicing scheme, or method of slicing the CAD model, that meets a user-defined tolerance. This tolerance, commonly referred to as a cusp, serves as an indication of the allowable deviation between the true CAD model surface and the physical surface of the prototype. The error associated with this deviation is present in all layer-based manufacturing technologies to one degree or another and is referred to as the stairstep effect. Separately, Dolenc and Mäkelä (1994) and Tata (1995) were some of the first researchers. They adaptively sliced parts that were represented using STL files. Other researchers, including Sabourin et al. (1996), Kulkarni and Dutta (1996), and Xu et al. (1997) have presented adaptive slicing methods that slice CAD part models represented by analytical surfaces. All approaches attempt to improve the geometric accuracy of the physical prototype by calculating the appropriate layer thickness based on the local geometry of the CAD model, which will minimize the error associated with the stairstep effect to an acceptable level as defined by the cusp. The effect of the adaptive slicing method is to reduce the layer thickness in areas of high vertical curvature. Generally, this work seeks to meet cusp specifications, while minimizing the time to build the prototype.

Marsan et al. (1997) take a broad view of the overall process planning and break process planning into four steps. The first step involves entering design data into a Solid Builder, used to generate a B-rep solid model. The next step is orienting the solid model in the Orientation Module, based on one of the following criteria: minimum build height, minimum support contact area, maximum area of base, minimum volume of supports, or minimum average surface roughness. The supporting structure is then automatically generated and passed on to an Adaptive Slicing Module, where it is adaptively sliced to minimize the error associated with the stairstep effect. The final module is Path Planning which is currently undertaken using commercial software. The process planning system outlined supports a variety of SFF technologies.

Research at Georgia Tech has focused on developing methods to facilitate trade-offs among build time, accuracy, and surface finish goals. McClurkin and Rosen (1998) developed a computer aided build style selection (CABSS) tool that aids users in making trade-offs among these goals. Only three variables were considered: part orientation (3 discrete choices), layer thickness, and hatch spacing. Lynn-Charney and Rosen (1999) extended this work by conducting a detailed study of SLA accuracy. That research presents a method where response surfaces are used to quantify the achievable accuracy for a set of geometric tolerances applied to a variety of surface types. The four build-style variables investigated in that research were fill-overcure, hatch-overcure, sweep period, and z-level wait period. West (1999) has significantly extended this work to incorporate adaptive slicing and more accurate surface finish models. His work will be presented in the first example in Section 5.

3. RTTB ARCHITECTURE

The architecture of the RTTB computing environment will be outlined. The long term vision of the RTTB is a distributed computing environment that supports the design and manufacture of prototype parts. The environment should be able to reconfigure itself to adjust to changes in computing resources. Additionally, it should reconfigure the organization of its software modules in response to the nature of a specific design-manufacture problem. That is, no strict design process is hard-coded into the RTTB; the design process adjusts to the starting information and the required output. Both commercial and research SFF technologies are being supported, as well as select rapid tooling technologies to produce multiple parts through injection molding.

The RTTB integrates design process and fabrication process models with product models to enable a designer to instantiate an approved design process with the appropriate tasks and resources (Allen and Rosen, 1997).

Selection, CAD, synthesis, analysis, and simulation software modules are integrated into the RTTB. The RTTB is implemented on top of the distributed computing environment called PRE from Sandia National Laboratory. We have developed the Fabrication Description Language (FDL) as the language in which fabrication processes can be described and process, material, and vendor capabilities can be encoded.

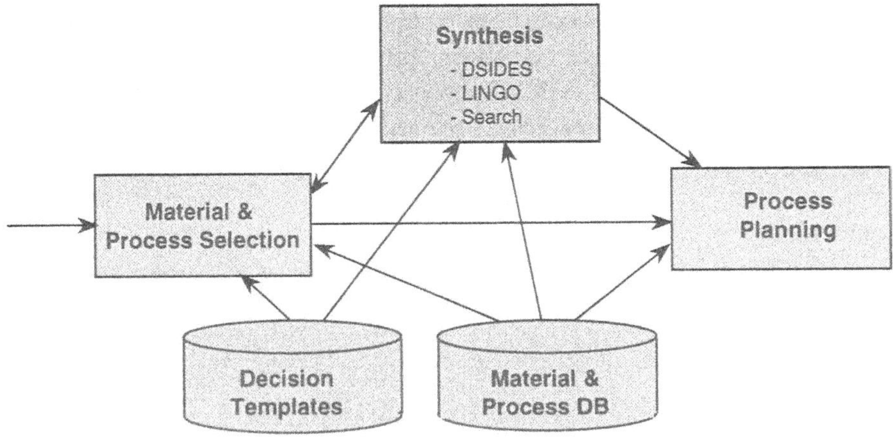

Figure 4. RTTB Architecture

To focus the presentation, only the subset of RTTB that is relevant to this paper is presented in Figure 4. Legacy codes such as ProEngineer and ANSYS have been wrapped so that they can be integrated into the RTTB. Additional software tools have been developed to perform other tasks and have been integrated as well. A more complete description of the RTTB architecture, focusing on its distributed computing nature, is provided in reference (Gerhard et al., 1999). To initiate RTTB operation, the designer provides a CAD model of his part, tolerances and surface finish specifications, preferences for prototype part characteristics (accuracy, finish, build time). Optionally, the designer may specify performance specifications, desired part characteristics, preferences for materials or fabrication processes, and preferences on other specifications and characteristics.

A web-based tool has been written in Java for coupled material and process selection (Herrmann & Allen 1999). Material property and SFF process capability descriptions reside in a relational database and provide this information to the selection tool. A process planning tool was written in C++ for the stereolithography process (West, 1999). Input to process planning consists of an ACIS solid part model with tolerances and surface finishes specified.

The synthesis module performs geometric tailoring. Two multiobjective optimization codes are currently integrated, DSIDES (Mistree et al., 1993) and LINGO (Nemhauser & Wolsey, 1988), as well as an exhaustive search code. At present, there is no elegant method of formulating and solving geometric tailoring problems, given only the RTTB input information from the designer. Compromise DSP templates must be constructed by hand and analysis codes must be written and integrated into one of the optimization codes. However, there is some promise of generating templates automatically, given the RTTB input information (see Section 4). Information can flow along any of the arrows in Figure 4, so that iteration among the major RTTB modules is possible. The selection and synthesis modules can be coupled to enable the solution of coupled selection-compromise Decision Support Problems.

With the RTTB architecture outlined, the stage is set to investigate the information modeling requirements to enable the RTTB to function.

4. INFORMATION MODELING

Information model requirements depend upon the design-manufacture transfer point, as presented in Figure 1. The earlier in the design process that the transfer is to occur, the greater the variety of information that needs to be transferred. Conversely, the later in the process that transfer occurs, the greater is the level of detail of information. In this section, some information modeling issues are raised and our approach to modeling a variety of information types is presented.

4.1 Information Requirements

Simply put, the information requirements for the RTTB include that information required to perform the activities in Figure 1. Nominally for process planning, a geometric part representation is required, as are a target fabrication process and material choice. The geometric model may be a solid CAD model, an STL file, or a part model in a data exchange language such as IGES or STEP. The advantages and disadvantages of each choice have been extensively debated, but this debate will not be addressed here (Kumar & Dutta, 1997). However, a widely held requirement is that this representation must be process independent. In Figure 2, several levels of geometric model decomposition are included (regions to be processes and base machine operations). It is not clear if any process independent decompositions exist, although for most commercial SFF technologies, decomposing a geometric model into slices can be accomplished without much process-specific information as mentioned in Section 2.2.

Our approach to transferring information to process planning is to use a solid model that is annotated with tolerances, datums, and surface finish specifications. We use the ACIS solid modeling kernel to facilitate our research, but Parasolids or other solid modeling would work equally well. Additionally, the STEP data exchange standard would be an equally good (perhaps better) choice.

Information requirements for geometric tailoring are much more extensive than for process planning. Again, both a target fabrication process and material are required, but it is also necessary to specify the design freedom allowed by the designer. A general solution to the specification of design requirements does not seem to be available; approaches to this problem are application or domain-specific.

Our approach to this issue is to utilize the Decision Support Problems as the framework for specifying design requirements to the manufacturer. Furthermore, the class of fabrication processes and materials under consideration is limited to SFF technologies. In this manner, problem descriptions can be limited to requirements on a limited set of part properties and these can be readily related to fabrication process capabilities and material characteristics. Process capabilities and material characteristics can be stored in a database, then made available when needed. For example, when a part material needs to be selected, designer requirements on part strength, durability, and weight, plus requirements on lead time and cost, can be compared to the characteristics of known materials and the selected fabrication process. This comparison is facilitated by treating process and material characteristics as attributes in a Selection DSP template. This will be explained further in the next sub-section.

4.2 Design Representations

As stated previously, our design representation for transfer to process planning consists of an ACIS solid model with tolerance, datum, and surface finish annotations. These annotations are implemented as user-defined attributes in ACIS and are attached to the topological faces in an ACIS model. This is sufficient as input to process planning, provided that the process planning module does not need material composition (of multiple materials) information. Since most of our target processes are commercial SFF technologies that process only one material at a time, material compositions have not been investigated. Our process planner can incorporate tolerance and surface finish requirements since these requirements can be evaluated using detailed process information (see Section 4.3).

Design representations for input to material & process selection and geometric tailoring are much more complicated. We utilize DSP templates as the information modeling medium for describing design requirements to the manufacturer. We have formulated generic templates for material selection, for process selection, and for coupled material-process selection. For geometric tailoring, we have developed several domain-specific templates for gears and gear trains using a general language of material and process attributes.

As one example, the process selection DSP is shown in Figure 5. Note that there is a one-to-one-correspondence to the general word formulation of the selection DSP of Table 1. Since all fabrication processes and materials are represented in a database, it is straightforward to update our set of alternatives if new processes are developed or capabilities are improved. Not all attributes are included in this list, but our database contains more than 30. The idea is that the designer will always select from this list those attributes that are relevant to his problem, then specify their relative importances. Additionally, the designer/manufacturer can specify the alternatives that should be considered, rather than including all in the selection problem. In this manner, the designer can communicate problem requirements to the manufacturer using the common problem description language provided by the DSP templates. A summary of the information sources for selection problems is given in Table 2.

Given: SLA-250, SLA-3500, SLA-5000, SLA-7000, SLS Sinterstation 2500, SLS RapidSteel, FDM 2000, Actua 2100, Zcorp 4206.

Identify: Key attributes from Accuracy, Surface Finish, Cost, Build Time, Post-Processing Time, Detail Capability.
Target values for each attribute.
Relative importances of attributes.

Rate: Alternatives with respect to each attribute.

Rank: Order the alternatives in terms of preference.

Figure 5. Word Formulation for the Process Selection DSP.

Table 2. Information Sources for Selection.

Designer Specified	RTTB System Provided
CAD Part Model	Material Properties
Tolerance and Finish Specs.	SFF Fabrication Processes & Capabilities
Target Values for Material Properties and Process Capabilities (Selection Attributes)	Ability to Rate Alternatives vs. Attributes
Preferences on Selection Attributes	Method and Software for Solving Selection Problem

For geometric tailoring, templates can be developed for specific types of problems, such as gear design, then applied to many different situations as needed. All templates are instantiations of the mathematical form of the compromise DSP from Figure 3. Users can adjust the problem definition by specifying importances on goals, converting a goal to a constraint, converting a constraint to a goal, and in other ways. However, it is not clear if a general geometric tailoring decision template can be formulated since domain specific analysis models are usually needed. For example, an analysis model for gear teeth strength is only applicable to gear design, but is irrelevant for cam-mechanism design.

How can designers communicate design freedoms to manufacturers so that the manufacturer can adjust the part without compromising designer requirements? Conceivably, analysis models, compromise DSP goals and constraints, and relative importances of goals can be communicated to the manufacturer to describe design requirements and specify freedoms the manufacturer has in adjusting the part design. With the general mathematical form of the compromise DSP, the structure of goals, constraints, system variables, bounds, and deviation functions has been specified, providing a language for defining decision problems. However, no general, computable format for this information has been developed. An interesting idea is to encode this information in Dynamically Linked Libraries and provide the protocol for extracting needed information (Storti et al., 1999).

A summary of the information sources for geometric tailoring problems is given in Table 3. Note that at present the designer has a much higher burden, as compared to selection problems.

Table 3. Information Sources for Geometric Tailoring

Designer Specified	RTTB System Provided
CAD Part Model	Material Properties
Tolerance and Finish Specs.	SFF Fabrication Processes & Capabilities
Performance Specs. (strength, weight, etc.)	
Analysis Models (embodied in a software module)	
Compromise DSP Template that Specifies Variables, Constraints, and Goals	Method and Software for Solving Tailoring Problems
Preferences on Specifications	

4.3 Manufacturing Process Information

Manufacturing process information of two broad types is needed to support the engineering activities of Figure 1:

- Detailed manufacturing process information and models to support process planning and geometric tailoring, and

- Simplified measures of process capability to support process selection and some geometric tailoring.

Each will be discussed in this subsection.

4.3.1 Detailed Manufacturing Models

Broadly, two types of information are critical to aiding process planning and geometric tailoring, analytical models for computing process capabilities and empirical models. Since we are supporting the stereolithography process, we have opted to utilize empirical models, rather than investigating the photo-chemistry basis of stereolithography. To date, we have developed three sets of empirical models for our SLA-250 machine:

- Geometric tolerance capability as a function of part orientation, scanning variables, and recoat variables;
- Surface finish capability as a function of part orientation, layer thickness, and surface type;
- Build time as a function of part orientation, layer thickness, and scanning and recoat variables.

More extensive and complete models are needed and can be developed, but these models are representative of the information types required for process planning and geometric tailoring. Each model will be briefly described.

Empirical models for accuracy were developed through extensive design-of-experiment studies to determine quantitatively the relationships between SLA-250 variables and geometric tolerance capabilities. Response Surface Methodology (RSM) comprises mathematical and statistical techniques to enable the construction of approximation models (Myers & Montgomery, 1995). RSM allows for a better understanding of the relationships between the inputs and the response, in this case between the build process variables and build goals, that can be written in the form of a polynomial function describing a surface, such as Equation 1. We use second order response surfaces in this work; k = 2.

$$y = b_0 + \sum_{i=1}^{k} b_i x_i + \sum_{i=1}^{k} b_{ii} x_i^2 + \sum_{i=1}^{k} \sum_{j=1, i \neq j}^{k} b_{ij} x_i x_j \quad (1)$$

Response surfaces are useful when detailed theoretical knowledge of the model does not exist, but the relationship between the input variables and the output variable is assumed to be smooth. This is the case for SLA machines. For instance, theoretical equations that give accuracy as a function of layer thickness and hatch spacing do not exist, but accuracy is likely to change continuously as layer thickness and hatch spacing are varied.

The accuracy models used in this work come directly from the response surface models developed by Lynn-Charney & Rosen (1999). By using a set of response surface models that relate four build process variables (hatch and fill overcure, sweep period, and z-level wait) with a specific type of geometric tolerance and a surface type, the obtainable accuracy for that tolerance may be predicted. Six types of geometric tolerances were considered in this work: positional, flatness, parallelism, perpendicularity, concentricity, and circularity. A total of thirty six different response surfaces were developed based on the type of surface, the orientation of that surface, and the type of geometrical tolerance. Given the tolerance type, orientation of the surface to which the tolerance is annotated, and the values of the layer and recoat variables, predictions of the achievable accuracy for every geometric tolerance can be made. One of the response surfaces for parallelism is shown in Figure 6. Deviation from perfect parallel planar surfaces is shown as a function of sweep period and z-level wait. As can be seen, deviation is mostly dependent upon sweep period; as sweep period decreases (sweep blade moves faster), deviations increase significantly.

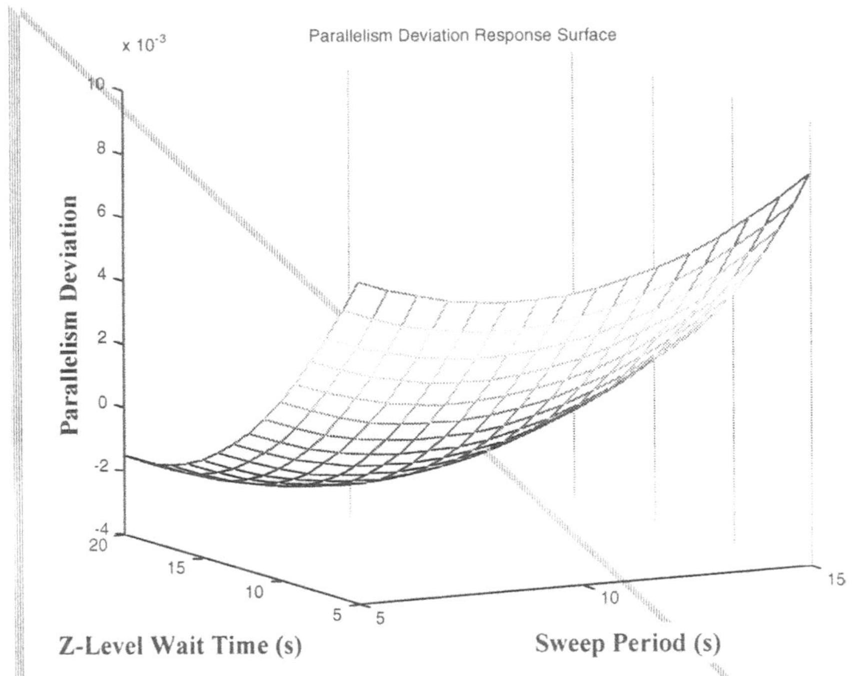

Figure 6. Parallelism Tolerance Response Surface

Surface finish capabilities may be predicted using a set of empirical roughness models (West, 1999) that are functions of layer thickness and surface orientation. In other research, Reeves & Cobb (1997) collected data in which the surface finish of a planar surface is measured for a series of different orientations. Similar experiments were performed in this work, but instead of associating the surface finish with the orientation, the cusp (which is a function of both layer thickness and orientation) is associated with the surface finish (roughness) as shown in the plots of Figure 7. In this manner the surface finish corresponding to a given cusp and layer thickness can be predicted for both planar and curved surfaces. Since surfaces are always composed of multiple layers, some of which may be at a different layer thickness, the average surface finish is used. Given the slice scheme for a CAD model, and the knowledge of the extents of the surfaces in the slice scheme, predictions of the surface finish may be made for every surface in the model.

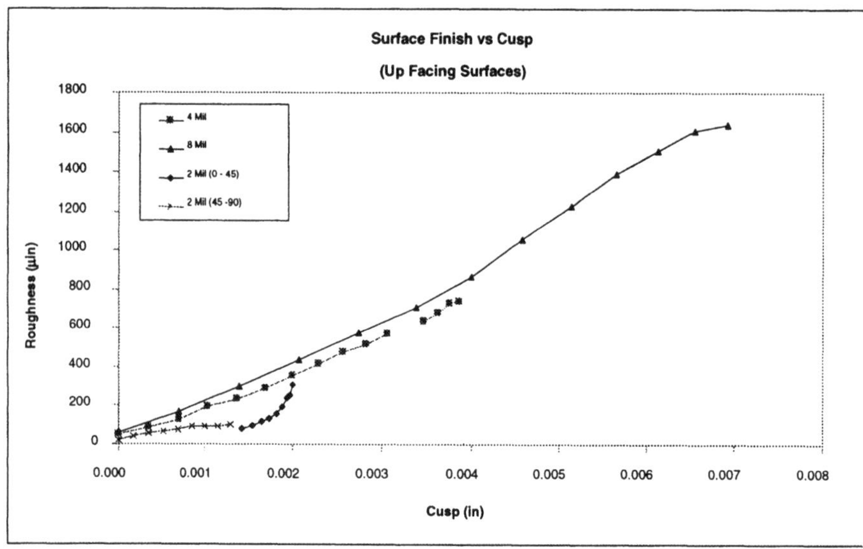

Figure 7. Surface Finish Empirical Model

In a similar manner, response surfaces were developed to predict build time. As part of our process planning method, part geometric models are sliced, enabling the slices to be used in build time prediction. Response surfaces were developed for different types of SLA scan vectors as functions of layer thickness and areas to be scanned. Again, extensive experiments were performed and actual scan times measured. Separate response surfaces were developed for border, hatch, and fill vectors. One response surface for hatch vectors is shown in Figure 8.

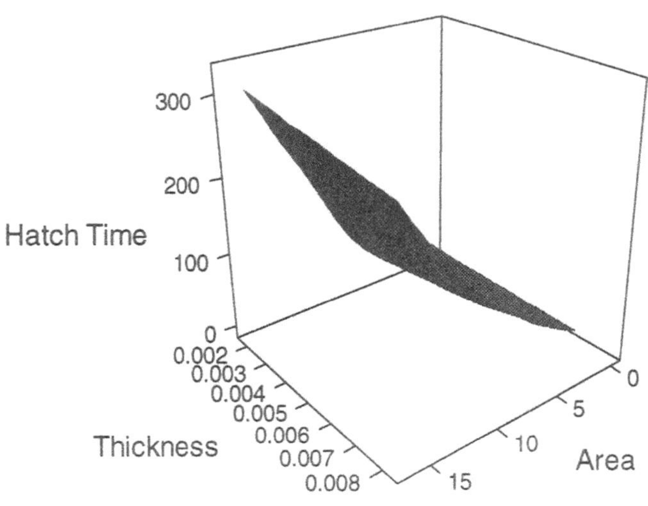

Figure 8. Build Time Response Surface for Hatch Vectors

4.3.2 Simplified Measures

To support material and process selection, and to enable some geometric tailoring, simplified measures of material properties and process capabilities are needed. We utilize information of the type supplied by machine vendors and MSDS material sheets, where for example, SLA-250 accuracy is given as 0.003/5 in. + 0.001 in. per additional inch. As a result, measures are given by individual values, ranges, or ratios.

MACHINE	**VENDOR**
Machine_name = SLA250	Company_name = 3D Systems Inc.
Technique_name=SLA	Address_Street = 26081 Avenue Hall
Build_time=20	Address_City = Valencia
Tolerance=0.001, 0.002	Address_State = California
Accuracy=0.005	Address_ZipNum = 91355
Detail_capability=HIGH	Address_Country = USA
Surface_finish=HIGH	PhoneNum = 805-295-5600
Support=NEED	FaxNum = 805-257-1200
Part_removal_time=45	Email = webmaster@3dsystems.com
Material_name=SL5220, SL5510, SL5520	WebSize = www.3dsystems.com
Vendor_name = 3D Systems Inc.	Contact_person = John Smith

Figure 9. SLA-250 and 3D Systems (vendor) FDL Files

We have developed a simple language, called Fabrication Description Language (FDL), to describe material, manufacturing process, and vendor properties, capabilities, and limitations. We are extending the language to also represent manufacturing processes, the sequence of operations required to fabricate a part. Figure 9 shows example SLA-250 and 3D Systems FDL files. There are three main entities in FDL: Machine, Material, and Vendor. Additionally, there are many other entities that represent attribute values (range, ratio, list, etc.).

5. DESIGN-MANUFACTURE TRANSFERS AND ACTIVITY FLOWS

As shown in Figure 1, three possible design-manufacture transfer points exist in the engineering practice under investigation here. Similarly, three different activity flows are possible. In this Section, three examples will be presented to illustrate several different combinations of transfers and activity flows. Broadly, the purpose of these examples is to demonstrate one approach to enabling design-manufacture transfer before design-for-manufacture has been completed. Each example is meant to illustrate some DFM capabilities that have been developed for the RTTB and highlight the information required for these capabilities.

In the first example, only the process planning activity is investigated, indicating design-to-manufacture transfer at point 1. Either activity flow A or B is consistent with this example. In the second example, the geometric tailoring activity is present, indicating design-manufacture transfer at point 2 and activity flow A. It is assumed that a material and process have already been selected. In the final example, iteration among the material & process selection and geometric tailoring activities is illustrated, indicating design-manufacturing transfer point 3 and activity flow C.

Two different parts are used in this section. For the first example, a bracket with some complex surfaces is used since process planning is non-trivial here. In the final two examples, a ring gear from a planetary gear train is used. Process planning for a gear such as this is straightforward, given the information of the first example.

5.1 Process Planning with Tolerances and Finish Specifications

The first example to be presented focuses on the process planning activity in Figure 1. Information being transferred from design to manufacturing includes solid geometry, tolerances, and surface finish specifications. Prior to process planning, a fabrication process and material were selected; they are the SLA-250 stereolithography machine and SOMOS

7110 resin. After briefly presenting the process planning method, the results are discussed of process planning on the part shown in Figure 10.

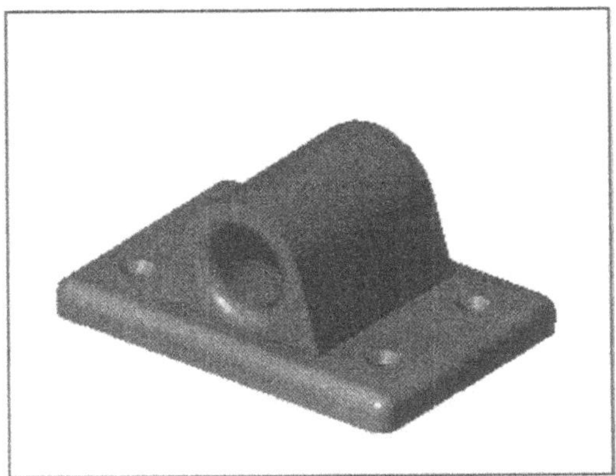

Figure 10. Bracket for the Process Planning Example

Our process planning method is intended to achieve the desired balance among the three build goals of accuracy, surface finish, and build time. This is performed by formulating and solving a Compromise DSP, where process variables are varied and an appropriate trade-off among the three build goals is achieved. The word formulation of the DSP for process planning is shown in Figure 11. The system variables consist of two part variables: the slice scheme and the orientation, two layer variables: hatch and fill overcure, and two recoat variables: sweep period and z-level wait. Part variables pertain to the build variables directly associated with the part. Layer variables pertain to the build variables that control how each layer is solidified in the vat of resin. Recoat variables pertain to the build variables that control how a new layer of resin is redeposited over the previously solidified layer. There are two constraints that are taken into consideration as well, the presence of large horizontal planes and the presence of support structures. The goals in the problem formulation consist of surface finish, accuracy, and build time.

At the heart of our process planning method is a series of three modules for orienting the part in the SLA machine, slicing the part, and selecting process variable values. All three modules are specific to the stereolithography process, although determining part orientation and slicing strategies are required in all layer-based fabrication processes.

GIVEN:
- CAD Model
- Surface Finish Specifications
- Geometric Tolerances
- Build Time target value
- SLA-250, SOMOS 7110 resin
- Goal preferences as weights

FIND:

System Variables:
Part Variables:
Set of Layer Thicknesses
Part Orientation
Layer Variables:
Hatch Overcure
Fill Overcure
Recoat Variables:
Sweep Period
Z-Level Wait

Deviation Variables: deviation of goal from target
Aggregate deviation of Finish
Aggregate deviation of Accuracy
Deviation from Build Time

SATISFY:

Goals: Surface Finish Specifications
Geometric Tolerances
Minimize Build time

Constraints: Large Horizontal Planes
Support Structures

MINIMIZE:
Deviation Function: Weighted sum of Goal Deviations

Figure 11. Process Planning Word Formulation

The selection of the best process plan is made by investigating the goal achievement of each of the three goals as indicated by the deviation values as well as the predicted values for accuracy, surface finish, and build time. In this formulation, the input is an ACIS based CAD model (.SAT file) with tolerances and surface finishes specified. Additionally, the user must supply measures of goal preferences. Generally, several scenarios (sets of preferences) are provided so that the user can better discern the trade-offs being made. Simple weights are used here, where the weights for accuracy, finish, and build time must sum to one. In this example problem, one set of goal preferences is investigated in depth and the results of several different sets of goal preferences are discussed briefly.

The set of layer thicknesses used for this example problem is 2, 4, and 8 mils, which are typical values for a SLA-250. The CAD model shown in Figure 10 is a bracket and provides a variety of interesting geometric shapes and surfaces. Four surfaces of this part are deemed to be critical. The inner cylindrical surface is to have a 2.5 micron surface finish. The two rounded edges on either side of the cylindrical surface have a surface finish requirement of 3.8 micron. The down facing planar surface at the base of the bracket is to have a 3.8 micron surface finish. The remaining surfaces are set to a default surface finish of 7.6 micron. Additionally, three geometric tolerances are specified. A cylindrical tolerance (0.0762 mm) is applied to the inner cylindrical surface. A parallelism tolerance (0.1016 mm) is applied between the down facing planar surface at the base of the bracket and the top up facing planar surface, and a flatness tolerance (0.1016 mm) is also used on the down facing planar surface at the base of the bracket. Six scenarios of goal weights were specified by the user and are shown in Table 4. Note that the weights in a scenario must sum to one.

Table 4. Scenarios for Example 1

Goal	Scen. 1	Scen. 2	Scen. 3	Scen. 4	Scen. 5	Scen. 6
Accuracy	0.9	0.05	0.05	0.6	0.2	0.2
Surface Finish	0.05	0.9	0.05	0.2	0.6	0.2
Build Time	0.05	0.05	0.9	0.2	0.2	0.6

Given this problem and the process planning method, the solution is computed by an exhaustive search method. Table 5 provides an overview of the resulting deviations for each of the different scenarios. The solutions that are shown in the table represent the process plans with the lowest overall deviations for the given goal preferences.

Table 5. Process Planning Results

Scenario	Weighting of Goals (AC, SF, BT)	Overall Dev.	Accuracy Dev.	Surface Finish Dev.	Build Time Dev.
1	(0.90, 0.05, 0.05)	0.30	0.31	0.07	0.21
2	(0.05, 0.90, 0.05)	0.04	0.31	0.01	0.32
3	(0.05, 0.05, 0.90)	0.07	0.68	0.36	0.02
4	(0.60, 0.20, 0.20)	0.24	0.31	0.09	0.19
5	(0.20, 0.60, 0.20)	0.13	0.31	0,01	0.30
6	(0.20, 0.20, 0.60)	0.15	0.31	0.23	0.07

As can be seen from the table, the weighting of the build goals has some affect on the resulting deviations. There are significant tradeoffs being made between the surface finish and build time goals, as one would expect. However, the accuracy goal does not appear to be significantly influenced by either of the other goals. Comparison of scenario 6 with scenario 3 provides the best example of the tradeoffs being made between the build time and surface finish goal. Both trials have a weighting scheme with the build time goal having the highest goal preference (0.90 for scenario 3 and 0.60 for scenario 6). The build time deviation is slightly higher for scenario 6 yet at the same time the surface finish deviation is also slightly lower. Thus it is evident that there is some degree of tradeoff being made between the build time and surface finish goal.

Although the goal deviations provide a summary assessment of a process plan, more meaningful information can be gained by examining the actual predictions of the surface and accuracy tolerances. Figure 12 shows the output from the process planning software for scenario 5, with all accuracy and surface finish requirements listed as well as their predicted values. Face 2 represents the inner cylindrical surface, while faces 0 and 3 represent the rounded edges on either side of that cylindrical surface. Thus in this process plan, most of the critical surfaces are meeting the specified surface finish requirements. Figure 13 provides a graphical representation of the slicing scheme for the process plan of trial 5. The darkest shading represents areas where the model is to be built with an 8 mil layer thickness while the lighter shading represents 4 and 2 mil layer thickness. As one would expect, the rounded edges on the bracket require the use of a smaller layer thickness to meet the surface finish requirements. By investigating the slicing scheme and the surface finish and accuracy predictions, a much better understanding of the given process plan may be developed. Armed with this type of information, the user can make much more informed decisions as to what process plan should be ultimately used for the fabrication of the prototype.

Accuracy Results:

Tol #	Face #	Tol Type	Desired Value (mm)	Actual Value (mm)
0	2	Cylindrical	0.0762	0.0762
1	19	Parallelism	0.1016	0.381
2	33	Flatness	0.1016	0.152

Surface Finish Results:

Face #	Desired Value (micron)	Actual Value (micron)
0	3.8	5.05
1	7.6	4.34
2	2.5	1.3
3	3.8	2.64
4	7.6	0.13
5	7.6	6.05
6	7.6	1.24
...		
31	7.6	1.24
32	7.6	1.55
33	3.8	1.24

Figure 12. Results of Scenario 5

5.2 Geometric Tailoring Example

For the next two example problems, the ring gear of the transmission of a cordless drill is investigated (Connor et al., 1999). The function of the transmission in the drill is to transmit power from the motor to the chuck and its associated planetary gearing. One stage of the planetary gear train is shown in Figure 14. As shown, the planetary gear train consists of a sun (2), an outer frame ring (1), and a number of planets (3).

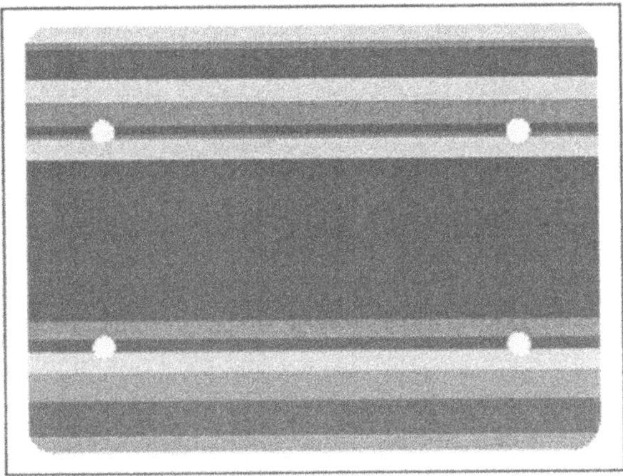

Figure 13. Slice Scheme for Scenario 5

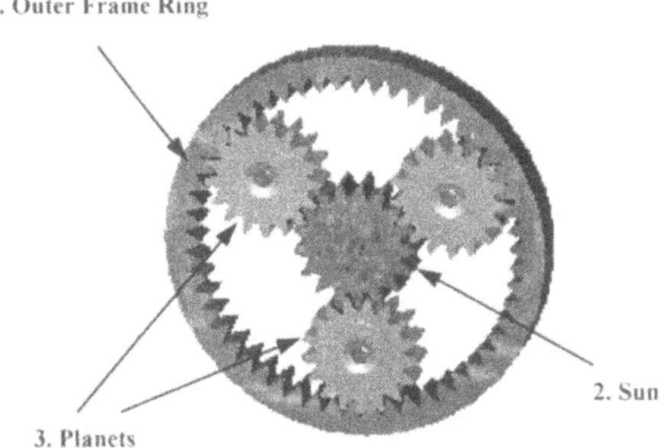

Figure 14. Planetary Gear Train - Subject of Examples 2 and 3

The purpose of this example is to investigate the geometric tailoring activity, illustrating typical decisions, and highlighting the information needed and the types of information produced. The key idea underlying geometric tailoring is that a part design must be adjusted for a prototyping technology such that some of the prototype's properties mimic those of the production part as well as possible. In this case, the production ring gear is nylon and injection molded. The designer desires a prototype gear, due to time constraints, that is fabricated on a SLA-250 using SL-5170 resin. The challenge is to adjust the dimensions and number of teeth of the prototype gear such that the same speed reduction is achieved and the teeth have the same bending strength as the production gear.

In the configuration assumed, the diametral pitch of the ring gear is 40 teeth/in, the face width is 0.11 in, and the number of gear teeth is 48. A maximum of 10% error is allowed in these dimensions for the final prototyped part. This error allows for redesign of the gear, without requiring redesign of the drill casing. The elastic modulus of nylon is assumed to be 300 ksi and the density is 0.040 lbs/in^3 (weight = 0.005 lb). The nylon gears are considered to exhibit fairly high accuracy and very good surface finish. Gear teeth must be designed to endure repeated loading, which results in bending stress. Bending failure normally occurs when the stress on a tooth exceeds the bending strength of the material of which the gear is made. The maximum load on the gear teeth is assumed to be 6.875 lb at a maximum working speed of 10,000 rpm and with four planet gears. The compromise DSP word formulation for this geometric tailoring problem is shown in Figure 15.

GIVEN:

- Parametrized CAD Model of Ring Gear
- Target values for variables
- Target value for gear weight
- Material Properties
- Goal preferences as weights

FIND:

System Variables:
Diametral Pitch
Face Width
Number of Teeth

Deviation Variables:
deviation of goals from target

SATISFY:

Goals: Meet target weight (0.005 lb.)
Meet target diametral pitch (40 teeth/in.)
Meet target face width (0.11 in.)
Meet target number of teeth (48)

Constraint: Bending Stress

MINIMIZE:

Deviation Function: Weighted sum of Goal Deviations

Figure 15. Geometric Tailoring Word Formulation

This problem was mathematically formulated, then solved using both the LINGO optimization code and an exhaustive search using a Matlab program. The solution for goal preferences of weight = 0.45, diametral pitch = 0.22, face width = 0.11, and number of teeth = 0.22 is shown in Table 6. For this solution, only the diametral pitch and number of teeth goals were met. Due to the lower yield stress of SLA resin, the face width increased slightly.

Also, due to differences in material properties and the face width, the gear weight was slightly greater than the production nylon gear. If preferences for the goals were changed, it is likely that different variations of system variable values would have been produced.

Table 6. Solution to the Geometric Tailoring, Ring Gear Problem

System Variable:	**Diametral Pitch**	**Number of Teeth**	**Face Width**
Value:	40 teeth/in.	48	0.111 in.
Stress Constraint	15,498 psi < 15,500 allowable		
Weight Goal:	Weight = 0.0051 lb	Deviation: 0.0001 lb	
Deviation Function Value:		0.0002	

5.3 Coupled Selection and Geometric Tailoring Example

The previous example can be generalized in several ways; of interest here is the integration of material and process selection into the geometric tailoring method. In the previous example, it was assumed that the SLA-250 and SL-5170 resin should be used to fabricate the ring gear prototype. However, it is desirable to consider alternatives before settling on a particular fabrication process and material. A coupled selection-selection-compromise decision problem is illustrated here to integrate the decisions surrounding the prototype. This example demonstrates that a manufacturer can successfully select a fabrication process and material, then perform design-for-manufacture, provided that the designer quantitatively describes the design freedom allowed the manufacturer.

Stated concisely, the objective in this example is to select the fabrication process and material that enables the prototype ring gear to have desired production-representative properties. Problem requirements remain the same as in the previous problem: the ring gear is to enable a specific speed reduction, gear teeth should be strong enough, and the gear must maintain dimensions as close to production dimensions as possible. For our purposes here, three stereolithography machines will be considered and six resins (material choices) will be considered. The machines are: SLA-250, SLA-3500, and SLA-5000. The resins are: SL5170, SL5210, SL5190, SL5510, SL5520, SL5195. Additional considerations upon which machine and resin selections are based include: accuracy, time, cost, surface finish, detail capability, and material properties of elastic modulus and density.

The word formulation of the coupled selection-selection-compromise decision problem is shown in Figure 16. In order to solve this problem, both additional information and the ability to solve a mixed-discrete, multiobjective optimization problem are needed. As opposed to the information level for process planning, the information level on process capabilities for evaluating accuracy, finish, and time are not nearly as stringent. In other words, it is possible to make good choices for fabrication process and material without detailed process capability information. In our work, we have used intervals, fuzzy sets, and crisp numbers to describe process capability and material properties (see Section 4.3). This enables a wider variety of processes and materials to be considered, even if one does not have access to detailed process models.

Compromise	*Material Selection*	*Process Selection*
GIVEN: Parametrized CAD Model of Ring Gear Target values for variables Target for gear weight	**GIVEN:** Set of alternative materials Desired material properties	**GIVEN** Set of alternative processes Desired process abilities
FIND: **System Variables:** Diametral Pitch Face Width Number of Teeth	**FIND:** **Attribute ratings for:** Elastic Modulus Density Accuracy, Finish, Build Time	**FIND:** **Attribute ratings for:** Cost Detail Capability Accuracy, Finish, Build Time
Deviation Variables: deviation of goals from target		
SATISFY: **Goals:** Meet target weight (0.005 lb.) Meet target diametral pitch (40 teeth/in.) Meet target face width (0.11 in.) Meet target number of teeth (48) **Constraint:** Bending Stress	**SATISFY:** **Goals:** Meet target elastic modulus Meet target density Meet targets on accuracy, finish, build time **Constraints:** Material / Process compatibility	**SATISFY:** **Goals:** Meet target cost Meet target detail capability Meet targets on accuracy, finish, build time **Constraints:** Material / Process compatibility
MINIMIZE: Deviation Function: Weighted sum of Goal Deviations		

Figure 16. Coupled Selection-Selection-Compromise Word Formulation

This problem was solved using both the LINGO optimization code and an exhaustive search in a Matlab program. For promising material-process combinations, LINGO performed an optimization to solve the compromise part of the problem, finding favorable dimensional values for the ring gear. In the Matlab program, all feasible material-process combinations were explored.

Without going into much detail, the solution to this problem is presented in Table 7. Notice that the SLA-3500 machine and SL-5510 resin were selected as the most favorable combination of material and process. Also notice that the ring gear dimensions are further from the targets of 0.11 in. (face width) and 0.005 lb (weight). SLA-3500 and SL-5510 were selected instead of SLA-250 and SL-5170 due to expected build time, cost, accuracy, and surface finish, even though the SLA-250/SL-5170 could produce a gear that is dimensionally closer to the production gear. This example demonstrates the trade-offs among various design and selection criteria that are frequently encountered in prototyping activities.

Table 7. Solution to the Coupled Material Selection, Process Selection, Geometric Tailoring, Ring Gear Problem

System Variable:	**Diametral Pitch**	**Number of Teeth**	**Face Width**
Value:	40 teeth/in.	48	0.1194 in.
Stress Constraint	14,395 psi < 14,400 allowable		
Weight Goal:	Weight = 0.0054 lb	Deviation: 0.0004 lb	
Goal Deviations:	**Compromise**	**Material Selection**	**Process Selection**
Value:	0.0013	0.6145	0.591
Deviation Function Value:	0.487		

6. CLOSURE AND OBSERVATIONS

In this paper, issues involved in transferring product information from design to manufacturing were described, in the context of designing and fabricating parts using Solid Freeform Fabrication (SFF) technologies. The focus of the presentation was on design methodology, rather than on the details of computable formats for representing information. Two design issues were explored: the point in the design process when the transfer occurs, and the routing of information flows through design and manufacturing activities. Three examples were presented that demonstrated information transfer and fabrication capabilities for combinations of transfer points and information flows. The main research question being investigated was: How early, and under what conditions, can design representations be transferred to manufacturing?

In answer to this question, such conditions were identified for SFF technologies in terms of information requirements and sources, including:

- For information transfer after design-for-manufacture to process planning, the designer must provide solid geometry with tolerances and surface finish specifications, as well as preferences for these requirements; doing so can result in very good process plans.

- For information transfer before geometric tailoring, the designer must provide parameterized solid geometry, performance requirements, fabrication process, material, and preferences among requirements are needed. Additionally, analysis models for evaluating performance requirements are needed. Utilizing a decision template with a common language (the compromise DSP was demonstrated here) enables all of this information to be transferred. The RTTB system must be able to interpret this information and solve the decision problem.
- For information transfer before materials and processes are selected, the designer must provide all the information for geometric tailoring plus suggestions for materials and processes. The RTTB system must provide materials and their properties and fabrication processes and their capabilities, in addition to selection solving capabilities.

Several unresolved issues were highlighted and lead to future research directions, including:

- Formal information models and representation formats are needed that enable general design requirements and freedoms to be communicated to manufacturers. It was suggested that the decision templates presented in this paper are promising information models.
- More complex design examples are needed to further explore the design methodology issues surrounding design-manufacture information transfer. The individual part design examples are interesting, but are lacking in the richness of assembly or product level problems.
- More comprehensive exploration of SFF technologies that includes research, not just commercial, technologies.

ACKNOWLEDGMENTS

We gratefully acknowledge NSF grant DMI-9618039. We also acknowledge the support from Rapid Prototyping & Manufacturing Institute (RPMI) member companies and Georgia Tech for partial support for the RPMI.

REFERENCES

Allen, J. K. and Rosen, D. W. (1997) "Design Methodology Issues in a Distributed Studio for Rapid Tooling and Molded Parts," CIRP International Design Seminar Proceedings: Multimedia Technologies for Collaborative Design and Manufacturing, Los Angeles, pp. 21-28, October, 8-10, 1997.

Bascaran, E., Bannerot, R.B., and Mistree, F. (1989) "Hierarchical Selection Decision Support Problems, in Conceptual Design," *Engineering Optimization*, 14: 207-238.

Connor, C.G., de Kroon, J.P., and Mistree, F. (1999) "A Product Variety Tradeoff Evaluation Method for a Family of Cordless Drill Transmissions," Proceedings ASME Design Automation Conference, paper DETC99/DAC-8625, Las Vegas, September 13-15.

Dolenc, A. and Mäkelä, I. (1994) "Slicing Procedures for Layered Manufacturing Techniques," *Computer-Aided Design*, 26(2):119-126.

Gerhard, J.F., Duncan, S.J., Chen, Y., Allen, J.K., Rosen, D.W., and Mistree, F. (1999), "Towards a Decision-Based, Distributed Product Realization Environment for Engineering Systems, Proceedings ASME Computers In Engineering Conference, paper DETC/CIE-9085. Las Vegas, September 13-15.

Hazelrigg, G.A. (1996) *Engineering Systems*, Prentice Hall, Upper Saddle River, N.J.

Herrmann, A. and Allen, J. (1999) "Selection of Rapid Tooling Materials and Processes in a Distributed Design Environment," Proceedings ASME Design for Manufacturing Conference, paper DETC99/DFM-8930, Las Vegas, September 13-15.

Kulkarni, P. and Dutta, D. (1996). "An Accurate Slicing Procedure for Layered Manufacturing." *Computer Aided Design*, **28**(9): 683-697.

Kumar, V. and Dutta, D. (1997) "An Assessment of Data Formats for Layered Manufacturing",*Advances in Engineering Software*, 28(3):151-164.

Lynn-Charney, C.M. and Rosen, D.W. (1999) "Accuracy Models and Their Use in Stereolithography Process Planning," accepted in *Rapid Prototyping Journal.*

Marsan, A., Allen, S.W., Kulkarni, P., Kumar, V. and Dutta, D. (1997). "An Integrated Software System for Process Planning for Layered Manufacturing." Proceedings from the 1997 Solid Freeform Fabrication Symposium, Austin, TX.

McClurkin, J. E. and Rosen, D. W. (1998) "Computer-Aided Build Style Decision Support for Stereolithography," *Rapid Prototyping Journal*, Vol. 4, No. 1, pp. 4-13.

Mistree, F., Muster, D., Shupe, J.A., and Allen, J.K., (1989) "A Decision-Based Perspective for the Design of Methods for Systems Design," *Recent Experiences in Multidisciplinary Analysis and Optimization*, Hampton, VA.

Mistree, F., Smith, W.F., Bras, B.A., Allen, J.K., and Muster, D., (1990) "Decision-Based Design: A Contemporary Paradigm for Ship Design," *Transactions, Society of Naval Architects and Marine Engineers*, 98:565-597.

Mistree, F., Hughes, O.F., and Bras, B.A., (1993) "The Compromise Decision Support Problem and the Adaptive Linear Programming Algorithm," in Structural Optimization: Status and Promise, AIAA, Washington, D.C.

Myers, R.H. and Montgomery, D.C. (1995) *Response Surface Methodology: Process and Product Optimization using Designed Experiments*, John Wiley & Sons, New York.

Nemhauser, G. L. and Wolsey, L. A., (1988) *Integer and Combinatorial Optimization.*

Reeves, P. E. and R. C. Cobb (1997). "Reducing the Surface Deviation of Stereolithography using In-process Techniques." *Rapid Prototyping Journal*, **3**(1):20-31.

Sabourin, E, Houser, S A, Bøhn, J H, (1996) "Adaptive Slicing using Stepwise Uniform Refinement," *Rapid Prototyping Journal*, 2(4):20-26.

Storti, D., Redl, C., Ganter, M., Turkiyyah, G., and Woo, T. (1999) "Encapsulated Transmission of Part Specifications for Distributed Solid Freeform Fabrication," Proceedings ASME Design Automation Conference, paper DETC99-DAC8617, Las Vegas, September 13-15.

Suh, N.P. (1990) *The Principles of Design*, Oxford University Press, New York.

Tata, K. (1995) "Efficient Slicing and Realization of Tessellated Objects for Layered Manufacturing," Masters Thesis, Clemson University, Clemson, SC.

West, A.P. (1999) "A Decision Support System for Fabrication Process Planning of Stereolithography," Masters Thesis, Georgia Institute of Technology, Atlanta.

Whitney, D.E., Nevins, J.L., DeFazio, T.L., Gustavson, R.E., Metzinger, R.W., Rourke, J.M., Selzer, D.S. (1988) *The Strategic Approach to Product Design,* NAS, Washington, D.C.

Xu, F., Y. S. Wong, H. T. Loh, F. Y. H. Fuh and T. Miyazawa (1997). "Optimal Orientation with Variable Slicing in Stereolithography." *Rapid Prototyping Journal*, **3**(3):76-88.

9

An Application of the Knowledge Intensive Engineering Framework to Building Foundation Design

Masaharu Yoshioka[1], Yasuhiro Shamoto[2], and Tetsuo Tomiyama[3]
1. Research and Development Department, National Center for Science Information Systems
2. Shimizu Corporation.
3. Research into Artifacts, Center for Engineering, The University of Tokyo.

Key words: Design Object Model Integration, Computer Aided Design, Building Foundation Design

Abstract: Because of increasing concerns about environmental problems and other economic and global issues, engineers are requested to evaluate their products from a wide variety of aspects. To support this, we proposed the concept of knowledge intensive engineering, in which various kinds of knowledge are used in a flexible and integrated manner aiming at generation of more added-value. In addition, we also proposed the Knowledge Intensive Engineering Framework (KIEF) that forms a computational framework of knowledge intensive engineering. In this paper, we describe the concept of knowledge intensive engineering and KIEF. Then, we apply KIEF to building foundation design to demonstrate the power of the system. To do so, we analyze knowledge that is used for building foundation design and discuss how to implement the knowledge on KIEF. Finally, we show some results of this application and discuss the capability of KIEF.

1. INTRODUCTION

During design of a new product, engineers evaluate it from various aspects, supported by computational tools with which a model represents the product. Since these tools represent and deal with an identical product, a change of the product, based on the evaluation results from one aspect, affects other models. To deal with these dependencies among models, it is necessary to have a framework that can integrate these tools. Speaking of mechatoronics design, for instance, design models, such as a geometric model, a kinematics model, an electric circuit analysis model, and a finite element model, are required to be integrated.

We have proposed knowledge intensive engineering that is a new style of engineering to assist engineering activities in product life cycle stages based on intensive use of various kinds of engineering knowledge (Tomiyama *et al.*, 1996). The Knowledge Intensive Engineering Framework (KIEF) system is a computational framework to support knowledge intensive engineering by integrating computational modeling systems for each activity.

This paper is intended to demonstrate the flexibility of the KIEF system by describing applications to a new engineering domain that is not an original target domain of the system. In Section 2, we briefly review our previous research about the knowledge base (Ishii *et al.*, 1995), (Sekiya and Tomiyama, 1997) and the pluggable metamodel mechanism (Yoshioka and Tomiyama, 1997) that are two basic elements of KIEF. In addition, we describe the architecture of KIEF. In Section 3, we argue that KIEF can be flexibly applied to designs in other domains than mechanical design for which KIEF was originally developed. To evaluate this idea, we demonstrate the result of applying KIEF to building foundation design domain as a case study and identify research issues for this application. Section 4 compares our approach with related work and Section 5 concludes this paper.

2. THE KNOWLEDGE INTENSIVE ENGINEERING FRAMEWORK

Engineering activities in various life cycle stages generate and modify information about the product. In KIEF, we formalize these activities as operations to computational models. This system supports engineers by integrating these computational models and managing their dependency and consistency.

KIEF has two basic elements (Figure 1).

- A very large scale knowledge base (VLKB):
  It gives ontological definitions of engineering knowledge that are used in various modeling systems.
- A model management mechanism called the pluggable metamodel mechanism:
  It provides the data sharing capability among various modeling systems and keeps dependency and consistency among them.

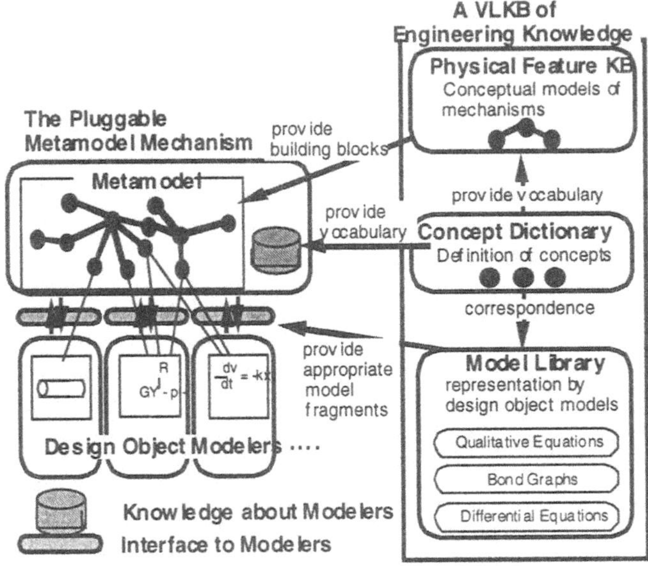

Figure 1 Knowledge Intensive Engineering Framework (KIEF) System

2.1 The Very Large Scale Knowledge Base

We have been working for developing an engineering knowledge base based on the concept of qualitative physics base (Ishii *et al.*, 1995), (Sekiya and Tomiyama, 1997). This knowledge base system has following three components.

- **Concept Dictionary**
  This dictionary gives ontological definitions of concepts used throughout the system. We classify these concepts into five categories: entity, relation, physical phenomenon, attribute, and physical rule.
- **Physical Feature Library**
  A physical feature is a piece of knowledge that represents a mechanism and related physical phenomena. This knowledge is used for two purposes. One is a building block to build a design object model, and the other is knowledge to reason out possible physical phenomena occurring on design object models. This is philosophically the same idea as embodiment in German systematic methodologies (VDI, 1977), (Hubka 1973). The difference is that this knowledge is a computational tool rather than just a theory or a textbook.
- **Model Library**
  This is a library of model fragments that is used for a particular modeling system. Model fragments are associated with a physical phenomenon, attribute, and so on.

In VLKB, the concept dictionary gives vocabularies used to describe knowledge in the entire system. We define physical features with combination of concepts that are defined in the concept dictionary and we also define the model library in association with the concepts in the concept dictionary. In KIEF, the user builds a design object model by selecting concepts from the concept dictionary and defines the relations among them. To support this modeling process, a physical feature is used as a building block. The model library is used for mapping a model to a particular modeling system. Figure 2 shows an example of physical features, concepts in the concept dictionary, and the model library in the system.

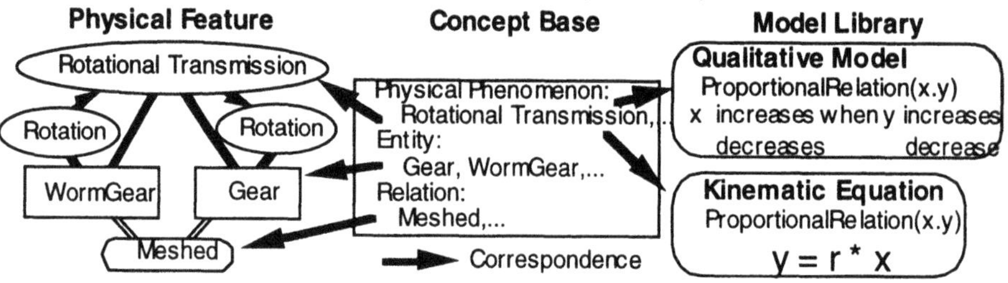

Figure 2. Examples of the Physical Feature, the Concept Dictionary, and the Model Library

When building a model for a particular modeling system, the system collects all related models from the model library. However, the assembling process of these fragments is not so easy in some cases. We also conduct a research to support this model building process (Sekiya *et al*, 1999).

2.2 The Pluggable Metamodel Mechanism

The pluggable metamodel mechanism is a computational system that integrates multiple computational modeling tools (called modelers in this paper) by using a metamodel and knowledge about each modeler. A metamodel represents relationships among physical concepts used for various design object models about an identical design object. VLKB gives definitions of the physical concepts and the relationships are described as links in the pluggable metamodel mechanism. The pluggable metamodel mechanism handles the following links.

- Causal link

  This link represents a causal relationship among physical phenomena.
- Occurrence link

  This link represents the relationship between a physical phenomenon and an entity.
- Attribute link

  This link represents the relationship between an attribute and an entity, a relation, or a physical phenomenon.

- Relation link
  This link represents the relationship between a relation and an entity. We use relation concepts associated with relation links to represent relationships among entities.
- Reason-from link
  This link represents the relationship between an attribute and other concepts that are used to reason out the attribute.

The pluggable metamodel mechanism maintains relationships and consistencies among these design object models and exchanges the information among them. It integrates existing modelers by defining the data exchanging interface and the knowledge about each modeler (Table 1).

Table 1. Knowledge about a Modeler

Name	Name of the modeler
Related concepts	Concepts that are relevant to the modeler
Usable concepts	Concepts that are used for making a model on it
Available concepts	Concepts that can be reasoned out by using it
Attribute Translation Method	Attribute relationship graph and translating method

The pluggable metamodel mechanism assists to build a model for each modeler based on the information provided by metamodel and information in other modelers. A modeling process with the pluggable metamodel mechanism consists of two steps.

1. Construction of a conceptual model
   a) Abstraction of a model
   Abstraction of a model is a process to map concepts in the metamodel to concepts used in a particular modeler. The pluggable metamodel mechanism first selects related concepts from the metamodel by using the related concepts definition in the knowledge about the modeler. Second, the user maps the selected concepts onto the concepts used in the modeler. For example, considering an analysis of distortion of a robot arm. The pluggable metamodel mechanism selects concepts such as force, robot arm, and connection in the first step. In the second step, designer maps the robot arm concept to a beam that is a usable concept of a distortion analysis tool.
   b) Simplification of a model
   Simplification of a model is a process to neglect some concepts of a model, considering the computational cost, computability, and so on. This operation is realized as selection of concepts that can be neglected. In the example of robot arm analysis, the following operations correspond to this operation; neglection of self-weight of

the robot arm when it is light, body of the robot if the user concentrates on the analysis of the robot arm.

2. Building a particular model
   In this process, the pluggable metamodel mechanism collects the necessary information by using the attribute translation method in the knowledge about the modeler. If the mechanism cannot find the information in the metamodel, the mechanism finds other modelers that can handle this information or asks the user to input the data. In this process, the mechanism tries to automatically collect as much information as possible, but there could be some that cannot be handled automatically. In the example of the robot arm, to calculate the length of beam, the metamodel mechanism asks the user to use a solid modeler or 2D CAD to input the data. In addition, it asks to input the location of the central axis of the beam to feed the information to the beam modeler.

The pluggable metamodel mechanism stores any information to build a model. This information, as a whole, is called modeling assumption and is connected to the resulting information with "Reason-from links". This information can be useful for checking the reliability of the computational result in later stages, and for maintaining the consistency.

2.3 The KIEF System

The KIEF system uses the pluggable metamodel mechanism as a core modeling system and VLKB as a source of knowledge. Building and evaluation of a product on KIEF proceeds as follows.

1. Create an initial metamodel by combining physical features.
   The user combines physical features to build a metamodel. The pluggable metamodel mechanism models the structure of the product and physical phenomena to achieve the functionality of the product. If the design problem is a typical routine design case, he/she just combines physical features to represent the design object. If the design problem is a new one, the FBS modeler (Umeda *et al.*, 1996) supports to build an initial model by functional decomposition and to map subfunctions to physical features.
2. Reason out possible physical phenomena that may occur on the product.
   We use a physical feature as knowledge that represents causal relationships between the structure of the product and the physical phenomena. A qualitative physics based reasoning system of KIEF reasons out possible physical phenomena with this knowledge.
3. Evaluate the product with other modelers.

The user evaluates the product from various aspects with modelers that deal with these aspects. KIEF also maintains the consistency of information by checking whether the modeling assumptions for a model are modified or not, every time the model is modified.

3. APPLICATION TO BUILDING FOUNDATION DESIGN

KIEF was originally developed for mechanical engineering design. However, since the system has a flexible framework to integrate different kinds of knowledge, we can apply KIEF to other domain by changing the knowledge base of KIEF.

To validate this idea, we apply the KIEF system to building foundation design domain. In this section, we describe an analysis of building foundation design and discuss a strategy to construct the knowledge base. Since we have not applied KIEF to larger scale problems, this discussion includes the scaling up problem of the system. Then, we illustrate an example of building foundation design with KIEF.

3.1 Knowledge for Building Foundation Design

In this research, we interviewed a researcher of a construction company to acquire knowledge about building foundation design.

Architectural Institute of Japan compiled a textbook that gives guidelines to design foundations of building (Architectural Institute of Japan, 1988). From the interview of the researcher, this type of textbook turned out to have the following problems.

- Knowledge is often a black box.
  Descriptions of each analysis method describe only how to use it without giving theoretical basis. This may cause inappropriate use of analysis methods.
- It is intricate to select necessary analysis methods.
  This textbook has a flowchart for selecting necessary analysis methods. However, in a real design process, the designers do not need to consider all of the considerations described in the flowchart.
- Information for selecting an appropriate analysis method is incomplete.
  This textbook describes various analysis methods used in the building foundation design process. In many cases, two or more analysis methods are listed for one problem, but there is not enough information how to select an appropriate analysis method from them.

To solve these problems, it is necessary to consider the following issues.

- Describe causal relationships of each analysis method.
  Since each analysis method is knowledge for evaluating some physical phenomena, and there exist causal relationships among these phenomena, we can describe the relationships among analysis methods with the causal relationship among physical phenomena. KIEF has a capability of describing them with the metamodel and physical features.
- Select necessary analysis methods based on an object model.
  The pluggable metamodel mechanism can reason out possible physical phenomena that may occur on a product. In order to select an appropriate analysis method for possible physical phenomena, we should describe knowledge about relationships between analysis methods and physical phenomena.
- Suggest an appropriate analysis method when two or more methods are applicable to one problem.
  It is necessary to have a scheme to describe features of each analysis method for selecting methods. Therefore, the knowledge about the relationships between possible physical phenomena and analysis methods should have a description for selecting an appropriate analysis method.

In addition, these analysis methods are described on different granularity levels; e.g., a building can be modeled as one mass or combination of floors, walls, and so on. Therefore, KIEF is requested to manage the consistency among different granularity levels.

3.2 A Building Foundation Design Support System on the KIEF system

Based on the discussion about the knowledge for building foundation design, we extend KIEF to deal with knowledge for selecting appropriate analysis methods and granularity modeling.

For dealing with different granularity modeling, we developed a mechanism to manage multiple metamodels for different granularity levels. In this metamodel, the designer defines relationships between one entity and its subcomponent model with the part-unit editor. Figure 2 shows an example of mapping different granularity levels. In this case, "Ground" is decomposed into "SoftClayStrata", "SoftSandStrata", and "StiffClayStrata". In addition, the designer also defines the relationships between "Ground" and the other entities in the decomposed level. By using these relationships, the system propagates physical phenomena occurred in the decomposed level to the "Ground" level.

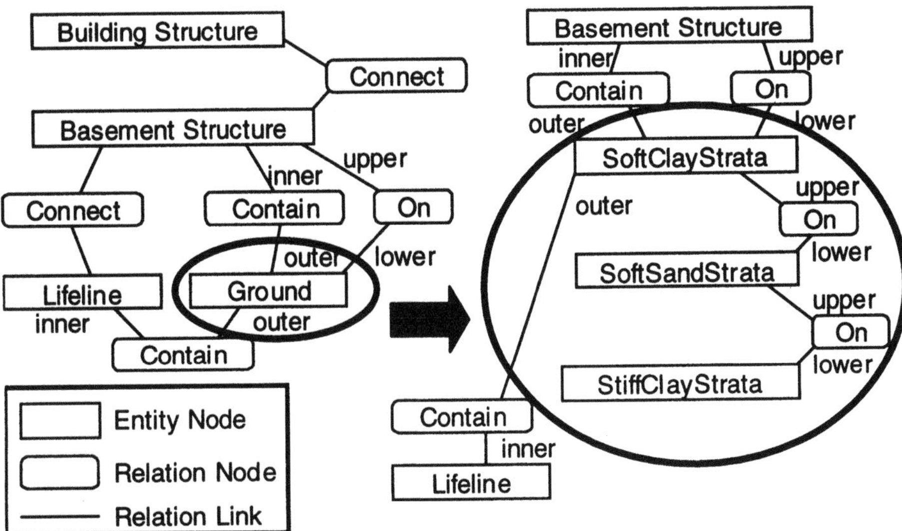

Figure 3. Relationships between Different Granularity Models

This granularity handling is also useful for other engineering domains including mechanical design. Therefore, we think this is an expansion not only for building foundation design but also of KIEF itself. In addition to this, it is better to give a guideline to make these different granularity models. However, this guideline requires understanding of all models that are used for the design and it is very difficult to make it. So we make these models based on the example at this moment.

For supporting selection of an appropriate analysis method from two or more methods, we define knowledge about analysis methods. Table 2 shows the scheme of the knowledge and Table 3 and 4 show an example of the definition for earthquake. Selection of an appropriate analysis method proceeds as follows.

1. Retrieve candidate analysis methods and check availability of the input attributes.
   KIEF retrieves candidate analysis methods by using knowledge about analysis methods. Then, the system checks whether or not information about each input attribute exists in the metamodel or not.
2. Select appropriate methods by the user.
   The user selects an appropriate method by using the descriptions about analysis methods and the input attribute information.

3. Suggest another analysis method to obtain input attribute information.
   If there is no input attribute information in the model, KIEF suggests another analysis method to obtain the information. This is done by comparing the concept of the information with the output attributes definitions in the knowledge about analysis methods.

Table 2 Knowledge about Analysis Methods

Phenomenon name	Name of physical phenomenon	
Analysis method (one or more)	Description	Description about the method
	Input attributes	Description about required attributes for the method
	Output attributes	Description about the result

Table 3 Example Definition for Earthquake (Simple)

Phenomenon name	Earthquake	
Analysis method SimpleMethod	Description	Use default variable This method can be used for simple design. Set Two levels for the earthquake. Maximum acceleration on the ground: Level 1: 250 Gal, Level 2: 500 Gal Maximum velocity on the ground: Level 1: 25cm/s, Level 2: 50cm/s
	Input attributes	None
	Output attributes	Maximum velocity on the ground Maximum acceleration on the ground,

Table 4 Example Definition for Earthquake (Use wave data)

Phenomenon name	Earthquake	
Analysis method WaveDataRetrieve	Description	Use earthquake wave data for design Use appropriate earthquake wave data for the place. This method is used for complex design
	Input attributes	Place
	Output attributes	Earthquake wave data(transition data of acceleration and velocity of the structure and the ground)

3.3 Example of Building Foundation Design

We demonstrate how KIEF works for an example of building foundation design. Before starting this design, we define concepts used in the building foundation design in the concept dictionary, and also define physical features to represent causal dependency knowledge of physical phenomena. Since mechanical engineering domain is so different from the building foundation design, we cannot reuse the knowledge, even though the knowledge is stored in the same knowledge base.

First, the designer selects an initial model of a typical building from the physical feature library (Figure 4). In order to evaluate a particular design case, he/she adds detail information to Ground with the part-unit editor (Figure 5).

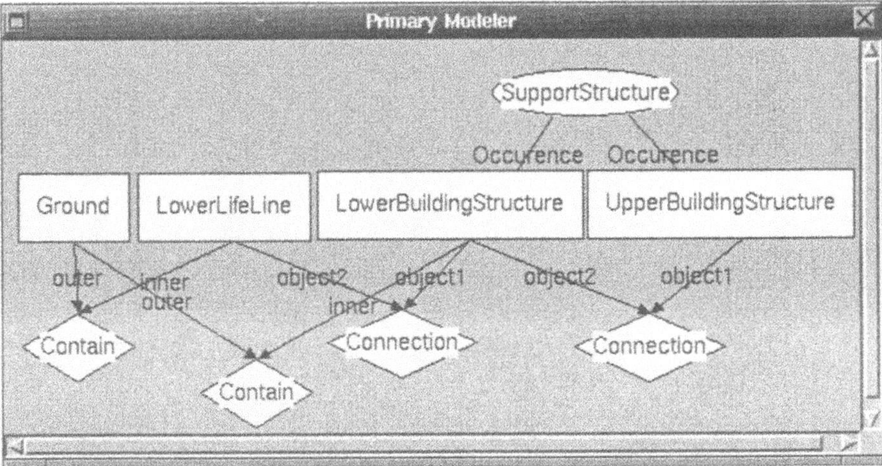

Figure 4. Initial Design Model

After building a decomposed model of Ground, KIEF reasons out the possible physical phenomena that may occur on this structure. In this case, KIEF reasons out earthquake, quick sand, liquefaction settlement, and so on. After reasoning out possible physical phenomena, the system suggests the necessary analysis methods for these phenomena (Figure 6) and evaluates whether or not the problems are critical.

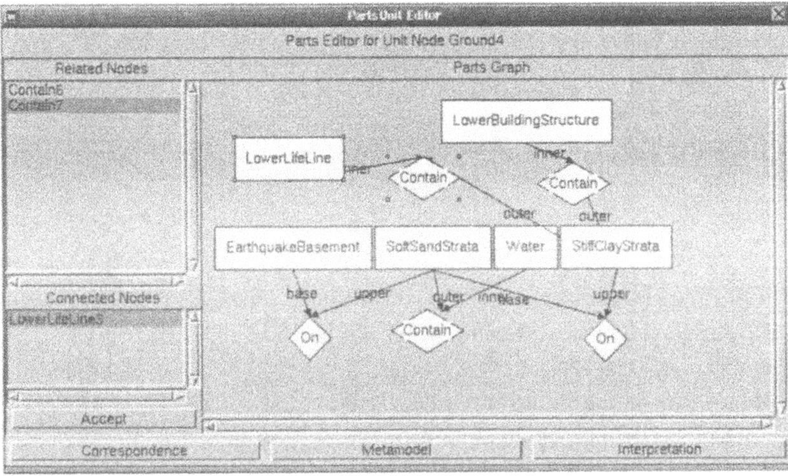

Figure 5. Decomposed Ground Unit

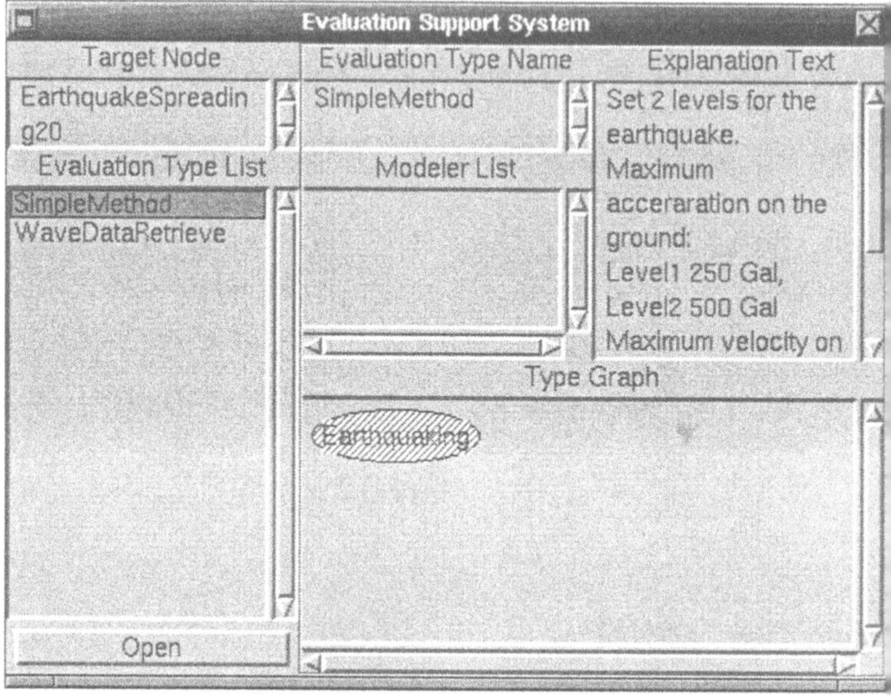

Figure 6. Suggestion of Evaluation Method

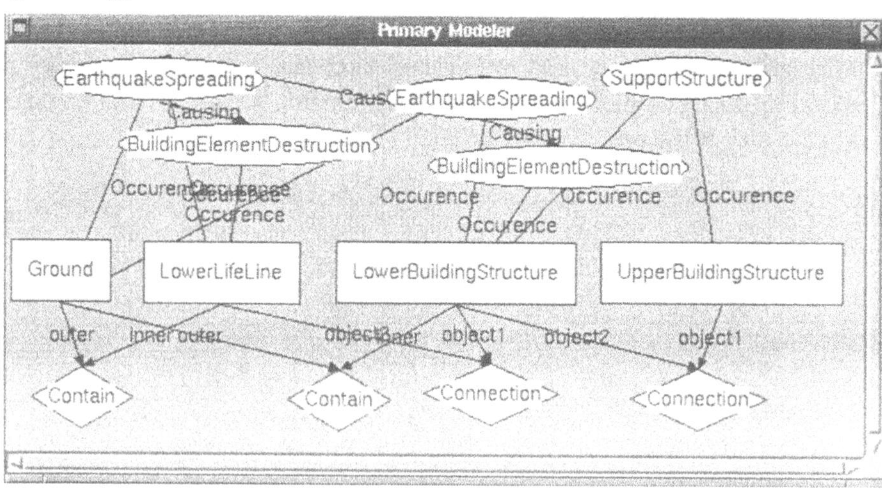

Figure 7. Physical Phenomena Occurred on the Top Level

When the phenomena are negligible, the designer specifies these phenomena to be neglected and propagates this decision to the unit level (Ground level). Figure 7 shows a propagated result. In this case, since quick sand is a negligible phenomenon, other phenomena caused by quick sand such as liquefaction settlement are also neglected. On the other hand, since earthquake is not negligible one, parts level physical phenomena such as EarthquakeSpreading and BuildingElementDestruction are propagated to the Ground level.

Next, the designer moves on to the design of the lower building structure and then to the upper building structure, and repeats evaluation for this building foundation in the same way.

3.4 Discussion

From this example, we conclude that KIEF has a capability of describing the knowledge of a typical engineering textbook (Architectural Institute of Japan, 1988). KIEF describes the causal relationships among physical phenomena and the relationships between physical phenomena and analysis methods.

Speaking of the analysis methods, most of them are just plain texts from the textbook. However, if we implement these analysis methods as computational tools, we can integrate them with the pluggable metamodel mechanism of KIEF. From these, we conclude that KIEF can be used as a kernel for an intelligent CAD system for building foundation design.

In this experiment, we only share the reasoning system and VLKB from the original KIEF domain and knowledge about physical phenomena is not reused for this design. This problem comes from the difference between mechanical engineering design and building foundation design. In order to discuss this cross-domain design issue, we need to try many other application domains.

From the viewpoint of the scaling up of KIEF, we have to deal with complex design object models. For managing this type of complexity, the building foundation designers set multiple granularity level for one design object and manage the relationship among them. This type of knowledge management can be seen in other engineering domains, too. Therefore, we believe that granularity handling mechanism of KIEF is also useful not only for building foundation design but also for other engineering design domains.

4. RELATED WORK

STEP (TC184/SC4, 1994) is a standard for sharing and exchanging product model data. STEP also tries to include different engineering domains such as mechanical design and ship design. However, STEP only focuses on data structure for representing products and does not explicitly mention knowledge used in these application domains.

In the SHADE project (McGuire *et al.*, 1993), they also propose framework to integrate various design tools. This approach is similar to our approach in that integrating models takes place through translating their knowledge in one format. While they use KIF (Knowledge Interchange Format) (Genesereth, 1992) as the format and Ontolingua (Gruber, 1992) to define ontology, we use the concept dictionary as the most fundamental description. However, since they try to integrate these tools automatically with KQML (Knowledge Query and Manipulation Language) (T. Finin *et al.*, 1992), they do not address the interaction between designers and the system during design. Therefore, the system cannot deal with knowledge for process management (e.g., selection of appropriate methods, supporting modeling process, etc.), although an intelligent agent oriented architecture is assumed.

SEED (Akin *et al.*, 1998) is an integrated application for building design. This system has an advantage of good integrity due to their particular modeling format. However, it has a difficulty to expand a system with existing computational tools. On the other hand, the main feature of KIEF is a flexibility to integrate new tools.

5. CONCLUSION

This paper described the architecture of KIEF that can be used as a kernel of intelligent CAD. In order to verify this concept, we applied the system to building foundation design. In this application, knowledge about causal relationships is described in the system and analysis methods are defined with regard to relationships among physical phenomena. Finally, we showed some results of the application and confirmed this framework can deal with most of the knowledge in the design of building foundations.

ACKNOWLEDGMENT

The work described in Section 3 was part of an international collaborative research project, GNOSIS within the Intelligent Manufacturing Systems (IMS) research program.

REFERENCES

Akin , Ö., Aygen, Z., Chang, T.-W., Chien, S.-F., Choi B. , Donia, M., Fenves, S., Flemming, U., Garrett, J., Gomez, N., Kiliççöte, H., Rivard, H., Sen, R., Snyder, J., Tsai, W.-J., Woodbury, R., and Zhang, Y. (1998) *A software environment to support early phases in building design.* International Journal of Design Computing (http://www.arch.usyd.edu.au/kcdc/journal/), Vol. 1.

Architectural Institute of Japan, editor. (1988) *Recommendations for Design of Building Foundations.* Architectural Institute of Japan.

Finin, T., Weber, J., Wiederhold, G., Genesereth, M., Fritzson, R., Mckay, D., McGuire, J., Pelavin, R., Shapiro, S., and Beck, G. (1992) *Specification of the KQML agent-communication language.* Technical report EIT TR 92-04, Enereprise Integration Technologies, Palo Alto, California.

Genesereth, M. R. (1992) *Knowledge interchange format.* In James Allen, Richard Fikes, and Erik Sandwall, editors, Proceedings of the Conference of the Principles of Knowledge Representation and Reasoning. Morgan Kaufmann Publishers.

Gruber, T.R. (1992) *Ontolingua: A mechanism to support portable ontlogies.* Technical report KSL91-66, Knowledge Systems Laboratory, Stanford University, Stanford.

Hubka, V. (1973), *Theorie der Maschinensysteme*, Springer-Verlag, Berlin.

Ishii, M., Sekiya, T., and Tomiyama, T. (1995) *A very large-scale knowledge base for the knowledge intensive engineering framework.* In KB&KS'95, the Second International Conference on Building and Sharing of Very Large-Scale Knowledge Bases, pp. 123-131.

McGuire, J. G., Kuokka, D. R., Weber, J. C., Tenenbàum, J. M., Gruber, T. R., and Olsen, G. R. (1993) *SHADE: Technology for knowledge-based collaborative engineering.* Concurrent Engineering: Research and Applications (CERA), Vol. 1, No. 2.

ISO TC184/SC4. (1994) ISO 10303-1 *Industrial Automation Systems and Integration - Product Data Representation and Exchange-, Part1: Overview and Fundamental Principles.*

Sekiya. T., and Tomiyama, T. (1997) *Case studies of ontology for the knowledge intensive engineering framework*, In Mäntylä, M., Finger, S., and Tomiyama T. editors, Knowledge Intensive CAD, Vol. 2, pp. 139-156, Chapman & Hall.

Sekiya T., Tsumaya, A., and Tomiyama, T. (1999) *Classification of Knowledge for Generating Engineering Models - A Case study of Model Generation in Finite Element Analysis -.* In Finger, S., Tomiyama, T., and Mäntylä, M. editors, Knowledge Intensive CAD-3, Preprints of the first IFIP WG 5.2 Workshop on Knowledge Intensive CAD-3, Kluwer Academic Publishers, 1999.

Tomiyama, T., Umeda, Y., Ishii, M., Yoshioka, M., and Kiriyama, T. (1996) *Knowledge systematization for a knowledge intensive engineering framework.* In Tomiyama, T., Mäntylä, M., and Finger S. editors, Knowledge Intensive CAD-1, Preprints of the first IFIP WG 5.2 Workshop on Knowledge Intensive CAD-1, pp. 33-52, Chapman & Hall.

Umeda, Y., Ishii, M., Yoshioka, M., and Tomiyama, T. (1996) *Supporting conceptual design based on the Function-Behavior-State modeler.* Artificial Intelligence for Engineering Design, Analysis and Manufacturing (AIEDAM), Vol.10, No. 4, pp. 275-288.

VDI-Gesellschaft. (1977) *VDI-2222 Konstruktion und Entwicklung*, VDI-Verlag, Düsseldorf.

Yoshioka, M., Sekiya, T., and Tomiyama, T. (1998) *Design knowledge collection by modelling.* In Jacucci, G., Olling, G. J., Preiss, K., and Wozny, M. editors, GLOBALIZATION OF MANUFACTURING IN THE DIGITAL COMMUNICATIONS ERA OF THE 21ST CENTURY Innovation, Agility and the Virtual Enterprise, pp. 287-298. Kluwer Academic Publishers.

Yoshioka M., and Tomiyama, T. (1997) Pluggable metamodel mechanism: A framework of an integrated design object modelling environment. In Bradshaw, A., and Counsell, J. editors, Computer Aided Conceptual Design `97, Proceedings of the 1997 Lancaster International Workshop on Engineering Design CACD'97, pp. 57-70, Lancaster University.

PART FIVE

KNOWLEDGE INTENSIVE DESIGN (KID)

10

Supporting Conceptual Design: A Model for Reflective-Interactive Design

Bill Chan[1] & Susan Finger[2]
[1] *Visionary Design Systems, Atlanta GA, USA*

[2] *Carnegie Mellon University, Pittsburgh, PA, USA*

Key words: conceptual design, computer-aided design, knowledge-intensive CAD

Abstract: In the process of developing a concept, a designer will view a design from multiple levels of abstraction, using mental simulation to verify the interaction between its different components. This interaction can be viewed as a conversation between the design and the designer, which is conducted in the languages of function, behaviour and form. A computational design tool that supports this conversation will both enrich the quality of the interaction, as well as provide a mechanism to capture the knowledge embedded within the discourse. Designers generate knowledge about aspects of the design artefact, other than its physical attributes, as part of the process in early design. This knowledge is valuable because it establishes the design context. Understanding of context is critical to guide downstream design processes such as model abstraction and evaluation. In this paper, we present a framework and initial computer implementation of a reflective-interactive design methodology. Using this framework, a designer can create and simulate incomplete and evolving designs using function, behaviour, and form concepts.

1. INTRODUCTION

The process of design is not function-driven *per se*; nor is it purely behaviour- or form-driven. In exploring possible design solutions, a designer tries to achieve function through some intended behaviour. Form acts to both enable and constrain the actual behaviour. Simulation of the design determines whether the actual behaviour is the same as the intended behaviour. The actual behaviours of complex systems are not known with certainty by the designer *a priori* and must be verified using virtual or physical prototypes.

Designers often use mental simulation to explore ideas at an early stage in their development, before details about structure or material properties have been defined. They use mental simulation to gain understanding the interaction between different parts of a design and between the design and the surrounding world. Yet predicting behaviour of complex systems mentally is often difficult and error prone. Computer simulation can be used to analyse the behaviour of completed designs; however, these simulations tend to be expensive, both in terms of the computational power and time needed to run the analysis, as well as in terms of the amount of time and effort needed to create a computable model of the design. For this reason, computational simulation is rarely used the way humans routinely use mental simulation.

We believe that the usefulness of such simulation is not limited to its analytical value. Rather, simulation is a mechanism through which the designer interacts with the design and explores the design space. It provides feedback to the designer about the consequences of a design move, and therefore increases the designer's understanding of the design problem. We believe that this interaction is an important aspect of the conversation between design and designer, which promotes reflection by the designer. A computational environment that allows the designer to interactively construct and simulate incomplete models of a design would enrich the conversation between the designer and the design.

Design knowledge created during the early stages of design can be used to advantage in the later stages of design. The task of capturing and organizing this design information should take place as part of the design process, not as a post-process after the design is complete. Design methods and tools need to be synchronized with the technical and social requirements of the design environment (Baya and Leifer, 1994). Rather than having separate models of a design during conceptual design and embodiment design, a single representation should provide continuity in the flow of design knowledge between the different stages of the overall process. A single design data-model should support the refinement of high-level abstractions of function and behaviour, through the addition of general characteristics of form during embodiment design, to the detailed specification of all its physical attributes in detailed design.

Existing CAD tools are not well suited for conceptual design because their functionality retains much from their origins in drafting and electronic storage of design geometry. Some proposed conceptual design tools have taken an analytical approach based on a systematic decomposition of an initial problem description. Others seek to automatically generate design solutions or to automate the exploration of the space of possible designs. Neither of these approaches is suitable for activities that are intrinsically synthetic and exploratory in nature. The lack of CAD support during early design isolates the early design activities from the later engineering activities and restricts the transmission of design knowledge between the different stages of the design cycle. Specifically, valuable design knowledge generated by the designer during early design is never captured for use in downstream processes.

2. REFLECTIVE-INTERACTIVE DESIGN

An important aspect of our work is the idea of design as reflective conversation. The phrase, "reflective conversation" was coined by Schön (Schön, 1983) in the larger context of reflection-in-action; his proposal for an alternative philosophy of practice. Reflection-in-action was Schön's response to what he felt were negative trends in professional practice that derived from ideas championed under the paradigm of Technical Rationality.

The reflective-interactive view of design holds implications for the practice of design and the tools that support it. Current prescriptive methodologies for design describe a process in which the designer acts on a design, effecting changes on a static representation without accounting for the designer's perception and reactions to the results of his actions. For example, simulation of a design's behaviour can expose problems that were not known beforehand or can provide insight to the designer about the design problem. This new knowledge can change the designer's formulation of the design requirements. Reflective-interactive design emphasizes the importance of the interaction that occurs between the designer and the design situation. The design situation includes the design and its relationship to the surrounding environment. Thus, the design environment must be able to communicate the effect that design moves have on the behaviour of the design and that the design representation support this functionality.

Based on the reflective practice model, our reflective-interactive model expands the scope of design to include the designer's situation, in addition to the design process oriented view taken in the rational problem-solving paradigm. In particular, the reflective-interactive view builds on the idea of reflective conversation as a metaphor for the mechanism whereby the designer interacts with the design situation.

Design methods and techniques must be built on three supporting structures: a model of the designer, a model of the design task, and a model of the dynamics of the design process. These three classes of models respectively define: the cognitive processes or mechanisms of action of the designer; the structure and methods within a particular design task; and the meta-level control structures and processes of design. In his comparison of rational problem solving and reflective practice, (Dorst and Dijkhuis, 1995) summarizes these three aspects for both paradigms. In the rational problem-solving paradigm, the designer is modelled as a finite-state machine, the design task is modelled as an ill-structured problem, and the design process is modelled as a generalized search. Under the theory of reflective practice, the designer is modelled as a person who constructs his or her own understanding of the world based on his or her perceptions. Each design task is essentially a unique construction of the designer, and the process of design is a reflective conversation with the situation.

The early stages of design involve a process of exploration in which the designer refines his or her understanding of the design problem through reflection and interaction with virtual and physical models of design concepts. Some researchers refer to this process as a meta-level search of the design space with the goal of obtaining knowledge for guiding further searches within the design solution space (Smithers and Troxell, 1990, Gero and Kazakov, 1996, Poon and Maher, 1997). Other use exploration in a purely generative manner (Faltings, 1992; Tanir *et al.*, 1993).

Knowledge about aspects of the design artefact, other than its physical attributes, is generated as part of the process in early design. This knowledge is valuable because it establishes the design context, and an understanding of context is critical in guiding downstream design processes such as model abstraction and evaluation. Support for this claim can be found in the recent literature. The work of (Allen, 1989, Tomiyama *et al.*, 1989, Ganeshan *et al.*, 1992, Subrahmanian *et al.*, 1993, Reddy, 1996, SEED, 1997) each include the idea that design creates and uses many different types of knowledge. To provide additional experimental support for this claim, we have analysed the content of design discourse between members of a team of six designers to determine the nature of the information that is created and used as part of designing. The results of this analysis are reported in (Chan, 1998, Reddy *et al.*, 1996).

A computational design tool that supports a reflective-interactive model of design provides an opportunity to capture the artefact knowledge that describes design context. The representation of the design model should also support the evolutionary refinement of the design after the early stages of design so that any additional knowledge generated is also captured. Existing and proposed product data-models are meant to capture product information for completed designs (Shaw *et al.*, 1989).

3. CHARACTERIZING DESIGN ARTIFACT INFORMATION

The knowledge that is created and used in the course of design can be differentiated as being concerned with the design process or the design artefact. Design process knowledge relates to the methods and practice of the design process. Examples of process knowledge include: the history of design decisions, the best formulation of a mathematical model for a class of problems, or a list of suppliers for a particular part. Design artefact knowledge relates specifically to the attributes, structure, and qualities of the artefact being designed. Within this research, we will only be concerned with knowledge about the design artefact that relates to design intent.

We partition the space of information about a design artefact into phases. The term "phase" is used exclusively in its chemical sense to identify a distinct region within a mixture, and not in its temporal sense. The process of design populates the solution space with information and organizes this information into the knowledge that defines the design intent of an artefact.

We use two basic structures to describe design artefacts: concepts and relationships. Because we are concerned with mechanical design, we assume that all concepts will be realized through physical means. Therefore, concepts possess physical form. Concepts can correspond to an entire design artefact, components in the artefact, parts of components, or regions of a part. In the early stages of design, however, a designer may think of a concept as an abstract entity without physical form. In this case, a concept is given form as part of the design process, through a process of refinement in which the design is fleshed-out. For example, a functional requirement that the height of an office chair seat be adjustable vertically can be instantiated as a behaviour where the seat translates in the vertical direction relative to the base of the chair. This behaviour links the motion of the chair seat with the position of the base. However, the specific geometry of a mechanism to achieve this behaviour can take on several different physical forms (*e.g.*, screw mechanism, four-bar linkage, rack and pinion, prismatic joint, *etc.*). Allowing the designer to defer commitment to a specific form until a later time in the design process ensures that the design solution space is not restricted before the designer has an opportunity to properly explore solution concepts. Most existing product models implicitly include information about form within the basic entity used to construct a design model. For instance, the design entity used with the SHADES framework (Hakim, 1993) includes knowledge about at least two design aspects (phases in our terminology).

3.1 Function, Behaviour and Form

In our research, we differentiate between function and behaviour. We define function to be the intended use of something. In the context of representation of design knowledge, function can be thought of as design intent. Behaviour is the manner in which something acts or reacts in the physical sense. Form refers to the geometry of a design as well as the physical properties of the material from which it is constructed. A common problem in design occurs when the actual behaviour of a design does not match its intended behaviour. Alternatively, an unexpected secondary behaviour might emerge in a design that violates an initial design requirement. In both cases, the design will not achieve its function.

Function encodes high-level knowledge about goal and context for an artefact. Behaviour complements functional information by defining the "how" for a design. Knowing what a design is supposed to do does not tell us how that goal is to be achieved. Knowledge about the behaviour of an artefact can be used to determine the interactions between parts of a design.

3.2 Concepts

Concepts are composed of elements from three phases in the design artefact information space. Each phase relates to a different aspect of the concept: its function, its behaviour or its form. Therefore, a concept, like the overall information space, is composed of three phases, each of which exists within the concept as a distinct part of the concept. Phases do not mix with one-another, however the state of one phase may have an effect on another phase. Therefore, relationships may exist between entities in different phases, as well as between entities within a phase. Some of the relationships within a phase, such as the part-of relationship, serve to define a hierarchy of abstraction within that phase. Relationships may also be topological (*e.g.*, adjacent-to) or causal (*e.g.*, enables) in nature. Figure 1 below illustrates the structure of design artefact information space, and the relationship between the phases within the total information space, and a single concept.

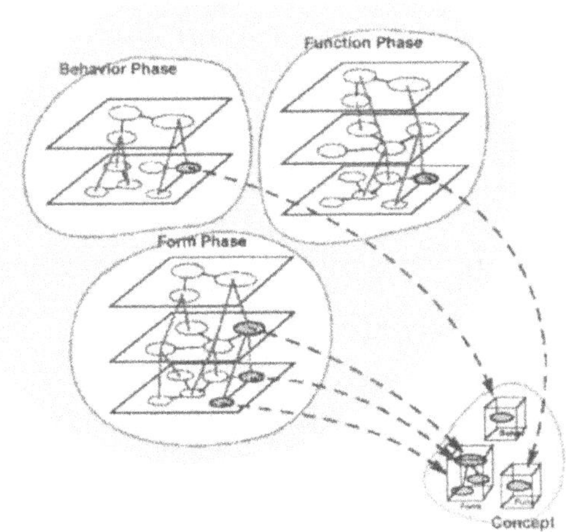

Figure 1. The structure of design artefact information space

3.3 Descriptors

Concepts are described by parameters or more generally, descriptors. Descriptors are typically associated with a particular phase. Therefore, descriptors describe a concept from the perspective of function, behaviour or form. The relationships among concepts are established between the concepts' descriptors. Relationships acting between descriptors in a phase relate concepts to one another and in this manner create the concept-relationship network that defines the design intent.

Each phase type has its own descriptors. Descriptors for the form phase include the geometric and material attributes inherent to the design artefact. Examples include geometric parameters such as length and width; topological primitives like face, edge, or vertex; and material attributes like density and Young's Modulus. Descriptors for the behaviour phase are derived attributes that involve an external disturbance acting on the concept. Examples of this type of descriptor include weight, motion, deflection, *etc.* Descriptors for the function phase describe the intended use of the concept and include machine element types such as lever, gear, bearing-surface, *etc.* Table 1 shows examples of descriptors for the three phases.

Table 1. Examples of descriptors for function, behaviour, and form phases

Form Phase	Behavioural Phase	Functional Phase
Inherent attributes	Derived attributes	Intended use
• length, diameter	• weight	• lever
• face, edge, vertex	• motion	• gear
• density, Young's Modulus	• deformation, temperature	• bearing-surface

3.4 Concept Structure

The concept structure is the basic building element used in the synthesis of a design solution. A concept entity can be thought of as a design feature in that it identifies a part or region of a design that has special significance to the designer. The specific nature of this significance is dependent on the context in which the design is examined. For instance, a concept might have significance related to its performance or ability to achieve its design functions. Examples of this type of design significance might include: resistance to plastic deformation under an applied load, rate of heat dissipation, or motion due to an applied force. Alternatively, a concept might be significant from the perspective of downstream considerations like manufacturing or assembly. Examples of concepts that are explicitly significant to downstream processes include locating-pins and bosses. A designer might create these features explicitly for the purposes of the downstream assembly process. More problematic are features related to downstream constraints that are emergent. These are features that are not explicitly created for downstream processes but rather emerge from the form associated with an existing concept or combination of concepts. Examples of emergent features can include undercuts or thin-walled sections that may pose problems for machining processes. The designer may not be able to recognize this type of feature a priori.

Since geometry and material properties are simply one aspect of a general concept entity (specifically that of form), and the operations of constructing geometric models and assigning material properties as instantiating relationships between concept entities, then the typical form-driven method of design can be understood as a process of instantiating and structuring concept entities. In our model of artefact information, a concept can be related to other concepts via relationships that act within one phase of the design artefact information space, as well as through relationships that act across different phases. In terms of its physical form, a concept is represented by its relationships within the form phase.

3.5 Relationships

Design is a process of generating knowledge. From an initial body of design artefact information, which might include design requirements and constraints, the designer creates new instances of artefact information and defines relationships between these information structures, to create knowledge about the design artefact. There are two types of relationships: inter-phasic and intra-phasic. While inter-phasic relationships only act within a concept, intra-phasic relationships exist both within concepts as well as across concept boundaries. An example of an inter-phasic relationship between the functional and behavioural phases would be several behaviours that combine to achieve a single function. An example of an intra-phasic relationship within a single concept would be several sub-functions that combine to create an overall function. An example of an intra-phasic relationship acting between two concepts would be the causal effect of the behaviour of one concept on the behaviour of another concept.

Figure 2 illustrates how inter- and intra-phasic relationships can be used to define more complex concept structures. In the example shown below, Concept-1 and Concept-2 are linked by two intra-phasic relationships, R1 and R2. Similar relationships are shown between Concept-1 and Concept-3. R1 is a causal relationship between a behaviour in Concept-1 and a behaviour in Concept-2, and R2 is a topological relationship between the two concepts' respective physical embodiments. In addition, similar relationships can be defined between Concept-1 and Concept-3. The resulting set of concepts linked by relationships creates a network. One interpretation for the concept-relationship network described is that of two linkages (Concept-2 and Concept-3) connected by a pin joint (Concept-1). Figure 3 depicts a possible physical embodiment for two simple linkages connected by a pin joint.

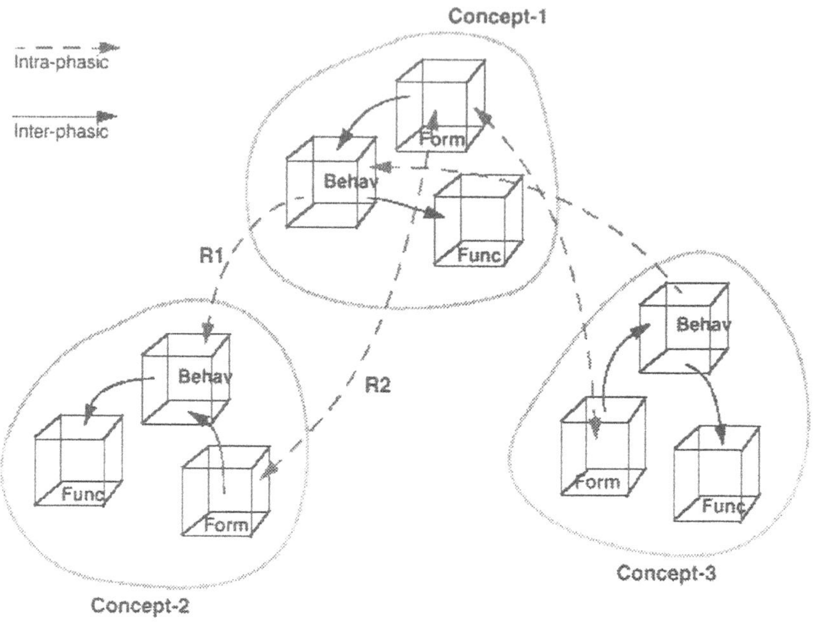

Figure 2. Intra-phasic relationships act between concepts as well as within concepts, while inter-phasic relationships act only within concepts

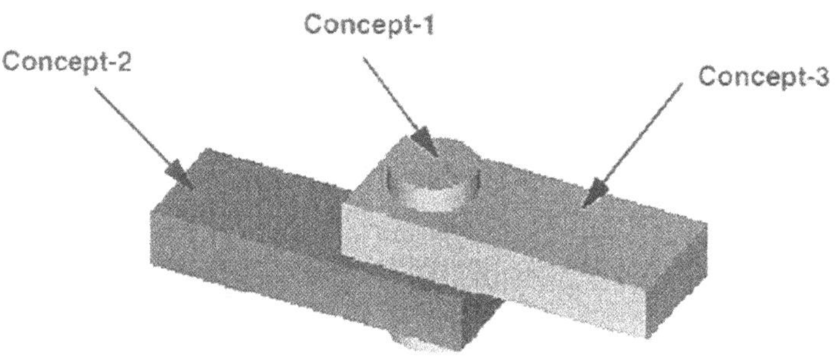

Figure 3. Two linkage arms connected with a pin joint, interpreted in terms of the concept-relationship network in Figure 2

The designer generates a concept to address a particular design requirement or constraint, and embeds the new concept within the evolving design context by defining its relationships to other concepts. As the design process proceeds, the designer refines and modifies the concept-relationship network, adding detail to concept descriptions and relationships. We have found that designers generate and work with concepts in a heterogeneous manner, in terms of function and behaviour, as well as form. These three aspects of the design are sub-sets of the information contained within three distinct phases of the total space of design artefact information. The relationships instantiated as part of design create a network of concepts across the different phases, as well as a hierarchy of abstraction within each phase.

4. IMPLEMENTATION

The architecture for our computational environment is built around a design modelling kernel, which plays the same role within the design environment as the solid-modelling kernel does within many existing CAD systems. The primary difference between the two kernels is that solid-modelling kernels are meant to model the geometry and topology of solids, whereas our design modelling kernel extends the capabilities of the solid-modelling kernel to model the knowledge about functional and behavioural intent that sets the context of a design. Simulation capabilities are provided by external modules that access the design data-model through its interfaces. For the initial prototype, only two interfaces are provided: a direct interface to the data-model through the public data members and methods of the object classes, and a formal application protocol interface.

4.1 The Modelling Kernel

The design modelling kernel provides a set of core object classes and interfaces to the data and methods within these classes. The object classes within the design modelling kernel include those that one would expect to find in a solid-modelling kernel (*e.g.*, object classes such as body, shell, edges, vertex, sphere, plane, and point). These topological and geometric classes provide the capabilities needed to describe the design in terms of its form phase, as well as the basic geometric functionality of the modelling kernel. The design-modelling kernel extends the solid-modelling capabilities with the addition of object classes for composing the functional and behavioural knowledge structures that define the intent behind the physical embodiment of the design.

In our prototype implementation, we use the ACIS solid-modelling kernel by Spatial Technologies, Inc. (STI, 1997). ACIS is based on a non-manifold boundary representation. We use ACIS's ability to represent bodies of mixed dimensionality to provide the capability of modelling the abstract knowledge structures alongside the physical form. Furthermore, the ability to represent non-manifold bodies is a requirement for a modelling environment that supports design at heterogeneous levels of abstraction.

A three-dimensional graphical interface for the design modelling environment is needed to support an interactive design experience that promotes exploration of design concepts. The current 3D mouse-based interface allows the designer to construct the design model within a GUI framework similar to the interface for existing 3D solid modellers. Standard views such as isometric and the different orthographic projections are provided, along with various camera tools for zooming, panning, and orbit. The design model can be either viewed as a wireframe or rendered object. (See Figure 4.) OpenGL provides the basic rendering functions (Woo *et al.*, 1997). The interface also allows the user to maintain multiple windows showing different views of the model space (*i.e.*, views of the form, function, and behaviour spaces) as well as views of results from multiple application modules (*i.e.*, views of results from the model construction and model simulation modules). Changes to the model space are automatically updated in all open views. Finally, a range of GUI tools for model creation, editing and manipulation are provided, including: selection, cut, paste, rotation, dragging, Boolean operations, blending of edges, and importing existing models.

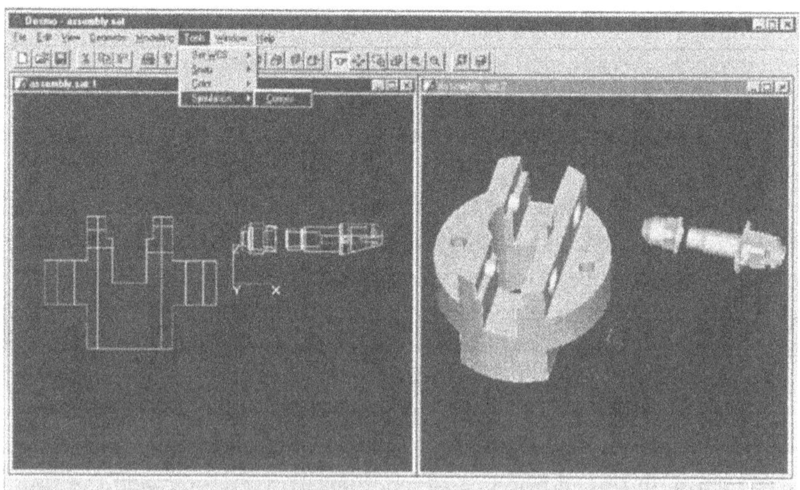

Figure 4. A graphical interface for model construction

4.2 Simulation Modules

The difficulty of creating an analytical model of a design from the knowledge available in existing design modelling frameworks (*i.e.*, solid-modelling information) remains an obstacle to the use of simulation for exploring concepts in early design. Our design modelling kernel supports simulation by representing the high-level knowledge about design intent needed to guide the process of abstracting from a geometric model to an analytical model. The knowledge is modelled by the designer as part of the design process because the designer is able to compose the design model in terms of function and behaviour as well as form.

Simulation modules have two roles: they provide an analysis of behaviour to allow evaluation of a completed design, and they provide the capability to increase the scope of the conversation between the design and the designer through interaction with an evolving design concept's behaviour. These two roles require a different degree of linkage between the module in the design modelling environment that handles model creation, and the module(s) that provide the simulation functionality.

Most modelling systems support only a uni-directional flow of information from the design data-model to the simulation data-model. In this case, the high-level knowledge within the design data-model facilitates the process of abstracting from the design model to the simulation model. The second type of linkage requires an interface that supports a bi-directional flow of information between the construction and simulation modules. The information flow is bi-directional because the simulation module must be able to retrieve current state information about a design from the design data-model and to effect changes to the design model based on the results of a simulation. The two scenarios for linking the design construction and simulation modules are shown in Figures 5 and 6 below.

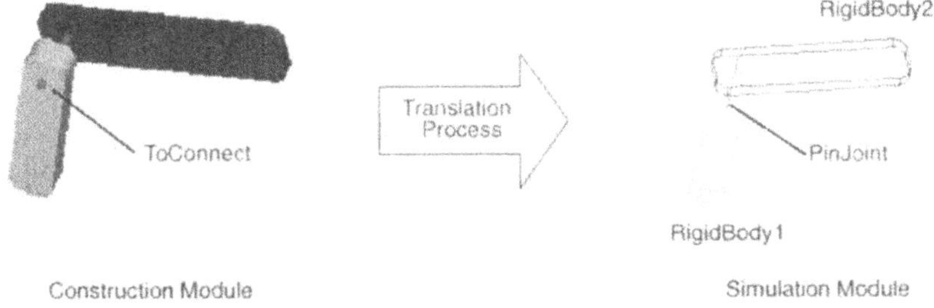

Figure 5. Capturing knowledge to facilitate intelligent model abstraction

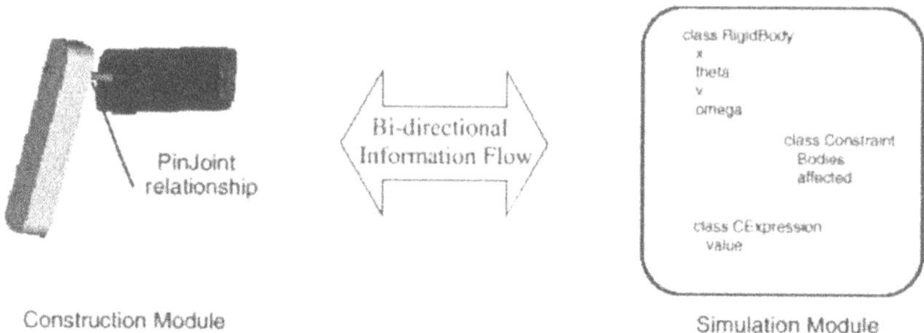

Figure 6. Supporting design within an active simulation

The data-model itself cannot guarantee the consistency of the knowledge structures created by the designer. Knowledge structures can be inconsistent and/or incorrect in a number of ways: a causal relationship may be incorrect (*e.g.*, a behaviour does not cause another behaviour), an implementation relationship may be incorrect (*e.g.*, a part cannot achieve an intended behaviour), and an accumulation may be incorrect (*e.g.*, a set of functions does not contribute to an overall function). It is expected that this type of analysis, to verify consistency, will be performed by one class of simulation module.

The rational for separating consistency checking from the basic modelling framework is that this arrangement most closely resembles the situation that occurs during mental simulation (unaided by computer). For example, in the case where a designer is working without the aid of a computer, a design concept that is generated remains untested (and essentially unproven) until it is physically realized. There the designer cannot know that the form of the design will behave as intended or that the given behaviour will achieve the intended function. The designer gains confidence in the correctness of the design as simulations at successively lower levels of abstraction are performed - from mental simulations through to testing on the final physical prototype. Similarly within a computational design environment, simulation is needed to verify the correctness of the design model.

4.3 A Data-model for Design Artefact Knowledge

Our data-model explicitly represents the functional and behavioural knowledge that defines the intent behind the physical embodiment of a design. Our design data-model represents the structure of the knowledge and the relationships between these structures, which are the basis of design intent. These structures and relationships are normally generated as part of the process in early design.

A design data-model is an improvement over existing data-models based on solid modelling because in the early stages of conceptualisation a design feature may exist in the mind of the designer as an abstract notion of desired functionality or behaviour. Solid modelling representations force the designer to commit to one physical interpretation of these concepts. Design concepts are generated in terms of function and behaviour as well as form. Our data-model allows the designer to model the intended function and behaviour of the design through composition of design features. Another benefit of a data-model, which is not based on a representation of solids, is more strategic. Specifically, knowledge about design intent is useful in all downstream activities that involve abstraction of the design model. By extending the representation of the design model to include intent as well as form, we provide the basic infrastructure to support knowledge intensive downstream processes.

In our data-model, a design model is composed of concepts (Concept_Entity). Concepts have three aspects, or phases that define the concept in terms of its intended function, behaviour and form. These are defined in the data-model as the Function_Entity, Behaviour_Entity, and Form_Entity object classes. Because the designer concepts design to address specific issues or requirements, concepts can be thought of as being analogous to design features. Like design features, concepts may address multiple functions. The different functions may be associated with different domains (*e.g.*, structural, thermal, kinematic domains). Since functions are realized through behaviours, concepts may therefore also possess multiple behaviours of interest from more than one domain.

4.3.1 Function Entity

Our representation for function has three requirements: it cannot be dependent on the pre-existence of a model of behaviour or form, it should relate to models of behaviour, and the individual function structures should be composable. Previous work in function representation has addressed some, but not all of the three above requirements simultaneously. Chandrasekaran's Functional Representation (Chandrasekaran, 1994) represents active functions in terms of state changes. However, little work has been done on its applicability to passive functions such as that of a column supporting a structural load. Furthermore, the Functional Representation framework models function at the device level and do not include the idea of functional composition. (Hodges, 1992) addresses part of the problem of creating more complex functions by assembling simpler functional entities, for certain classes of devices. He classifies functions in terms of a hierarchy of general machine elements like linkage, lever, wheel-axle, and gear. However, because his scheme defines functions as sequences of behavioural primitives, the approach requires that a behavioural model of the design be created prior to the functional model.

Our design data-model for representing functional knowledge assumes that, at a high level of abstraction, relationships can be specified between functions and between functions and concepts. At lower levels of abstraction, the interaction between concepts may be specified to occur through regions of space defined by abstractions of form. Because these regions of space are abstractions of physical form, they are not necessarily manifold. Yet, even at this relatively high level of geometric abstraction, sufficient information has been specified to transform a strictly functional concept into one that includes an aspect of behaviour. For example, the control function of a component that allows a chair-back to tilt relative to the seat may act on the chair-back through a shared axis of rotation. The axis of rotation might be represented by a topological entity such as wire or edge. As such, an axis of rotation would be part of the form aspect of a concept. The specification of the axis of rotation assumes a behaviour (*i.e.*, revolute) that is intended to achieve the controlling function. For this reason, the function class object maintains only direct links to other function objects or concepts.

At a high level of abstraction, relationships between functions are of two types: hierarchical and temporal. Hierarchical relationships are maintained through parent and children descriptors. Temporal relationships are maintained through the antecedent and subsequent descriptors. Relationships between functions at lower levels of abstraction, where form comes into play, occur through the function's associated behaviour instance. We will elaborate on these regions of interaction later in this chapter when we discuss representation of the behaviour entity.

4.3.2 Behaviour Entity

A Behaviour Entity object models a part of the intended behaviour of a particular design concept. It is possible for a design concept to have multiple behaviours belonging to different domains and appearing under different conditions. A behaviour entity is meant to support an arbitrary description of behaviour. Like the Function Entity, a model of behaviour should not be dependent on a pre-existing functional model of the design. This allows the design to move forward in a heterogeneous manner. However, since designed behaviour is the mechanism by which a function is achieved, behaviour's relationship to its associated function needs to be maintained. In mechanical artefacts, behaviour is closely tied to form. We need to be able to identify the parts of the form that are associated with a behaviour. These parts may or may not be physically realizable depending on the current level of development of the design. Behaviour is described both in terms of state transformation between initial and final states, as well as in terms of information flow given by the direction of the relationships joining the different entities within the concept/relationship structure.

A behaviour interacts with external entities (other concepts) through its form phase. The interface for this interaction within the behaviour object is provided by the Region Entity object. Instances of the Region object describe the source and destination regions of interaction for a behaviour. The distinction between source and destination regions allows a causal relationship to be created in those cases where a direction of flow exists in the model of the behaviour. For example, Figure 7 below shows a revolute kinematic behaviour entity connecting two links. If link-A is driving link-B, the source region for the revolute behaviour is the interface between link-A and the revolute. Depending on the level of abstraction, the region of interaction may be a common axis of rotation or the mating faces between the hole in link-A and the surface of the revolute. Similarly, the destination region is the interface between link-B and the revolute.

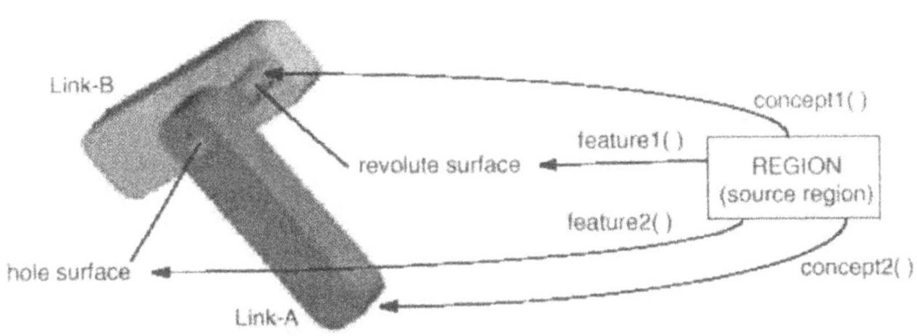

Figure 7. Link-A driving Link-B through a revolute behaviour entity

The Behaviour Entity also maintains a description of its initial and final states using a State Entity object. A State Entity contains the set of parameter and value pairs used to describe a behaviour. Parameter/value pairs are stored as a linked list of instances of classes derived from a common base class, which provides the basic naming and linking methods. The derived classes enable multiple types of parameters to be stored on the same list. The each State Entity has a pointer back to its owning behaviour.

4.3.3 Form Entity

The Form aspect of a concept is based on a boundary-representation topological model. The B-rep model specifies the spatial relationships of geometric elements used to represent the boundary of an object. Using the topological elements of the B-rep model, the geometry of physical and non-physical features within the design can be represented within the same model. Examples of non-physical design features of interest are:

- centre-lines - *e.g.* for locating centres of holes, axes of rotation,
- paths - *e.g.* for defining motion paths, sweep,
- faces - *e.g.* for indicating contact surfaces or regions of interaction.

The top-level object within the form aspect of a concept is the Body Entity. Starting from the root body, the B-rep hierarchy can be traversed to locate the position of all the geometric features of the model in space.

5. DEMONSTRATION OF CONCEPT

The construction of a revolute joint connecting two links is used to illustrate how the functional and behavioural model can be built alongside the geometric model of a design concept. The process begins with the designer creating three concepts: one for the revolute behaviour and two for the links. (See Figure 8.) Initially, the concept entities have no form, behaviour, or function associated with them. The designer is free to develop each aspect of a design concept in a heterogeneous manner. As shown in Figure 8, the designer may choose to refine the form aspect of the link concepts, without refining that of the third concept entity. One possible reason for this may be that the designer is primarily concerned with the length of the links and wishes to ensure that they do not interfere with other objects in the surrounding area. At this point in the process, the designer is not concerned with the form of the design concept connecting the links. Rather, he/she is solely interested in the connecting concept's behaviour as a kinematic pair. The designer adds a kinematic behaviour to the third concept entity (Figure 9) and further defines its relationship with the two links.

Specifically the designer identifies the lines-lines for axes of rotation on the two links as the source and destination feature regions for the kinematic pair, and adds a Control function to the concept entity. At this point, the designer is able to start a kinematic simulation tool (Baraff, 1995) attached to the modelling environment and to load the design model into the simulation module. The simulation module creates a specialized simulation model from the design data-model using the knowledge about function and behaviour, which is represented along side the form elements.

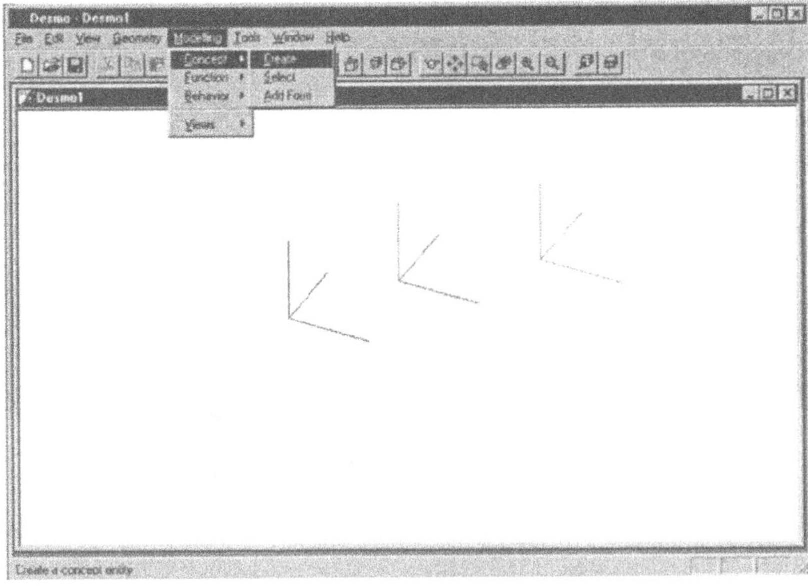

Figure 8. Three concept entities, each represented by a local coordinate frame

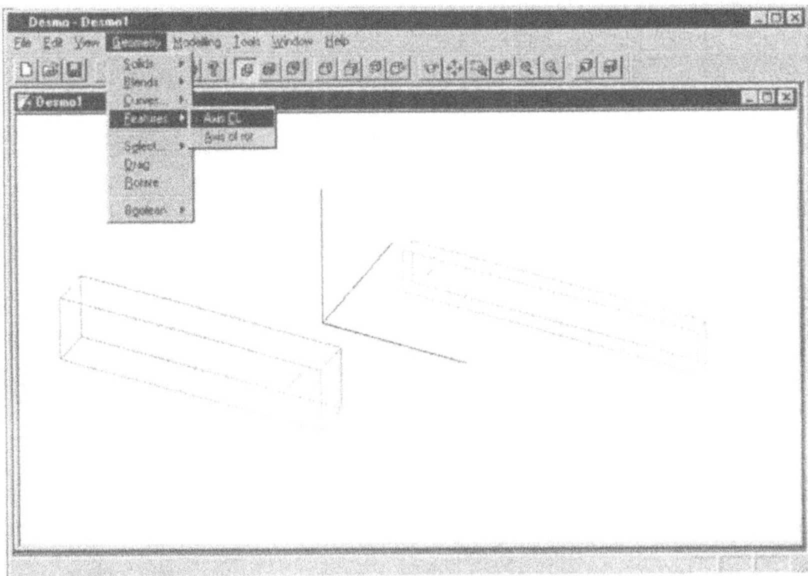

Figure 9. Form refinement of the two concepts representing links

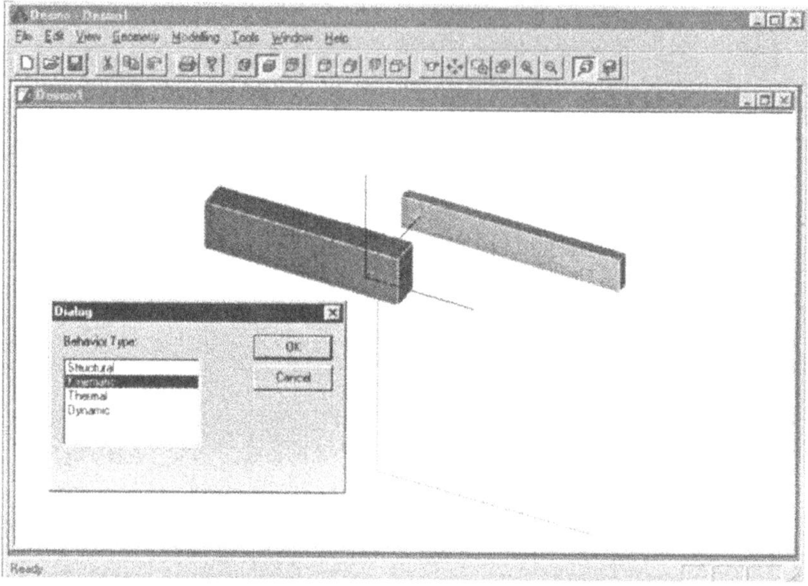

Figure 10. Adding kinematic behaviour to the third concept and making relationships to the link entities

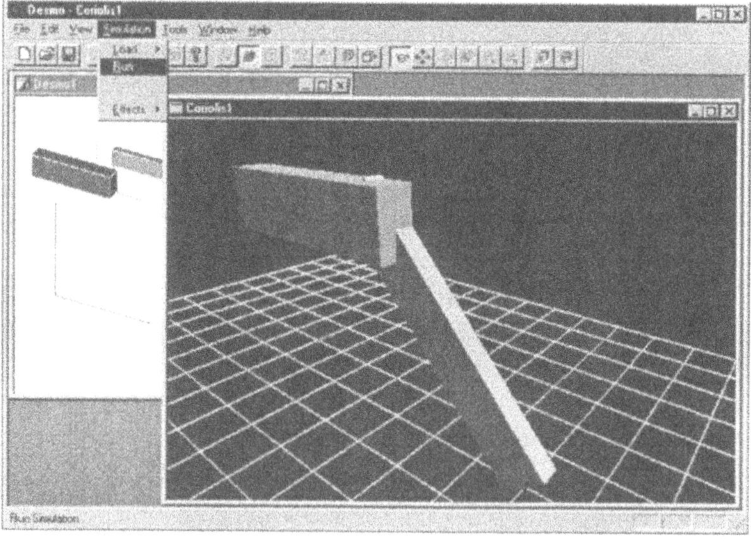

Figure 11. Running a Coriolis simulation

6. CONCLUSIONS

We note that among existing computer-aided engineering tools, the purpose of CAD tools is to construct the geometry that is used as input to downstream analysis tools. For this reason, the capabilities of current CAD tools are not suited for exploring concepts in the early stages of design, and their underlying data-models of the design artefact do not support the explicit representation of knowledge that describes the function and behaviour of a design. To address this deficiency we have developed a data-model and an architecture for a computational design environment that support the modelling of explicit high-level knowledge about design artefact function and behaviour and the reuse of this knowledge by downstream processes.

A reflective-interactive methodology for design leads to a set of requirements for design tools that are not met by current CAD systems. These requirements include the ability to model knowledge that describes the design context, a closer relationship between the construction and simulation of a design model, and a relaxation of the manner in which design models are constructed. The reflective-interactive methodology offers the opportunity for, and a mechanism through which, design context can be captured as part of the normal process of designing. The framework for capturing and representing the functional and behavioural knowledge consists of a data-model. The basis for the methodology is a synthetic and exploratory model of reasoning in design. The synthetic model explains the process for formulating an initial problem statement, it is better suited to early design when the problem and the solution space are ill-defined, and it fits in within the broader theory of knowledge building as the primary product of the design process.

REFERENCES

Allen, C., (1989) "Situated Design," Master's thesis, Design Studies, Carnegie-Mellon University, Pittsburgh, PA.

Baraff, D., (1995) "Interactive Simulation of Solid Rigid Bodies," *IEEE Computer Graphics and Applications*, Vol. 15, No. 3, pp. 63-75.

Baya, V. and Leifer, L. J., (1994) "A Study of Information Handling Behavior of Designers During Conceptual Design," *Design Theory and Methodology - DTM'94*, American Society of Mechanical Engineers, Minneapolis, MN, pp. 153-168.

Chan, B., (1998) Supporting *Conceptual Design: A Methodology and Infrastructure for CAD*, PhD dissertation, Civil Engineering, Carnegie Mellon University, Pittsburgh, PA.

Chandrasekaran, B., (1994) "Functional Representation: A Brief Historical Perspective," *Applied Artificial Intelligence*, Vol. 8, pp. 173-197.

Dorst, K. and Dijkhuis, J., (1995) "Comparing Paradigms for Describing Design Activity," *Design Studies*, Vol. 16, No. 2, pp. 261-274.

Faltings, B., (1992) "Supporting Creativity in Symbolic Computation," *Proceedings of the 2nd International Conference on Computational Models of Creative Design*, J. S. Gero and F. Sudweeks, ed., University of Sydney, Sydney, Australia, pp. 191-206.

Ganeshan, R., Garrett, J. and Finger, S., (1992) "A Framework for Representing Design Intent," *Design Studies*, Vol 15, No 1, pp. 59-84.

Gero J. and Kazakov V. A., (1996) "An Exploration-Based Evolutionary Model of a Generative Design Process," *Microcomputers in Civil Engineering*, Vol. 11, pp. 211-218.

Hakim, M., (1993) Modeling *Evolving Information about Design Engineering Products*, PhD dissertation, Civil Engineering, Carnegie Mellon University, Pittsburgh, PA.

Hodges, J., (1992) "Naive Mechanisms," *IEEE Expert*, pp. 14-27.

Poon, J. and Maher, M. L., (1997) "Co-evolution and Emergence in Design," *Artificial Intelligence in Engineering*, Vol. 11, No. 3, pp. 319-327.

Reddy, J. M., (1996) Building *and Reuse of Artifact Theories: A View of Design and its Implications for Computational Environments*, PhD dissertation, Civil & Environmental Engineering, Carnegie Mellon University, Pittsburgh, PA.

Reddy, J. M., Chan, B. and Finger, S., (1996) "Patterns in Design Discourse: A Case Study," *Knowledge Intensive CAD*, Volume 1, Chapman & Hall, London, 1996, pp. 265-283.

Schön (1983) Schön, D. A., *The Reflective Practitioner*, Harper-Collins, New York.

SEED (1997) SEED, "SEED: A Software Environment to Support Early Phases in Building Design," *International Journal for Design Computing*.

Shaw *et al.* (1989) Shaw, N. K., Bloor, M. S. and de Pennington, A., "Product Data Models," *Research in Engineering Design*, Vol. 1, No. 1, pp. 43-50.

Smithers and Troxell (1990) Smithers, T. and Troxell, W., "Design is Intelligent Behavior, But What's the Formalism?" *Artificial Intelligence for Engineering Design, Analysis and Manufacturing*, Vol. 4, No. 2, pp. 89-98.

STI (1997) STI, "ACIS 3D Toolkit – Modeling Primer, Version 3," Spatial Technologies, Inc., Boulder, CO.

Subrahmanian, E., Konda, S. L., Levy, S. N., Reich, Y. and Westerberg, A. W., (1993) "Equations Aren't Enough: Informal Modeling in Design," *Artificial Intelligence in Engineering Design, Analysis and Manufacturing*, Vol. 7, No. 4, pp. 257-74.

Tanir, O., Agarwal, V. K. and Bhatt, P. C. P., (1993) "System Design Exploration in a Specification Driven Simulation Environment," *Proceedings of the 1993 European Simulation Symposium*, Verbraeck, A.; Kerckhoffs, E. J. H., ed., Society for Computer Simulation, Delft, Netherlands, pp. 591-596.

Tomiyama, T., Kiriyama, T., Takeda, H., Xue, D. and Yoshikawa, H., (1989) "Metamodel: A Key to Intelligent CAD Systems," *Research in Engineering Design*, Vol. 1, No. 1, pp. 19-34.

Woo, M., Neider, J. L. and Davis, T. R., (1997) OpenGL *Programming Guide*, 2nd Edition, A-W Developers Press.

11

A Knowledge Based Engineering Application to Support Weight Distribution Analysis for IRL Cars

L. Susca[1], F. Mandorli[2], C. Rizzi[1], and U. Cugini[1]
[1]*Dipartimento di Ingegneria Industriale, Universita' degli Studi di Parma*
[2]*Dipartimento di Meccanica, Universita' degli Studi di Ancona*

Key words: Knowledge based engineering, configuration system, weight distribution

Abstract: Knowledge based engineering is a technology whose aim is to provide tools to develop vertical applications which can integrate different types of knowledge representation within a common model and carry out model evaluation, modification and updating. This paper presents a knowledge based engineering application to support the design of Indy Racing League (IRL) cars. The IRL Championship is regulated by a very strict set of technical specifications, which limit the designer as far as car structure and sizes of the parts are concerned. For this reason it is very important to evaluate the effects of modifying main design parameters on the car configuration. The first part of the paper describes how Dallara's know-how on IRL car design has been re-organized with specific reference to the problem of weight distribution. This has led to the definition of a hierarchical IRL car model containing the fundamental parameters for weight computation. In the second part the use of examples highlights that different types of knowledge representation are necessary to compute weights distribution. The final part contains the description of the prototype implemented by using results from the previous phases. Comparing the results obtained with experimental data has validated the application.

1. INTRODUCTION

In mechanical engineering various design problems can be seen as configuration tasks, i.e., the overall structure and the design/manufacturing process of a family of products is already known, but, time after time, the designer has to select the right solution among possible alternatives in order to define the family member which meets specific requirements.

The designer has to quickly and accurately select the most desirable choices from hundreds or thousands options and instantly understand the implication on the final product of each selection in terms of cost, component incompatibility, mandatory requirements, performances, and manufacturing and delivery constraints.

In general, to evaluate several possible alternatives, the designer has to manage different information typologies, concerning many product aspects (e.g., machining processes, marketing perspectives, physical resources, properties of materials, engineering design). Thanks to personal expertise and knowledge about the problem the designer is able to evaluate the best solution intuitively; this solution then needs to be verified before it can become operative.

While developing a decision support system for a configuration problem (AIEDAM 1998), a key aspect is the definition of a suitable knowledge base containing all the different types (declarative, procedural, control) and forms (tables, geometry, functions, etc.) of the knowledge required, organized into a structured product model. This product model becomes the kernel of the system and the designer can inquire it in order to have feedback on feasible alternative solutions.

In this work we describe a system which supports a configuration problem related to the design of Indy Racing League (IRL) cars. The developed knowledge-based application is able to evaluate different configurations of the car and resulting distribution of weight, a key parameter to evaluate car performances.

The paper presents underlying philosophy and motivations that guided the development of the system; it also describes how Dallara's know-how on IRL car design has been re-organized with specific reference to the problem of weight distribution. This phase of the analysis has led to the definition of a hierarchical IRL car model where atomic components have been described in terms of a set of significant properties, and grouped to form hierarchical sub-assemblies.

Examples are also utilized to show how different types of knowledge representation are necessary to compute weight distribution. The final part is about the prototype implemented by using results from the previous phases. The prototype was developed using Selling Point by Concentra (Concentra

1995) and validated by comparing the results obtained with experimental data.

2. MOTIVATIONS AND OBJECTIVES

A new racing car championship was introduced in 1996: the Indy Racing League (IRL) championship is held on oval circuits in the US. Its aim is to allow teams with a limited budget to participate in the race. A very strict set of technical specifications was established (Indy, 1996), and the number of car producers has been limited to two engine producers, two tire suppliers, and two manufacturers for the chassis and the bodywork. Dallara, an Italian company involved in the production of racing cars, is one of the chassis and bodywork producers.

In order to beat competitors, designers have to define specific sub-goals that directly concern some product features and guarantee the achievements of the original aims. For example, in order to improve car performances in acceleration and deceleration the designer can work on brakes and engine power, or he/she can lighten the car. The two alternative solutions produce the same main result, but in very different ways and with different secondary consequences (e.g., changing the material to lighten a part requires verifying that new mechanical properties assure structural resistance under stress conditions). Moreover, other constraints must be verified, such as functionality of the part, compatibility between the new material and other ones used, relationships among parts, machining and so on.

In this paper we have focused the attention on the critical problem which deals with the impact of design decisions on the car weight distribution.

Traditionally design alternatives are evaluated by performing simulation on a scale model of the car. It is evident how expensive and time consuming this solution is in respect with car weight distribution analysis (all parts should be included in the model).

On the other hand, CAD systems are useful for detailed and realistic geometric representation of one o more parts, but they are not suitable for complex structures involving "fusion" of different knowledge contexts (geometric, functional, technological...). For these reasons, the designer usually evaluates different car configurations relying on his/her own experience and knowledge of car structure and the effects of modifying design parameters on all sub-assemblies.

In such a context our objective has been the development of a decision support system able to evaluate the weight distribution for different design solutions of an IRL car. The system should support the designer and allows him configuring the car and evaluating consequent weight distribution.

The interaction between the system and the designer generates a loop (Figure 1), in which the operator provides alternative ideas (possible car configurations) and the computer evaluates car asset and weight distribution of the current solution. The output from the designer (values of independent parameters) is the input for the computer, which uses the data to configure the model. At the same time the output from the computer (car asset) is the input for the designer, who interprets the results and re-considers the initial hypothesis to move towards an optimum solution.

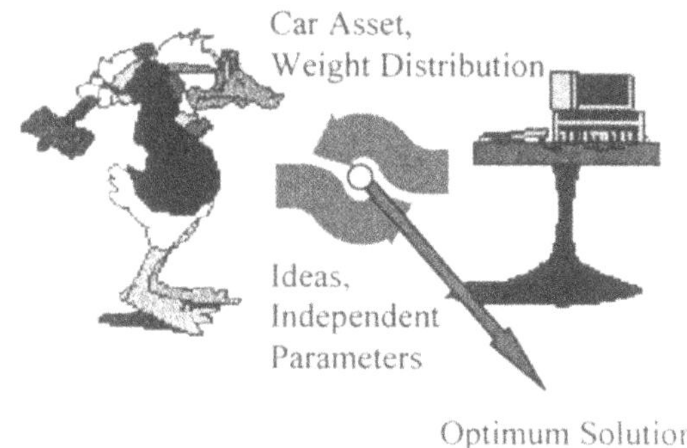

Figure 1. Computer-man interaction

To address such a problem, different types of knowledge need to be managed and related to each other. Knowledge based engineering technology can be used since it provides the tools to represent the designer's decision making process, integrate different types of knowledge within a common model and carry out model evaluation, modification and updating (Cornet 1991, Kariko-Buhwezi 1995, Di Lecce 1997, and Mandorli 1997).

A KBE shell is a development tool made of: a proprietary Object Oriented (OO) language to define the product model, a tracer to support the debugging activity, a set of drivers to communicate with external data base, and a set of libraries to integrate the model within other available tools for the user interface development (e.g. Visual Basic, Visual C++).

Libraries of basic objects are supplied with the shell in order to provide basic functionality to the language. These libraries contains objects that can be roughly grouped into the following categories: objects to handle series of clones, objects implementing methods to access external data bases, objects implementing calls to a geometric modeler and objects to handle input/output functionality.

The OO language allows the user to define models, which represent the product in terms of its basic components and their following aggregation in functional sub-systems down to the complete system. Each model component is defined by its name and a set of property/expression couples representing respectively the name of a property and the property value. The expressions can be any valid sentence of the language. These expressions are usually called "rules", but notice that in KBE context, the word "rule" does not have the traditional meaning used in Artificial Intelligence, but it is considered as a symbolic relationship among several properties of the parts).

These symbolic expressions (that can represent appropriated dimensioning, positioning, analyses relationships among properties of the model components) represent the model parameterization and define the model behavior when a property changes.

The shell provides the mechanisms, which update and check properties consistence. These mechanisms are called *Demand Driven Processing* and *Dependency Backtracking* (notice that a KBE does not have an inference engine). The Demand Driven Processing mechanism checks that the properties of a model are calculated only when they are explicitly required. The Dependency Backtracking mechanism automatically updates all the properties that depend on a modified one.

The kernel of a KAE application is then a hierarchical structure representing the product model in terms of its part and sub-parts defined by all their significant properties, related to each other by appropriated symbolic expressions. It is important to notice that, thanks to the flexibility provided by the KAE shell, a KAE application can represent the product related knowledge in all of its required forms (See Figure 2).

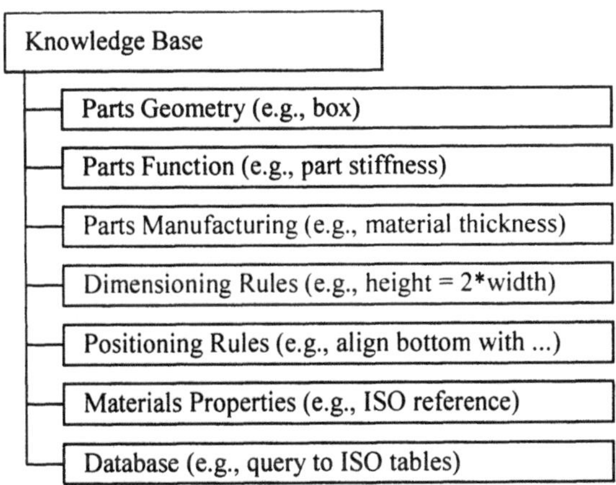

Figure 2. Different forms of Knowledge representation in a KAE application

Following sections contain a detailed description of the knowledge required to address the problem of weight distribution, and how it has been structured into the developed KAE-based model.

3. STRUCTURE OF THE IRL CAR MODEL

A hierarchical model of an IRL car, containing all types of data (shapes, materials, part positioning, standard components) which are relevant for the correct computation of weight distribution, has been defined.

The IRL car structure has been studied in order to identify sub-assemblies and parameters that are significant for the weight evaluation. This activity was carried out in close collaboration with Dallara engineers who provided their know-how on the problem.

The model hierarchy reflects the functional sub-assemblies, which constitute the car. The parameters needed to carry out the correct evaluation of weight distribution have been identified for each sub-assembly and related to each other.

Several sub-systems have been analyzed: the bodywork, the chassis, the front and rear wings, fuel, water, oil and exhaust systems, pedal, steering and wheel assembly, etc. (see Figs. 3-5).

One of the most important parts is the chassis. It is made of composite material and its shape is defined by the geometry of four bulkheads (Figure 4), dimensioned and positioned within ranges imposed by the league's technical specifications.

The shape of the four bulkheads also defines the main cross sections of the chassis: the first bulkhead (front bulkhead, Figure 4-1) is positioned as interface between the front part of the chassis and the front wing. The second bulkhead (pedal bulkhead, Figure 4-2) is positioned close to the pedals. The technical specifications place constraints on the minimal cross section in this area and the distance from the front bulkhead.

The third bulkhead (dashboard bulkhead, Figure 4-3) is positioned close to the dashboard area. The dashboard bulkhead has a central cut for the driver's legs. The dimensions of this cut are fixed by the league's specifications. This bulkhead also provides support for the steering column. The last bulkhead (seatback bulkhead, Figure 4-4) is positioned behind the driver's seat.

The tank is located behind the seatback bulkhead, into the space between the seat and the engine. The back part of the chassis is constrained by the shape of the engine and there are no particular specifications for this part, as just two types of engine are allowed.

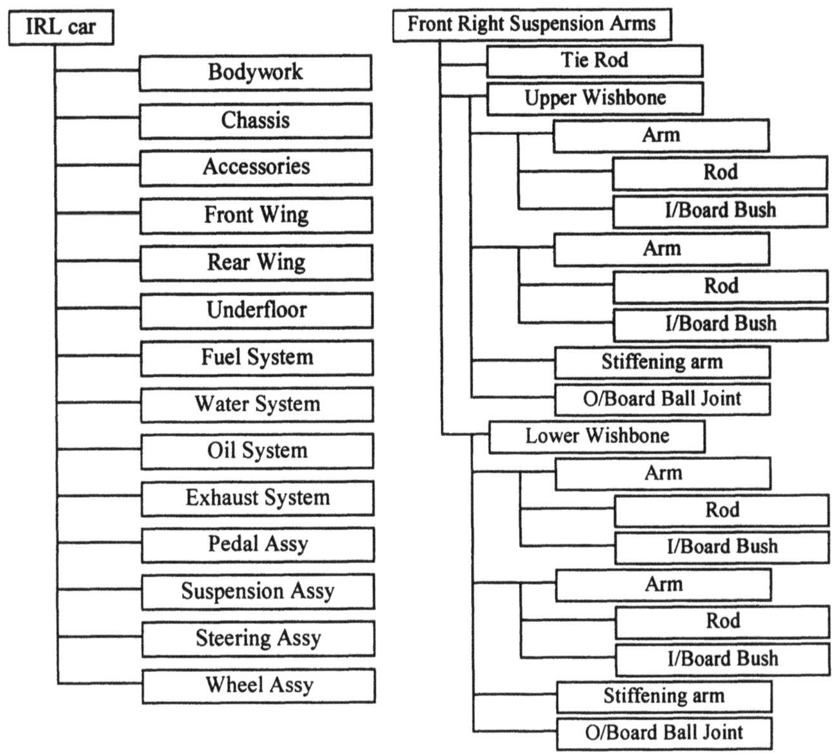

Figure 3. First level of car hierarchical structure and suspension arms assembly structure

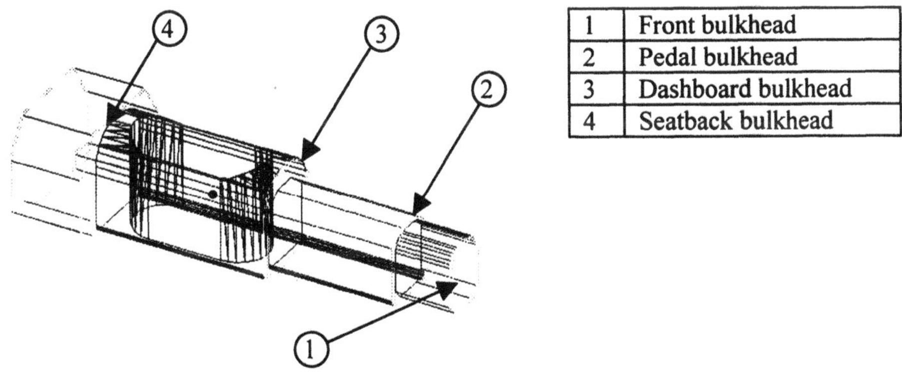

Figure 4. Chassis structure with bulkheads

However, there are specifications to constrain the shape of the underfloor, which must be flat, at least 1778 mm long, with a maximum angle of 5° from the engine interface to the pedal bulkhead and 10° from the pedal bulkhead to the car nose.

The engine, the bellhousing and the gearbox make up the back part of the car. Those parts also provide interfaces to connect other sub-assemblies, such as the suspensions.

Suspensions have been carefully analyzed because different suspension configurations may generate different weight distribution and therefore different car attitudes.

A tie rod and a couple of wishbones make up the suspension arms. The base vertices of the wishbones are fixed with spherical joints respectively to the chassis (front suspensions) and to the bellhousing and the gearbox (rear suspensions); the opposite vertex is fixed to the hub carrier. The front suspension arms have an additional stiffening rod located between the wishbones.

Notice that the bases of the upper and lower wishbones of the front suspension arms may be different in size. However, the wishbone vertices need to be aligned because they define the wheels' vertical axis of rotation for the steering and the toe-in. The damper and the antirolling systems are directly connected to the suspension arms' assembly.

Figure 3 (tree on the right) shows the hierarchical structure of the sub-assembly representing the front right suspension arms.

4. WEIGHT AND CENTER OF MASS COMPUTATION

The weight of the different components that make up an assembly or sub-assembly can be computed in different ways: from data bases storing sizes of standard parts (e.g., spherical joints) provided by external suppliers; from data bases containing experimental results; from the computation of formulas containing references to the size, material, and position of other parts.

In the following we report, as an example, the weight computation of some of the components mentioned in the previous section.

Theoretically, the weight of the chassis is computed as follows:

$$P = \int_S \left[\left(d_{\mathrm{honeycomb}} \cdot s_{honeycomb} \right) + \left(d_C \cdot s_{C1} \right) + \left(d_C \cdot s_{C2} \right) + d_{glue} \right] \cdot ds + \\ + P_{stiffening}$$

where:

P	=	computed weight of the chassis
$P_{stiffening}$	=	total weight of additional stiffening parts (retrieved from a data base)
$d_{honeycomb}$, d_C, d_{glue}	=	density of the honeycomb, carbon fiber and glue
$s_{honeycomb}$, s_{C1}, s_{C2}	=	thickness of the honeycomb and internal and external carbon fiber
ds	=	infinitesimal surface element

In practice, the weight is computed by approximating the previous formula, i.e., it is calculated for each one of the four sections defined by the bulkheads and a sum is applied as follows:

$$P = \sum_{i=1}^{4} P_i + P_{stiffening}$$

$$P_i = C_i \cdot \left[\left(d_{honeycomb} \cdot S_{hi}\right) + \left(d_c + S_{c1i}\right) + \left(d_c \cdot S_{c2i}\right) + d_{glue}\right] \cdot Sup_i \,,$$

where:

P	=	computed weight of the chassis
P_i	=	weight of each section
$d_{honeycomb}$, d_C, d_{glue}	=	density of the honeycomb, carbon fiber and glue
S_{hi}, S_{c1i}, S_{c2i}	=	thickness of the honeycomb and internal and external carbon fiber for the i-th section
Sup_i	=	area of the i-th section

The weight of the suspension components (wishbones and stiffening arms) can be computed from their volume and density. The volume depends upon the dimensions of the components; these are based on the dimensions and position of the spherical joint. The joints are selected from a database of standard parts, depending on the strength required (See Table 1).

As for the joints, the weight of other standard parts (dampers) can be retrieved from databases too. Regarding the wheels, the technical specifications limit their dimensions and therefore the resulting weight.

Table 1. Table of standard joints (values are in mm and g)

Code	D int	D ext	Radius	Thickness	Weight
3	4.826	15.875	11.0998	8.3058	14.075
4	6.35	15.875	11.0998	8.3058	14.074
5	7.9375	17.4625	11.0998	8.0518	15.89
6	9.525	20.6375	12.7	10.3124	27.24
7	11.1125	23.8125	14.2748	11.2268	36.32
8	12.7	25.4	15.875	12.827	45.4
9	14.2875	28.575	17.2212	13.6144	61.29
10	15.875	30.1625	19.05	14.4018	72.64
12	19.05	34.925	22.225	16.002	108.96
14	22.225	41.275	22.225	19.177	158.9
16	25.4	53.975	34.925	25.527	440.38

The car's center of mass is computed with respect to a reference co-ordinate system. The X-axis of this system coincides with the car's longitudinal axis and is oriented in the direction of its motion. The Z-axis is the vertical axis and its origin is located in the intersection between the longitudinal axis and the front wheel axis. The XY plane coincides with the underfloor, as the XZ plane defines the car symmetry plane.

The distribution of weight at the front and back can be computed from the car's center of mass as follows:

$$P_{front} = \frac{P \cdot d_{back}}{D}$$

$$P_{back} = \frac{P \cdot d_{front}}{D}$$

where:

P_{front}, P_{back} = load respectively on the front and back car axle

P = total car weight

d_{front} , d_{back} = center of mass distance from the front and back car axle respectively

D = car axle base

5. DEFINITION OF THE IRL CAR MODEL

Some fundamental functionality is required in order to implement an automatic application which supports the evaluation of different configurations and corresponding weight distribution. These include the possibility to:

- represent the hierarchical structure of the car in terms of parts, sup-parts and related properties (as required by the analysis performed);
- represent relationships among properties of the different parts and re-compute the whole model as a consequence of modified properties;
- link external data bases;
- generate geometric models of parts and sub-parts (to compute volumes, weights and centers of mass).

Selling Point by Concentra is a KAE development shell, which provides mentioned functionality. This tool has been used to implement the prototype.

The car model is defined as a tree where the root represents the whole car, nodes represent sub-assemblies and leaves represent atomic components. The root stores general parameters, which have an impact on the whole car configuration, and nodes and leaves store local parameters, which have an impact on specific sub-assemblies.

The components whose weight and center of mass need to be computed starting from their shape (e.g. wishbones and stiffening arms) are represented by leaves, which inherit mass properties from linked solid models. These leaves must also store parameters, which represent the appropriate positioning of the solid model.

Components whose weight is known and which contribute to the total car weight, with (e.g. engine) or without (e.g. liquids) a significant geometric representation, are represented by leaves, which are linked to external databases storing their weight values.

Figure 5 shows the geometric representation of the car in standard configuration.

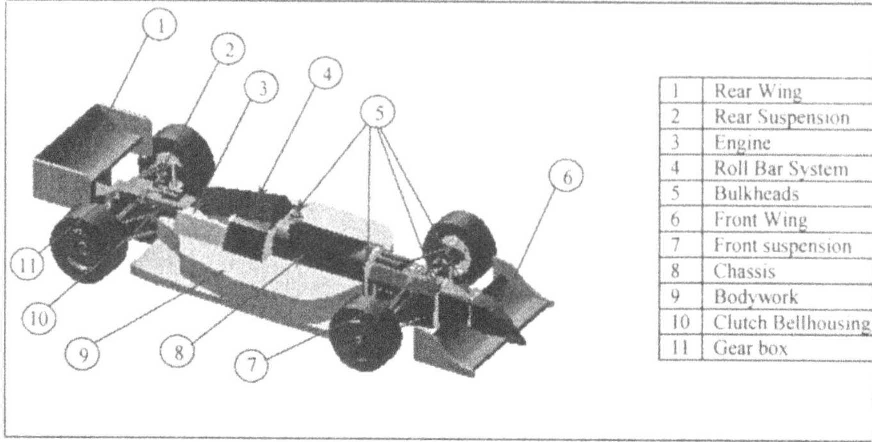

Figure 5. Geometric representation of the car in standard configuration

The user interacts with the system modifying general and local parameters and looking at the resulting configuration. Computed results are reported to the user in both graphic and numerical representation. The main general parameters, which the user can set, are shown in Table 2, together with an indication of the impact they have on the configuration of the car.

Table 2. General model parameters and related impact on model configuration

Parameter	Impact
front, back track	position and dimension of suspensions
rear wing height from reference plane (constrained by safety specifications)	vertical dimension of wing support
underfloor height and angle from the ground	front wing and suspension configuration
ballast position	weight distribution
Weight of the driver	weight distribution
Percentage of tank filling	weight distribution

Different configurations, related to different values of the front track, are shown in Figure 6. Notice that in the picture on the right, the ARB system center of mass (small dot in the center of the ARB system) is located behind the axle, whilst in the one on the left it is located on the axle.

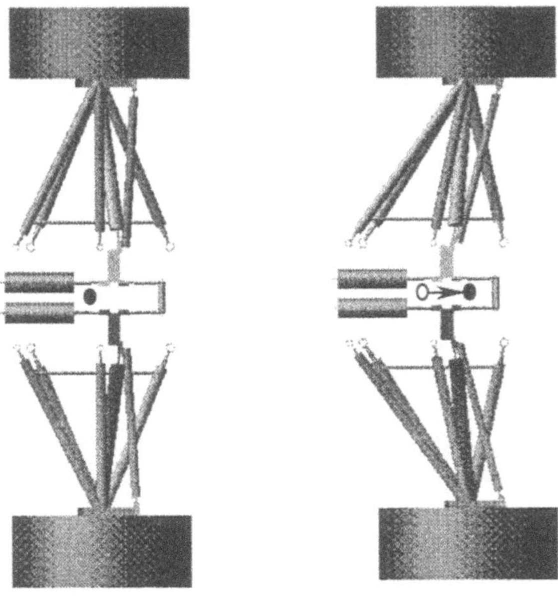

● Current center of mass position ○ Old center of mass position

Figure 6. Top view of front suspensions in different configurations

The system can be upgraded by changing the declarative knowledge stored in the external database. Due to the nature of the configuration problem considered, an upgrading of procedural knowledge is not generally required but, if necessary, it can be done by changing the model structure.

6. EXPERIMENTS AND RESULTS

Front and back loads have been computed for different car configurations and different tank load situations, i.e., three conditions (93.5%, 39% and 0%, respectively 35, 15 and 0 gallons), with and without driver, and three wheel base configurations.

The experimental data related to the car base configuration (named wheel base 2998) without driver were available. These data (values in brackets in Table 3) were provided by the racing teams and compared with computed data (Table 3). Approximations are due to the fact that the geometry of some parts is not precise (e.g., the shape of the chassis) but was approximated.

Table 3. Computed loads for different car configurations

Tank Load %	Driver's Weight (Kg)	Front Load (%)		
		Wheel base 2998	Wheel base 3048	Wheel base 3098.8
93.5	0	41.39 (41.43)	40.85	40.33
39	0	40.90 (40.96)	40.4	39.92
0	0	40.41 (40.18)	39.91	39.43
93.5	68	43.03	42.44	41.89
39	68	42.67	42.12	41.60
0	68	42.37	41.81	41.29
Difference Full/Empty (%)		0.66	0.63	0.60

Table 3 shows how the car's center of mass moves to the back as fuel is consumed; this situation is reflected in a different performance of the car attitude during the race. The difference in the front load between the conditions of full and empty tank can be taken as a measure of the center of mass variability, and must be minimized.

The car's center of mass moves because the tank's center of mass is not located in the same X position of the car's total center of mass (Figure 7 and Table 4 show how the location of the center of mass of the tank/fuel system depends on the fuel load).

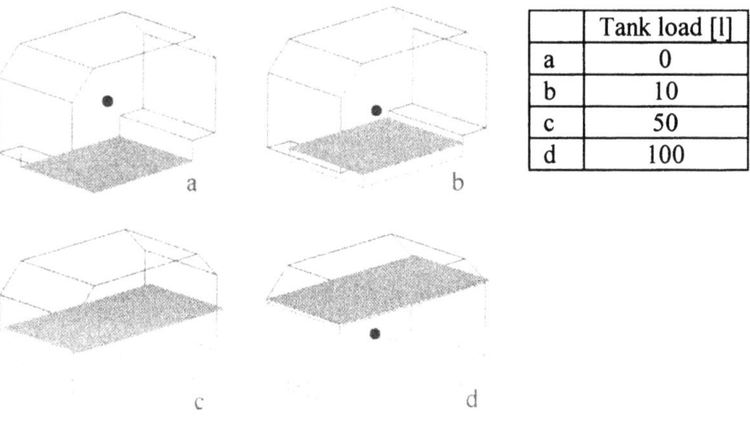

	Tank load [l]
a	0
b	10
c	50
d	100

Figure 7. Location of the tank's center of mass for different load conditions

Table 4. Center of mass co-ordinates values

Tank Load		Center of mass location [mm]		
%	l	X	Y	Z
0	0	-1578,5	0	22,88
10	12,5	-1562,1	0	16,57
20	25,9	-1556,9	0	14,4
30	41,7	-1557,4	0	14
40	57,1	-1559,1	0	14,66
50	71,6	-1562,2	0	15,81
60	85,1	-1566,5	0	17,12
70	98,74	-1569,8	0	18,66
80	112,4	-1572,5	0	20,36
90	124,4	-1574,5	0	22
100	135,2	-1576	0	23,56

One possible solution of the problem is to move some parts (e.g. battery, electronic components, and radiator) to the front of the car so that the car's center of mass may coincide with the tank's center of mass.

Of course, functional components are not always easy to move, due to other considerations such as bounding volumes, functionality, etc.

The ballast is the easiest component to locate, however within constraints imposed by technical specifications. Computing the car weight in standard configuration (empty tank and no driver) and then subtracting it from the minimum allowed weight (734 Kg) sets the weight of the ballast. It is evident that the lighter the car is, the heavier the ballast must be, in proportion to the weight, which is necessary to move the center of mass.

A new car configuration has been worked out, by modifying many parameters in order to reduce weight, and the ballast has been located as near as possible to the front of the car.

In the new configuration, with a wheel base set at 3048 mm and a driver weighting 68 Kg, the front load distribution varies from 44.78% (full tank) to 44.47% (empty tank), thus the front load difference between the two conditions is 0.31%, i.e., about half of the value computed for the configurations previously presented.

Figure 8 shows the car's and tank/fuel centers of mass for both the standard and the new configurations. Notice how the two center of mass are closer to each other in the new car's configuration.

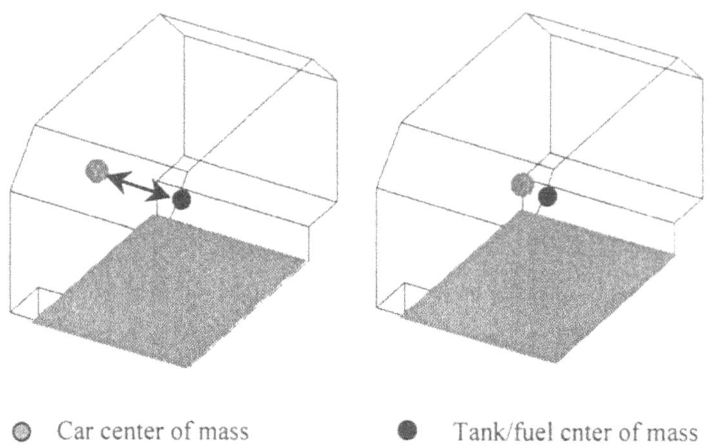

Figure 8. Car's center of mass compared to the tank's center of mass for two different car configurations

7. CONCLUSIONS

A prototype application for the evaluation of weight distribution in IRL cars has been studied and implemented within a KBE environment. The application is based on a hierarchical model containing different types of engineering knowledge.

Many kinds of data have been used to represent all information involved in weight computation: constant values (to represent input parameters), formulas (to represent evaluated parameters), SQL strings (to represent queries to external databases), geometric models (to represent shape of the components), and constraints (to represent relative positioning of components). Notice that all pieces of information are related to each other, in the sense that the procedure to compute one value may refer to other computed values (e.g., the dimensions of components, needed to compute weight and center of mass, may depend on properties of the material or applied loads).

The comparison of computed data with experimental ones provided by the racing teams validated the model. After the tuning activity, the difference between the computed values of total weight and center of mass and the experimental data is less than 0.57%.

The prototype has been used to study a new car configuration that allows reducing the changes in the car's center of mass as the fuel is consumed in the race.

The objective is not to produce detailed models of car sub-systems; however, the design parameters and related data provided can be used as an input to other specific software tools, like traditional CAD systems, which can perform this job. Moreover, it is possible to achieve kinematics analysis, FEM analysis, etc, starting from the geometric models of car sub-assemblies, generated automatically by the prototype. In this context, the possibility of re-using car prototype information in commercial CAD/CAE systems has been tested. In particular we have verified two different integrative solutions:

- the first one is about the automatic generation of 3D CAD model of car components;
- the second one concerns the possibility of exporting and re-using geometric elements produced by the prototype in a simulation environment; the objective has been to analyze dynamic and cinematic behavior of the car and of the front suspension assembly.

Future developments are as follows:

- extension of the model parameters for the computation of moment of inertia;
- implementation of a user-friendly interface for the final user (at present model parameters are set by the user interface of the development tool);
- porting on an equivalent development tool with higher capabilities for surface representation (at present the bodywork is approximated with a set of extrusions with constant cross sections).

AKNOWLEDGMENTS

We would like to thank staff from Dallara, and in particular Ing. Andrea Toso e Ing. Davide Seletti for their collaboration and for the information provided. A special thanks to all reviewers for their valuable suggestions.

REFERENCES

Concentra Corporation (1995), Selling Point reference guide.

Cornet, P., Elu, P., Dossier, G., (1991), Systemes de conception a base de connaissance: une application industrielle, Acte de MICAD, pp. 598-608.

Di Lecce, B., Tagliabo', F., Mandorli, F., Accornero, B., Strata, A., (1997), A Knowledge-Based tool for automatic generation of wire harness design and schematics, 6th European Conference, Lightweight and Small Cars, the Answer to Future Needs, V: 2, pp. 987 - 998.

Kariko-Buhwezi, B., Cugini, U., (1995), A Knowledge Based Computer Programming for the Automatic Design of a Gear Pump, Preprints of the First IFIP WG 5.2 Workshop, Knowledge Intensive CAD-1 (KIC '95), T. Tomiyama, M. Mantyla and S. Finger eds.., 421-434.

Indy Racing League (1996), Division Technical Specifications.

Mandorli, F., (1997), Customized Product Design: Shearing Dies Test Case, 10th ADM Conference, Design Tools and Methods in Industrial Engineering, pp. 189 - 198.

AIEDAM, (1998), Special Issue: Configuration Design, William P. Birmingham, Editor, V. 12, N. 4, ISSN 0890-0604.

12

Lens Barrel Design Based On Distributed Knowledge-Base

Kiso Bok[1], Sehyun Myung[2] & Soon-Hung Han[2]

[1]LG Electronics Inc., Republic of KOREA

[2]iCAD Lab., Dept. of Mechanical Eng., Korea Advanced Institute of Science and Technology, Republic of KOREA

Key words: Distributed knowledge-base, CAD, Collaborative design, CORBA, Design expert system

Abstract: Engineering designers use computers for their daily work; with their CAD systems, they define their own features, and reuse them to reduce the development cycle time of products. These features can be implemented on a knowledge-based system which automatically creates geometric models or checks their validity. Further, user-defined features which take the form of a *macro* or a *procedure* can be shared by other designers. Company design offices are physically scattered, yet logically connected through the Internet. To improve design productivity, design information about CAD data that is scattered across design offices must be shared among participating designers. This paper explains a collaborative design environment and proposes a product design environment based on distributed knowledge-bases. Such an environment integrates OMG's CORBA (Common Object Request Broker Architecture), Microsoft's OLE (Object Link and Embedding), WWW (World Wide Web) as network architecture, a 3D CAD system, and an expert system shell. A design example of the lens barrel of a projection television is implemented to verify the idea.

1. INTRODUCTION

1.1 Motivation

CAD systems have become essential tools in the industry, while the design environment continues to change. First, design offices are connected to Internet. The network model is changing from a central host/terminal type to a distributed client/server type. Second, design paradigms are evolving to a concurrent engineering concept. The sequential and procedural design process is inefficient in the present market situation, where continuous development of new products is required. Engineers are asked to develop new products by simultaneous processes. The concurrent engineering must enhance designer efficiency; efficient product development can reduce both development cycle time and cost.

Design engineers can reduce product development cycle time by sharing and reusing design results. The *design by editing* system, based on a computer network environment, can achieve this goal. This system reuses existing designs and parts data, which are stored in a remote server. As more design offices are equipped with network environments with Internet access, efficient distribution of design information-including the design knowledge and sharing the information using computer network- are required.

Two important aspects of design information sharing are data sharing and knowledge sharing. Current *design by editing* systems is more oriented to data sharing; however, design knowledge should also be shared among design engineers. Knowledge of a specific domain is mostly used within that domain, and heuristic knowledge continues to change in response to technology development. Therefore, it is desirable that a domain expert manages the knowledge of the domain, and that design information be shared in a distributed environment.

1.2 Literature survey

One method of sharing design information is to express design knowledge with a rule-based expert system. An efficient means of using distributed rule-bases is to control the expert system remotely. The *XpertWeb* project (Belo & Ribero, 1996) has integrated the World Wide Web and an expert system. The *XpertWeb* system controls the remote expert system using RPC (Remote Procedure Call) communication technology. The basic structure of the systems is client/server; the server has a knowledge-base and an expert system shell. The expert system shell generates HTML (Hyper Text Markup Language) documents to display the inference results after processing requests from clients. The server is a RPC server and the client is an web browser (RPC client). The client uses the CGI (Common Gateway Interface) to verify data during communications with the server.

JESS (Java Expert System Shell) is an expert system shell programmed in JAVA language (Sandia National Laboratories 1998). It is a JAVA version of the expert system shell Clips which was developed by NASA. *JESS* is an expert system which can be downloaded as a JAVA applet; the applet is controlled by a web browser through the Internet. The server is not burdened with inferencing of a large local knowledge-base, because the client performs inferencing after downloading the applet.

Several studies about Internet-based collaborative CAD are being conducted, because of the potential of Internet technology (Regli, 1997), among them the ACORN (Adaptive, Collaborative, Open Research Network) (Michael, 1996) project. The aim of the project is to construct a design and manufacturing architecture based on Internet, with the WWW used as the user interface.

Design agents can be combined with expert systems. The agent is software with an active communication feature (Pak et al., 1996). Research on agents has been performed based on JAVA and KQML, and a collaborative design system implemented through the WWW (Ahn et al., 1998). A knowledge-based expert system, that is a multi-agents system, has been studied in the electronic commerce area (Lee et al., 1995, Lee et al., 1997).

A design expert system controlled through Internet and integrated with a CAD system visualizes the product shape (Choi & Lee, 1997) ; a Concept-Modeler, an expert system shell with a CAD ability, has also been used. The interface between the expert system shell and the web was developed by CGI script using Pearl (Christiansen, 1996). VRML (Virtual Reality Modeling Language) (VRML Consortium, 1998) is used for visualization and HTML is employed to display product information. However, the VRML is used only for viewing shapes; for a *design by editing* system, a more tightly coupled system is required.

A distributed design expert system should use an expert system shell and provide information related to design and manufacturing through Internet and multi-agents. However, the current distributed design expert system is not based on distributed design knowledge, but is limited to an expert system shell remotely operated through the Internet. A multi-agents system using JAVA and KQML is difficult to integrate with existing CAD systems, because such CAD systems which are fully JAVA based or support KQML are not yet available.

1.3 Research questions

This paper introduces a system of sharing design information which is distributed on the Internet. The shared design information includes not only geometric data but also heuristic design knowledge. Figure 1 shows the framework of the design information sharing system. The system consists of 3 layers: local servers to store design results of individual designers; domain servers to store design information on standard parts and frequently used parts within a specific design domain or office; and a central server to store standard design information within a department.

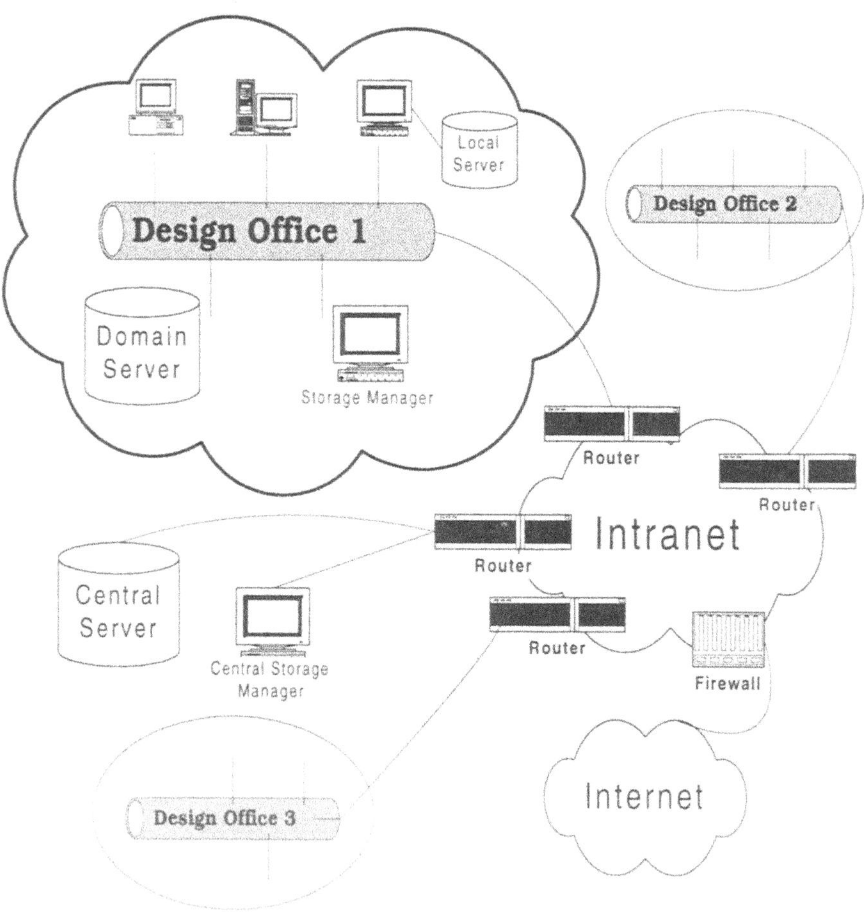

Figure 1. Sharing system of distributed design information

The proposed system can interoperate independent of computing environment. Two components are examined in this paper to establish the framework of the system. The first is the distribution of design expert systems around the network; the method of controlling the remote knowledge-base and the inferencing engine through the Internet is also described. Second, we will address organization of the clients. A client controls the CAD system of an individual designer, the remote CAD data, the knowledge-base, and the remote inference engine.

2. DISTRIBUTED DESIGN EXPERT SYSTEM

In order to distribute the knowledge-base of design information, a communication method is required. It is a difficult task to construct a low-level communication interface, because a low-level interface requires complicated programming work when the specifications of its interface are changed. Such programming adjustment may bring about consistency and adjustment problems. To prevent these problems, a standard method is required such as KQML, CORBA, or DCOM, which use a high level interface of communication.

KQML (Knowledge Query and Manipulation Language) is a language designed by the External Interface Working Group of ARPA Knowledge Sharing Effort which works for communication between software agents (DARPA, 1993).

2.1 CORBA

CORBA (Common Object Request Broker Architecture) is an open distributed object infrastructure being standardized by the OMG (Object Management Group). It allows applications to communicate with each other regardless of their location or designer. CORBA defines true interoperability by specifying how ORBs (Object Request Broker) from different vendors can inter-operate (Kim et al., 1998).

ORB is the middleware that establishes client-server relationships between objects. Using ORB, a client can invoke a method on a server; the client need not be aware of the server object's location, operating system, or programming language.

2.2 OLE/COM and DCOM

Whereas CORBA is considered an industry standard, OLE (Object Linking Embedding) / COM (Component Object Model) is a standard from Microsoft (Brockschmidt, 1995). The OLE/COM runs only on MS

Windows, and OLE objects are integrated based on COM architecture, which is similar to the CORBA.

OLE supports frameworks to create, manage, and access object-based components which serve other objects or applications on Windows. On the other hand, COM is a protocol for communication among objects; OLE is a COM object. Because Microsoft Windows™ is popular, COM can be regarded as a standard for personal computers.

A COM object consists of member data and member functions. In COM terminology, a set of such member functions is called the interface, in which methods of object-oriented programming are included. COM supports interface pointers to invoke these methods.

DCOM is a network version of COM. While COM runs on a single machine, DCOM supports communications with processes of different machines. The architecture of COM and DCOM is similar to that of CORBA; however, COM does not support the concept of inheritance as does CORBA. It is inconvenient if inheritance is used to implement multiple inheritance. Further, COM runs only on Microsoft operating systems.

2.3 Product design environment and CORBA

The process of product design can utilize characteristics of objects. During the product development process, objects are created as the design proceeds. These objects may be parts of a product or the product itself. For the former, attributes of the part are dimensions and material properties. These attributes are usually determined by the designer's knowledge; the knowledge comes from a mathematical theory or the designer's experience.

If a product itself is an object, each part and the relationship among the parts become the member data, which is also determined by the designer's knowledge. It is well known that engineering artifacts are well represented by object-oriented methodology. Figure 2 shows the object representation of a product.

Each design object is represented with user-defined design features (Shah & Mäntylä, 1995). If the design features of similar products are distributed over several offices and each designer can access the design features repository, designer efficiency can be improved. If the design features or design units are implemented as CORBA objects, a distributed design system environment (shown in Figure 3) can be constructed. Individual designers have their own design data and a design expert system on the local server. If the design expert system runs as a CORBA server, it becomes a CORBA object. Using this CORBA object, clients can share the design information stored in the individual CORBA servers.

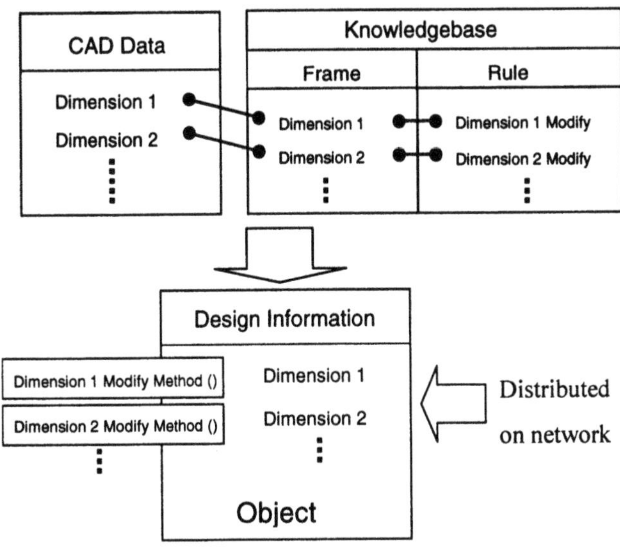

Figure 2. Object modeling of a product

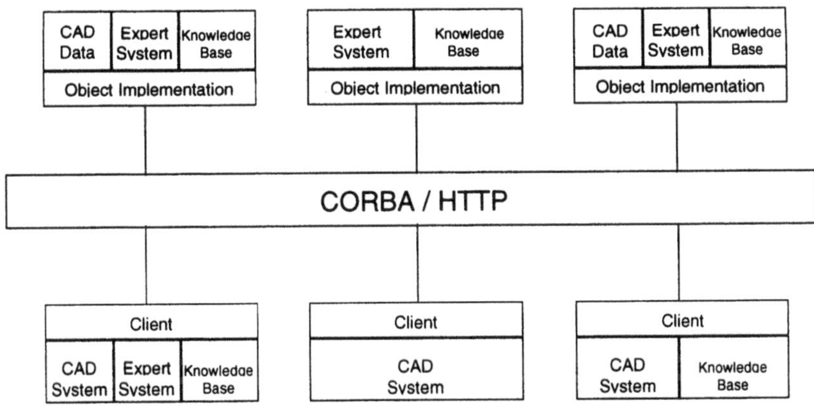

Figure 3. Object architecture of distributed design environment

2.4 Distributed design expert system

The task of product design is to determine the geometry and relationships of its parts. That of product design is to determine system configuration. Parts of a system and its own composition have geometric information. A design expert system is software which aids in the design task with heuristic knowledge. There are various kinds of design expert systems according to their target domains; expert system should have knowledge about geometry, and the geometry should be visualized to users; this geometric information can be shared by designers who are connected on the Internet. Expert systems can show the product geometry by controlling a CAD system, because CAD systems are generally used for product design.

CAD systems and expert system shells have been integrated through the network (CORBA). Distributed design data at client sites can be utilized by expert system. It is assumed that designers use the same CAD system. The expert system which controls design results from the CAD system behaves as a CORBA server. Clients are distributed on the network, and downstream designers access the CAD data through the client. They remotely control the expert system, and modify the CAD data using design methods such as parametric design.

3. SYSTEM ARCHITECTURE AND EXPERIMENT

One efficient way to implement the distributed design expert system is using a web browser. CAD data and the client applet can be transmitted according to the HTTP. The design information sharing environment such as that shown in Figure 3 can be established by applying methods of system integration; when implemented on the intranet, it can meet the requirements of the *sharing environment of domain sever layer* of Figure 1.

3.1 Experimental design task

To verify the design information sharing environment, an experiment was performed with the lens barrel design of a projection TV. The lens-CRT assembly consisted of a CRT, a cooling system, and lenses. The lens was the core component; the barrel controlled and supported the lenses.

Figure 4 shows the configuration of the lens barrel which was prepared by 2D CAD. The design expert system determined the shape, dimensions, and configuration of each part; parts 1~4 of Figure 4 were re-designed using the design expert system. Part 3, the inner barrel, enforced the light axes of lens 11 and 12 are coincident. Part 4, the spacer, left a space between the lenses 11 and 12. Part 1, the F-clamp, fixed the two lenses and the spacer to the inner barrel. Part 2, the outer barrel, fixed this lens system. Parts 1~4 were the main parts of the barrel, and were dependent on the configuration of the lenses.

The basic shape of a product depends on the engineer's experience. The design expert system is useful for engineers who have little experience in barrel design. It helps to produce the basic shape and configuration of the barrel model suitable for the lens data. This barrel can be used as the final design or can be changed by downstream engineers.

Figure 5 shows the hierarchical structure of a projection TV, which consists of electrical, optical, and mechanical parts. Electrical parts include audio, video, and the power system. Optical parts are comprised of a screen, a lens CRT unit, and a mirror. Mechanical parts are made of a case, a screen frame, a back cover, etc. The lens CRT unit contains a CRT, a lens unit, and a coupler. The lens unit is subdivided into lenses and a barrel.

In this experiment, the knowledge-base is consisted of 9 rules and 5 objects which corresponded to 5 parts. Dimensions of the parts were stored in the slots of objects. Each rule checked the changes of slot values of the lens object, and modified the slot values of the part objects accordingly. Special method of knowledge acquisition was not used, as the authors are domain experts.

The following illustrates a rule in the knowledge-base..

```
IF ( lens.dist1_2 • lens.dist1_2_dum ) AND
   ( lens.dist1_2_dum • 0 )

THEN
   ASSIGN ( lens.dist1_2_dum+0.96 ) TO ( in_barrel.ofront )
   ASSIGN ( lens.dist1_2_dum ) TO ( spacer.tot_length)
   ASSIGN ( out_barrel.tot_length + ( lens.dist1_2_dum - lens.dist1_2 ))
          TO (out_barrel.tot_length)
   ASSIGN ( lens.dist1_2_dum ) TO (lens.dist1_2)
```

The above rule changes dimensions and composition of the parts when the air gap between lens 11 and lens 12. *lens.dist1_2* is a slot corresponding to the air gap in the knowledge-base; its initial value is 16.9mm. The above rule is performed only when the slot value of *lens.dist1_2_dum* changes. *lens.dist1_2_dum* is a slot for the air gap value which can be changed by the user. If the air gap is changed, the length of spacer (*spacer.tot_length*) and the length of the inner barrel are changed accordingly. The slot *in_barrel.ofront* controls the length of the inner barrel. The length of the outer barrel (*out_barrel.tot_length*) which supports and controls the inner barrel is also changed.

The Following explains the THEN phrase of the above rule. First, 0.96 is added to the slot value of *lens.dist1_2_dum* and the sum value assigned to the slot *in_barrel.ofront*; the slot value of *lens.dist1_2_dum* is assigned to slot *spacer.tot_length*. The value 0.96 which is determined based on the experience of the domain expert. The slot value of *out_barrel.tot_length* is updated by adding the changing value of air gap. Finally, the changed value (*lens.dist1_2_dum*) is stored in *lens.dist1_2*.

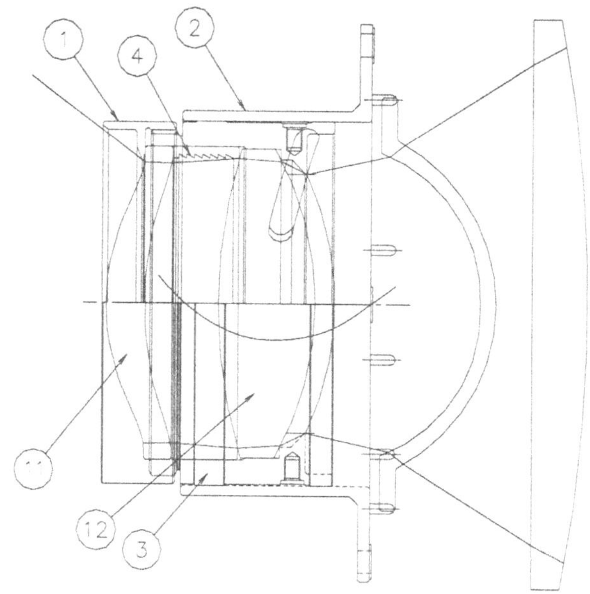

Figure 4. Lens barrel Composition

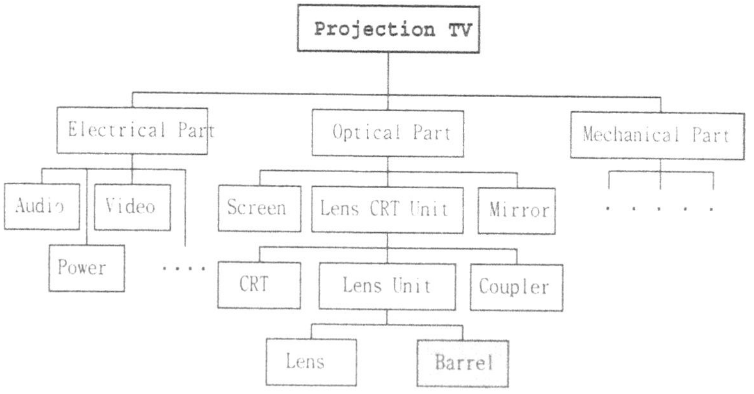

Figure 5. Hierarchical structure of a projection TV

3.2 System integration

The distributed design expert system was implemented by integrating the component technologies. The system is consisted of the following components.

- An expert system shell (Intelligent Rules Element) with its API and a knowledge-base.
- A CAD system with modeling data (SolidEdge).
- CORBA (Orbix), CORBA/OLE object broker (Server/Client Interface).
- MFC (Microsoft Foundation Class), OLE automation server, Microsoft COM.
- A web server (Microsoft Personal Web Server) and a web browser (Microsoft Internet Explorer).
- A design expert system client (ActiveX Document server).

Neuron data's Intelligent Rules Element, a commercial expert system shell, was used for the construction and control knowledge-base (Neuron Data, 1996). Intergraph's SolidEdge (now, Unigraphics Solutions) (Unigraphics Solutions, 1998) a Microsoft Windows 95/NT-based 3D CAD System was utilized to supports the OLE for DM (OLE for Design and Modeling, Manufacturing) (Design and Modeling Applications Council association, 1998) and Visual Basic objects (Microsoft, 1997). Iona's Orbix was used for the CORBA implementation (Iona Technologies, 1996).

For the user convenience the client program was executed on a web browser; ActiveX, Microsoft's component technology, made this possible (Integraph, 1997). An application can contain other application's document using ActiveX Document technology. An application containing documents is termed an ActiveX Document Container, while the contained document is the ActiveX Document Server (Anderson, 1997). The Microsoft's web browser, Internet Explorer, is a typical ActiveX Document Container. The client of the design expert system is constructed as ActiveX Document server. Engineers who have a web browser can use the design expert system from a remote site.

The status of the server and client before they are connected is shown in Figure 6. The expert system on the server was transformed into an OLE Automation Server and registered on the system registry. The CORBA interface, which is the CORBA/OLE object broker, was registered on CORBA ORB. The web server provides CAD data, the design expert system client, and client's CORBA/OLE object broker ActiveX Document format. The web server also provides guideline information in the form of HTML documents.

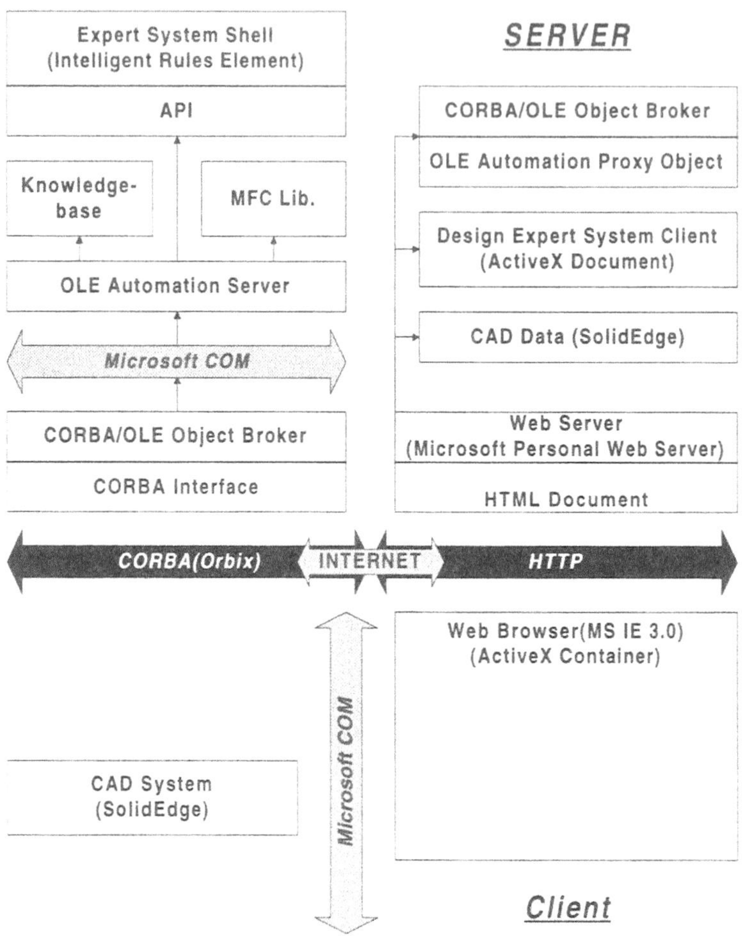

Figure 6. Status of server and client before connection

A client requires a web browser, a CAD system, and the CORBA client module which is downloaded from the server at the moment of connection. It is assumed that CORBA environment has already been prepared. Further, any client can take the role of server.

A client connects to the web server with HTTP. Users can download the CAD data according to guideline information written in HTML format. At this time, the communication protocol is not CORBA, but HTTP. The web browser contains the design expert system client as an ActiveX Document server. The web browser ascertains whether the client system has the CORBA/OLE object broker, GUI module, and other elements that are needed to run the design expert client; if not, the web browser installs them. The communication protocol is still HTTP.

The design expert system works when the server and client are connected. It consists of a server, a client, and communication components (See Figure 7). The server component is the expert system converted into a CORBA skeleton. Client components are the client program, CAD data, CORBA stub, a CAD system, and a web browser. Communication components are Microsoft COM and CORBA run-time environments.

When the client program is executed on the web browser, communications between the components establish the CORBA/OLE object broker as shown in Figure 7. The expert system runs at the server. Using the inference results of this expert system, the CAD data at the client side can be modified.

The control flows between the modules are as follows. The design expert system client (Figure 7, ②) within the web browser (Figure 7, ①) controls the expert system at the server in addition to the CAD system at the client. The design expert system client (Figure 7, ②) calls the CORBA OLE Automation proxy object (Figure 7, ⑤) through the Microsoft COM (Figure 7, ③). Then, the OLE Automation proxy object calls the CORBA/OLE object broker (Figure 7, ⑥) through the CORBA(ORB) environment (Figure 7, ⑦).

Properties and methods of CORBA/OLE object broker (Figure 7, ⑥) and the OLE Automation server (Figure 7, ⑨) are bound with Microsoft COM (Figure 7, ⑧). Finally, the OLE Automation server (Figure 7, ⑨) performs inferencing using the run-time module of expert system and the knowledge-base (Figure 7, ⑪). The client program (Figure 7, ②) receives these reasoning results and calls the CAD system (Figure 7, ④) to modify the CAD data (Figure 7, ③). The CAD data at the client side is independent of the CAD data at the server side because it is downloaded to the client.

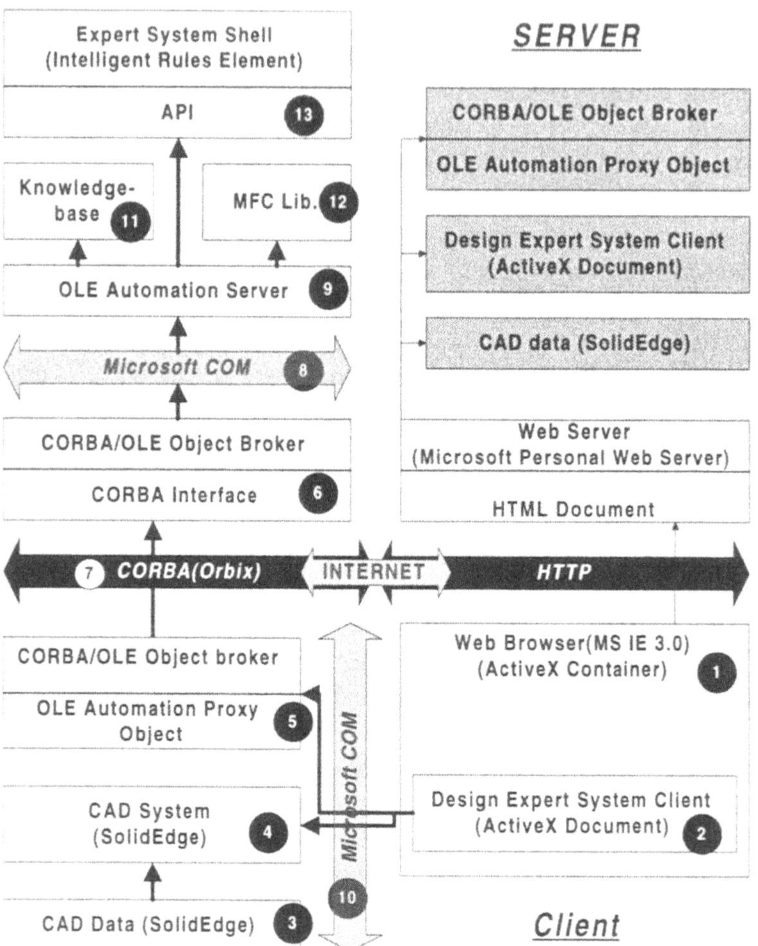

Figure 7 Control flows between components after connection

3.3 Results of the experiment

A sharing system of design information has been implemented by integrating component technologies. Using a web browser, users can connect to the server which has the design data, and obtain the parts and assembly information in HTML document format

When the client program is loaded in a web browser, it connects to the expert system and shows the initial data loaded from the knowledge-base of the server (See Figure 8). If a user changes the lens data and transfers it to the expert system located at the server, the design expert system modifies the design. Figure 9 shows the modified design model after design change.

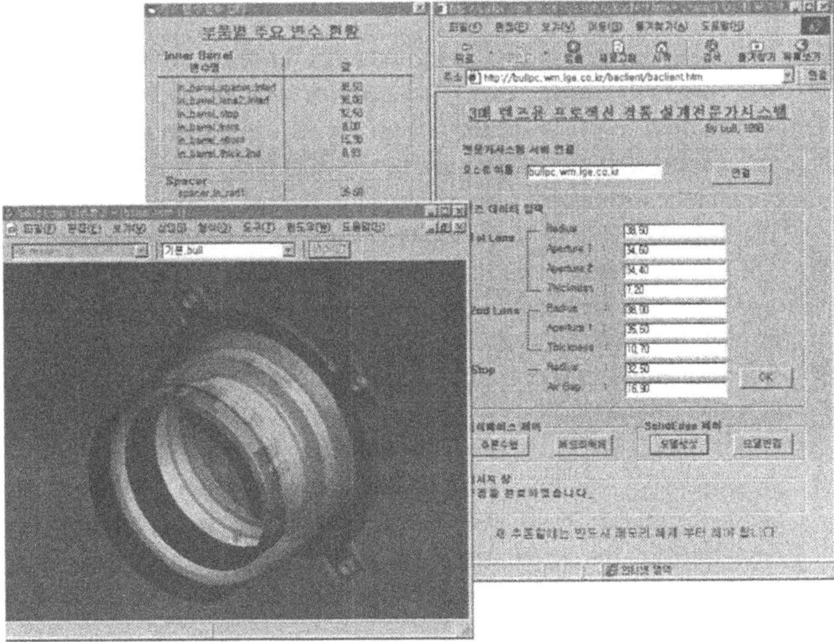

Figure 8 Creation of a model by default values

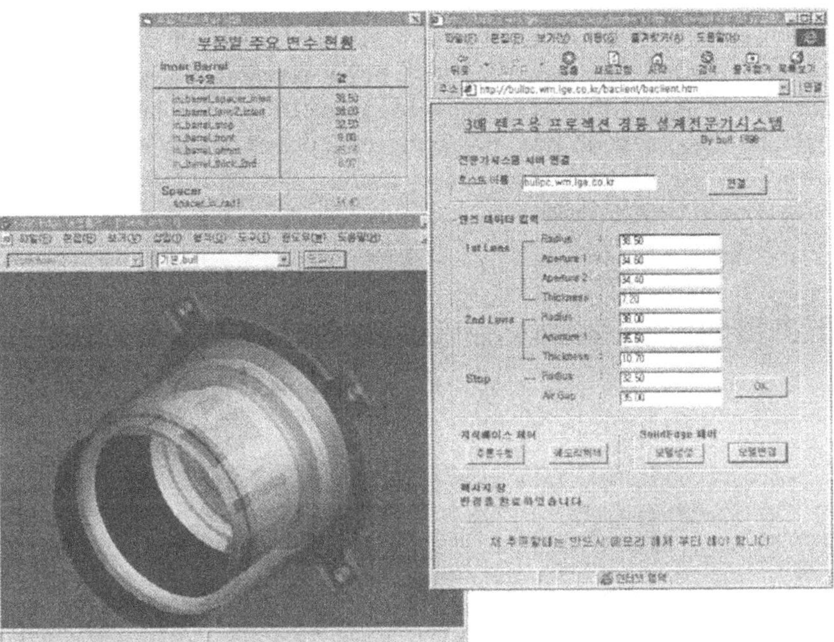

Figure 9 Modified model after inferencing

4. CONCLUSION

The following benefits can be identified from the results of the research;

- The product design expert system is constructed as an OLE Automation server using the API of the expert system shell. Because this expert system is integrated with CORBA, not only the OLE containers within the system but also remote Unix-based CORBA clients can control the expert system through network access.
- The expert system client has been implemented and can control the CAD system and can remotely control the expert system server through the CORBA stub.
- The distributed expert system is easy to use because it is embedded in a web browser.

The following observations are made from the research;

- A prototype of the collaborative design system which shares geometric information and design knowledge has been proposed. And through the implementation process, OLE object technology, CORBA technology, an expert system, and the web have been integrated.
- While the prototype system has been tested with the SolidEdge CAD system, the proposed prototype can be applied to any CAD application which works with MS Windows, COM, and CORBA

An expert system efficiently utilizes knowledge of human expert. However, use of the expert system by a practicing engineer can be problematic due to difficulty in knowledge acquisition. The knowledge-base should be easy to build and efficiently maintained. If the domain expert knows how to describe knowledge pieces, the knowledge acquisition bottleneck can be alleviated.

REFERENCES

Ahn, Sang Jun, Lee, Soo Hong (1998), "Agent-based Collaborative Design Environment using WWW" (in Korean), *Transactions of the Society of CAD/CAM Engineers*, 3(1):31-39.

Anderson, Jerry (1997), *ActiveX programming with Visual C++5.0*, Que Corporation.

Belo, Orlando, Ribero, Antonio (1995), "A Web-based framework for distributed expert systems", *1st Portuguese WWW Conference (CNW3)*, *http://www.di.uminho.pt/~anr/PAPERS/WWW95/www95.html*, html.

Choi, Hae-Jin, Lee, Soo-Hong (1997), "A Development of Ship-Block Cutting CAD Module Connected to WWW" (in Korean), *Proceedings of the Society of CAD/CAM Engineers Conference*, pp. 16-25.

DARPA Knowledge Sharing Initiative External Interfaces Working Group (1993), "Specification of the KQML Agent - Communication Language (draft)".

Design and Modeling Applications Council association (1998), "What is OLE for Design and Modeling?", *http://www.dmac.org/whatis/whatis.htm*, html.

Intergraph Corporation (1997), *SolidEdge programming users guide.*

Iona Technologies Ltd. (1996), *Orbix2 : Desktop programming guide*, pp. 4-9.

Kim, Joon Hwan., Han, Soon-Hung, Han, S. B., Kim, H. (1998), "Retrieving a STEP Database through the CORBA on the Internet" (in Korean), *Proceeding of the Society of CAD/CAM Engineers Conference*, pp.24-29.

Kraig Brockschmidt (1995), *Inside OLE*, second edition", Microsoft Press.

Lee, S. K., Lee, Jae Kyu, Lee K. J. (1997), "Customized Purchase Supporting Expert System: UNIK-SES", *Expert Systems with Applications*, 11(4), pp. 431-441.

Lee, W. K., Lee, Jae Kyu (1995), "Intelligent Agent Based Electronic Marketing: UNIK-AGENT", *Proceedings of Korean Expert Systems Society '95 Spring Conference*, pp. 179-180.

Microsoft Corporation (1997), "Microsoft COM", *http://www.microsoft.com/com/*, html.

Neuron Data Inc (1996), *Neuron Data Elements Environment: Intelligent Rules Element V4.0 - User's Guide*, 1996.

Pak, S. C., Choi, J. M., Lim, Y. H., Chang M. W., Park, S. K., Lee, K. R. (1996), "Interaction Contortion a Distributed Multi-agent System" (in Korean), *The Transactions of Korea Information Processing Society*, 3(7):1803-1811.

Regli, William C. (1997), "Internet-Enabled Computer-Aided Design", *IEEE Internet Computing*, 1(1), pp. 39-51.

Sandia National Laboratories (1998), "Jess: the Java Expert System Shell", *http://herzberg.ca. sandia.gov/jess/*, html.

Shah, Jami J., Mäntylä, Martti (1995), *Parametric and Feature-Based CAD/CAM*, John Wiley & Son Inc., New York, pp. 259-266.

Terk Michael (1996), "Changing Priorities of Research on WWW-Based Engineering Services", *Workshop Proceedings of Network-Centric CAD : A Research Planning Workshop*, pp. 169-185.

Tom Christiansen (1996), "What is Perl?", *http://language.perl.com/info/synopsis.html*, html.

Unigraphics Solutions (1998), "SolidEdge", *http://134.244.209.21/Default.htm*, html.

VRML Consortium (1998), "What is VRML?", *http://www.vrml.org/consort/FAQ.html*, html.

PART SIX

KNOWLEDGE REPRESENTATION FOR KIC

13

Guiding Agent Learning in Design

Dan L. Grecu & David C. Brown
Worcester Polytechnic Institute, Worcester, MA 01609, USA

Key words: machine learning, multi-agent systems, expectations

Abstract: In this paper we discuss the need for learning in multi-agent design systems, and the variety of forms it might take. We propose a particular method of guiding learning in these systems, describe an architecture for its implementation, and discuss how the learning should be evaluated.

1. INTRODUCTION

This paper is concerned with the use of Machine Learning techniques in Multi-Agent Design Systems (MADS). It is clear that designers who are attempting to solve large and complex design problems require computational support, and that some aspects of these designs might be fully automatable. MADS have been proposed as a viable approach to building such design systems. They offer a variety of advantages, including extensibility, the potential for parallel activity, and the capability of acting in a distributed manner (Lander 1998).

In this paper we discuss the need for learning in MADS, and the variety of forms it might take. We propose a particular method of guiding learning in a MADS, and describe an architecture for its implementation.

2. LEARNING IN A MULTI-AGENT DESIGN SYSTEM

2.1 Opportunities for learning

Multi-agent design systems (MADS) are similar to organisations: their performance can be improved. Two characteristics of performance in organisations are *effectiveness* and *efficiency* (Etzioni 1964). Effectiveness is the degree to which the goals of the system are attained, i.e., the quality of the solution. Efficiency refers to the amount of resources used to produce the result.

In a MADS, effectiveness is affected by the amount, distribution and use of the knowledge in the system, as well as by the accuracy and completeness of information exchange. Efficiency is affected by the details of the process used, including the number of conflicts, the amount of communication, the reasoning approaches selected, and the quality of conflict resolution strategies.

It would be nice if systems that were both highly efficient and highly effective could be developed from scratch. However, this is rare. As design systems move from addressing small and 'neat' design problems towards real-world design tasks, it becomes harder at development time to address the range of efficiency and effectiveness issues that the system will encounter at run-time.

Ideally, we would like to have a system where design agents base their decisions on all the knowledge that is available in the design system, and where they know the possible consequences of every potential decision. The utilities associated with these consequences would drive the decision selection, and would allow agents to precisely respond to design goals.

The truth is that agents have only limited information about how other agents operate, about their knowledge, and their internal reasoning strategies. Within a multi-agent system, it is not possible to anticipate all possible interactions between agents *a priori*. Furthermore, agents typically see only the part of the design covered by their domain competence.

As a result, agents support their decisions based on *the knowledge they have*, and not on *the knowledge that is available in the system*. Furthermore, an agent may *sometimes* know *some of the consequences* of a decision it has made, but it cannot know or compute all the consequences of its decisions. Decisions can be made based on *heuristic criteria*, and consequences can be *evaluated*. The difference between the ideal and the real setting opens opportunities for improvement through learning.

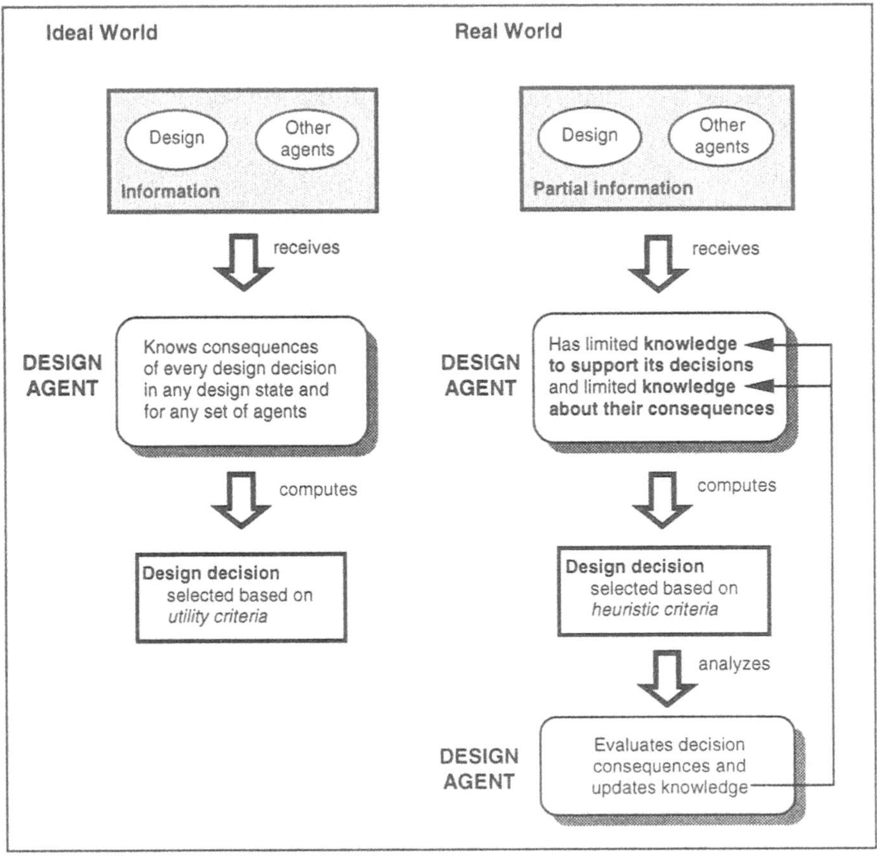

Figure 1. Agent decision-making in design

2.2 Dimensions of learning

In a multi-agent design system there is no single place where learning might occur, and no single time for it to occur. Such a system is complex, with many types of knowledge and reasoning, many types of interaction, and many roles for agents to play. This complexity provides a myriad of opportunities for learning (Grecu and Brown 1998a).

There are several "dimensions" of learning in a design context. For example, the *triggers* of learning might include failure, success, expectation violations or a perceived need to improve some aspect of the system. Different types of information may support learning. Some of it might be available while designing (e.g., critiques), and some after a design is produced (e.g., feedback about the design's quality). Some of it is communicated directly to the learner (e.g., another agent's design decision), while some is collected and available for retrieval (e.g., design traces).

Perhaps the most variety is found in what gets learned, i.e., the targets of the learning process. These include constraints, dependencies between design parameters, plans, preferences, and the consequences of design decisions.

3. FLEXIBLE AGENT LEARNING

Human problem-solvers do not persist with the same learning task forever. They start by identifying areas where they need to change their approach to the problems they face. Then they use learning in an attempt to acquire knowledge that will allow them to be better at the task. In time, the acquired knowledge will lead the problem-solvers to different decisions in situations similar to the ones that triggered the learning process in the first place.

The temporary nature of the learning process is highlighted by two observations: First, the improved results achieved by the problem solver will presumably reduce the need for learning in a specific area, and other areas of concern in the problem-solving process may become more important for learning. Second, the learning environment changes, as the learned knowledge is used. Therefore, the learner will only have a finite opportunity to learn from a specific context.

These observations establish several requirements and constraints for learning design agents. We will refer to them interchangeably as learners and agents, to stress their role as both design problem-solvers and adaptive entities.

First, an agent should be able to determine *on its own* that a specific need for learning has occurred. For instance, a design agent may decide that it needs information about how particular design and manufacturing choices influence the cost of a product, to reduce the number of times products are rejected based on cost criteria. While the types of learning needs may be pre-defined by the implementer of a MADS, for example, “The agent needs to learn in response to conflicts”, the occurrence of a learning need at run-time has to be determined by the agent itself.

Second, given that the learning scenario is no longer pre-scripted, design agents are themselves responsible for identifying the ‘ingredients’ of a learning process: *the learning target*, e.g., the cost of a component; *the sources that will provide information to support the learning process*, such as design and design process parameters, dependencies, and constraints; and, *the learning strategy*, e.g., inductive learning or explanation-based learning.

Finally, an agent needs to recognize when a learning process should be stopped. This may be because no further improvements are achieved through the learning process as it is, or because the information acquired through learning does not produce reliable or desired results.

In summary, agents, like humans, have to display flexibility in learning if they are to prove efficient in constantly changing environments. The ability to determine the need for learning, the parameters of learning, where and what to learn, and the possibility of refocusing on new learning tasks are essential for multi-agent design systems. This is especially true when attempting to scale up to new problems: sooner or later the system will have to operate with knowledge and contexts that were not anticipated when the design system was developed.

In the following we will propose to use expectations as a basis for flexible learning in design. We will show how expectations can be acquired dynamically, to respond precisely to the requirements we have enumerated above. Before we focus on the learning process itself, let us first define expectations in the particular context of design, and how expectations are used in design.

4. EXPECTATIONS IN DESIGN

4.1 The observable world of a design agent

Design agents have knowledge about the problem domain in which they operate and about the agent environment in which they find themselves. The very idea of using agents in problem-solving suggests that agents are *specialized.* In mechanical design, for example, an agent's *domain* can be restricted to materials and their physical properties, to assembly operations, or to product marketing. The agent's *tasks* can range from making decisions about the design, to critiquing design aspects, or to evaluating design parts.

Within its 'society' an agent may know about the roles or specializations of the agents with which it interacts, about when to act, how to communicate, and how to solve conflicts with other agents. However, a realistic approach which considers the resources available to an agent would not be able to anticipate or to compute the behavior of all the other agents in the system (Cherniak 1986; Russell and Wefald 1991).

We define the *observable world* of an agent as the collection of features, in the design domain and in the agent environment, that the agent can 'perceive'. The observable world of an agent is delimited epistemologically and by the physical nature of the access to information.

Epistemologically, the observable world of an agent is constrained by the agent's specialization and by its limited ability to infer new knowledge. An agent that is specialized in material selection may have no use for information about the impact of color on product aesthetics or on marketing. Therefore, color aspects of the designed product may not be part of the set of concepts used by the material selection agent. Alternatively, even if the agent may have the knowledge to reason about how colour impacts aesthetic aspects, it may be time constrained in executing a task that has a relatively low priority, or requires extensive processing.

Physical access to information depends on two main factors. If the design agents are physically distributed over a network, relevant design or process information, such as agent behavior, that may be typically monitored if the agents were co-located, may become available only through communication with other agents. Second, even if the agents are located on the same machine, the notion of agency implies an encapsulation of information that makes it invisible outside of an agent, unless deliberately exposed through posting or communication.

4.2 Defining expectations

Expectations express the belief that an event will happen. More precisely, not only *that* an event might happen, but also *the circumstances* or *conditions* under which the event will happen.

Expectations are typically created because limited resources prevent the holder of the expectation from establishing a proven causal relationship between the set of conditions and the ensuing situation. The considerations outlined in discussing the observable world of the agent – time, the factual information about the conditions that predict the situation of interest, or the knowledge needed to establish the causal connection between the conditions and the situation to which the expectation refers – provide the reasons for these limited resources. If agents were omniscient and had unlimited computational power, expectations would not be needed, since events, values and outcomes would be computable in advance.

In our multi-agent design paradigm, expectations represent the knowledge of agents that events will occur in a pre-defined way: design parameters will be within specific ranges, responses from other agents will arrive within a given amount of time, or decisions will lead to given outcomes. Figure 2 shows an example of an expectation, expressed as a rule. The conditions for the cost expectation include conditions related to the design and to the design agents.

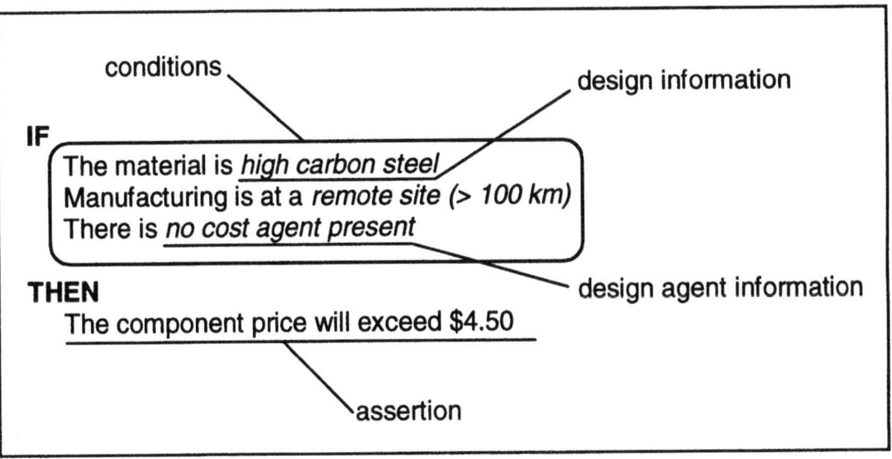

Figure 2. Design expectation example

Expectations have an *empirical character*, in that often there is no deductive connection between the conditions that are observed and the situation that is asserted. The absence of the deductive connection is either due to the absence of the knowledge that allows to make the necessary inferences, or to the unavailability of the resources to carry out the computation.

Expectations are a *tentative* form of knowledge, which has to be acquired dynamically. Consequently, they have to be set up based on the learning requirements described in section 3, they have to be monitored and updated, and eventually they have to be validated or rejected.

4.3 Expectation-based design decision making

In our approach to multi-agent design, expectations are used when a design decision is being proposed, and when its consequences are evaluated (figure 3).

Using an expectation while taking a design decision is necessary when a piece of information that is a precondition for that decision cannot be or has not been inferred. For example, an agent may need to know whether the material that will be used in a component is resistant to corrosion. However, it may be the case that the agent holds an expectation that provides the required information, such as:

IF

The material is steel

The component is chrome plated during manufacturing

THEN

The component is corrosion resistant

If the conditions for the expectation hold, then the agent can use the assertion as a basis for the decision it is about to take.

Once a decision has been selected, the design agent will evaluate its consequences. Again, expectations will bridge the gap of unavailable knowledge. An agent may have expectations about the cost range of its solutions, and use them to verify that at that point the solution it is about to propose will not drive the overall cost above a given limit. If the expectation indicates that the constraint will not be satisfied the agent will revise its design decision, to prevent a later constraint violation or a conflict.

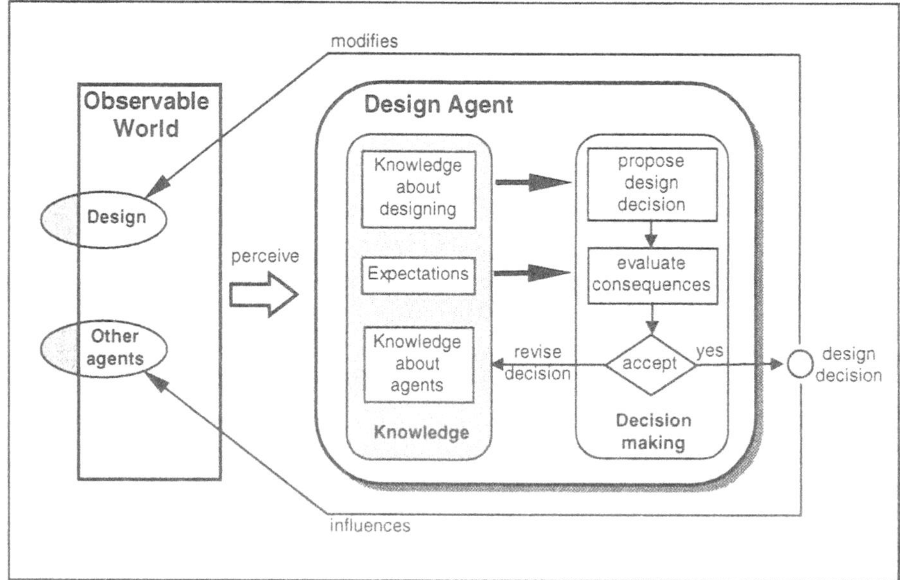

Figure 3. Using expectations in design decision-making

5. EXPECTATIONS AS A BASIS FOR AGENT LEARNING

In this section we will describe how agents acquire expectations. An agent initiates an expectation learning process when it determines that it needs information about a design or a design process element. As described in the previous section, the need may occur when the agent tries to determine whether the conditions for a specific decision are met, or when it tries to evaluate the consequences of a decision. The need for information defines the assertion of the future expectation, that is the event or parameter that the expectation will predict.

Once the agent decides to acquire an expectation, it proceeds through two major phases: learning an initial expectation and monitoring/updating the expectation.

5.1 Learning expectations

5.1.1 The learning process

To learn an expectation an agent identifies the conditions that predict the event on which the expectation focuses, i.e., the assertion of the expectation. This amounts to a causal reasoning process, in which the design agent searches its observable world for conditions that might influence the assertion. Recent research in understanding the mechanisms that underlie causal reasoning has identified two major stages within this process: the use of causal mechanisms to delimit a set of candidate of conditions, and the use of covariational principles to extract from the candidate conditions the subset that is relevant for predicting the assertion (Koslowski 1996).

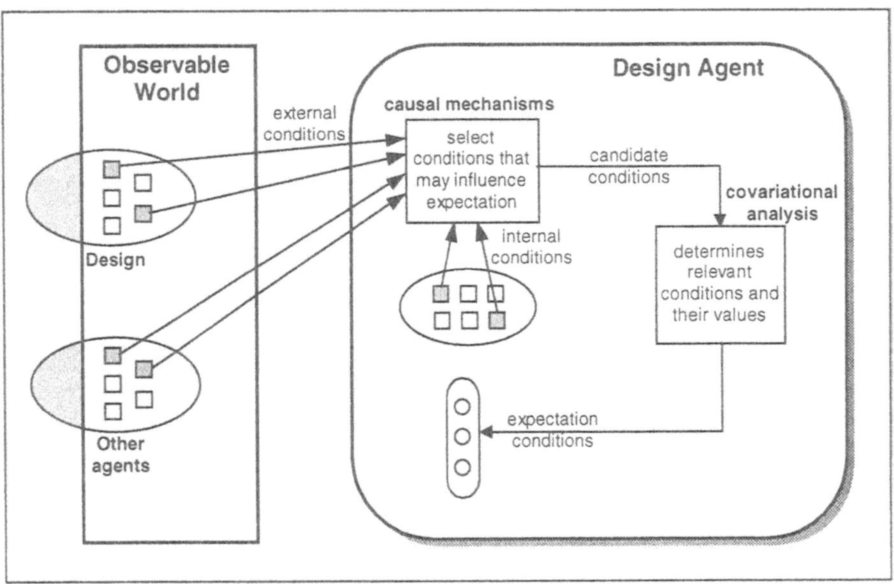

Figure 4. Learning expectations

Accordingly, a design agent implements a two-stage expectation learning (figure 4). In a first stage, the agent uses **causal mechanisms** to select from the external world and from its own domain specific knowledge candidate conditions that, in some combination, might affect the expectation assertion. Subsequently, these conditions are submitted to a **covariational analysis** to construct a subset of relevant conditions that are the ones that indeed impact the assertion.

To illustrate this process, figure 5 provides an example of a spring design agent that, in the context of deciding the diameter of a spring, needs to anticipate the range of the cost of this component. This knowledge need triggers the learning of an expectation, which will make an assertion on the cost of the component. The agent's causal mechanisms will first set-up a list of possible factors (the expectation's conditions) that may impact the cost. In doing so, the agent selects its own choice of material – an internal design condition, the range of stress and the manufacturing site – external design conditions determined by other agents, and the presence of a cost critique agent – an external condition that refers to other agents.

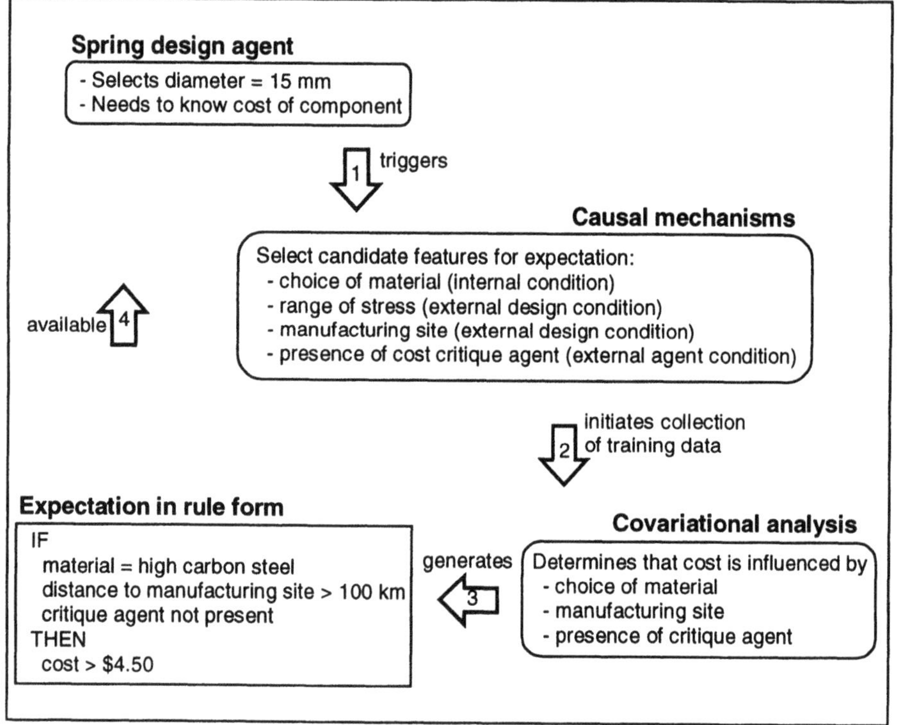

Figure 5. Expectation learning example

Once the candidate conditions are selected, the agent will collect training data for the covariational analysis. The training data is obtained from subsequent design sessions in which the design agent records values for the expectation conditions, as well as for the expectation assertion, i.e., the cost. Based on the training data, the agent eliminates redundant and irrelevant conditions, and generates an expectation in rule form, that now becomes available to the design agent.

5.1.2 Causal mechanisms and covariational analysis

The causal mechanisms involved in the first stage of the expectation learning process play a fundamental role in focusing the learning process. A pure covariational process would be simply overwhelmed by the number of influence factors it would have to consider. It has been argued that people rely only on statistical associations to identify causes and explain events, and deviations from this behavior were regarded as cognitive biases (Tversky and Kahneman 1974). A significant body of evidence indicates that this is the case only when any other evidence or information is lacking. However, domain experts tend to go through a causal attribution stage in which they use domain specific knowledge to reason about possible causes for an event (Hilton 1990; Koslowski 1996; Shultz et al. 1986).

Design agents being domain experts have access to knowledge that allows them to hypothesize possible causes for an event. Dependencies between design parameters, either explicitly represented, or represented implicitly as constraints represent one source of causal attribution. Actions or attributes of agents that include in their domain of expertise the parameter to which the expectation assertion refers are another important source. A task that computes the parameter present in an expectation assertion can also provide causal information, and even more so when the task was divided into sub-tasks.

The covariation analysis is an inductive learning stage in which expectations are seen as concepts. The expectation conditions are the concept features, while the ranges for the expectation assertion, such as the component cost in the previous example, represent the concept classes. The inductive learning algorithm attempts to learn a representation for the concept. The features of the resulting concept description are the *relevant* conditions that the agent has identified as influencing the occurrence of specific assertion ranges, i.e., classes.

To achieve this learning goal, agents use wrappers for relevant condition selection (figure 6). Wrappers (Kohavi and John 1998; Liu and Setiono 1998) apply an induction algorithm to a training data set. The experiments are run by eliminating different sets of features from the training data instances. Specifically, wrappers eliminate conditions from the candidate condition set. The wrapper method proposes a subset of features that are relevant for the identification of a given class. Features are considered relevant if their "values vary systemically with category membership" (Gennari, Langley, and Fisher 1989).

The learner performs a search in the space of subsets of features to identify one subset that allows for both a reduced description and good prediction of the new expectation that is being learned. The wrapper maintains several subsets of candidate features. An accuracy testing component determines the performance of each subset, and eliminates or adds new subsets of features, by providing information to a feature selector.

Wrappers have the major advantage of being able to work with different learning algorithms, as long as the algorithms have the same interface. Therefore, the approach provides flexibility in choosing and testing different learning algorithms without affecting the agent or the multi-agent system. They have also been proven to be effective in pruning large initial sets of features (Kohavi and John 1998). Therefore, even if the agent does not have a strong set of causal mechanisms for setting up a new expectation, and producing a small set of candidate conditions, the wrapper technique can partially compensate for this weakness.

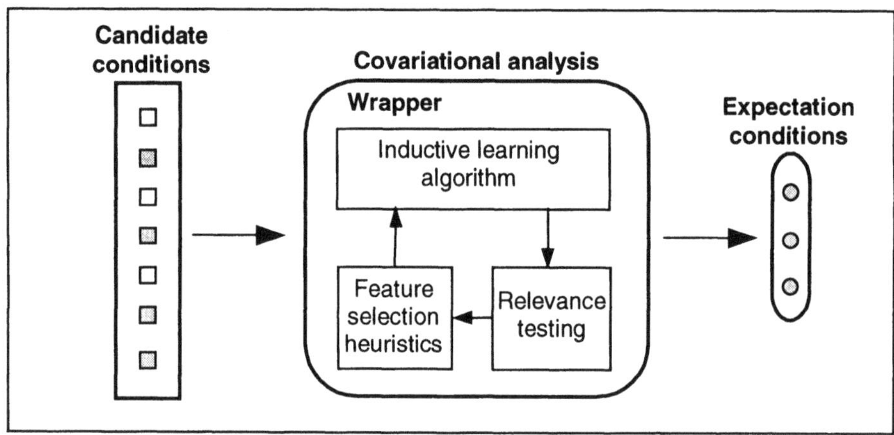

Figure 6. Selection of relevant expectation conditions

5.2 Monitoring expectation validity

Given the fact that expectations are set up empirically, design agents need to validate them before using them (figure 7). During the validation process an expectation is used to make predictions wherever the expectation assertion is needed. The value that was predicted by the expectation is then compared with the final value resulting from the design process. If the expectation is violated, that is, if the resulting value does not match the predicted assertion, the agent needs to review the expectation.

Reviewing an expectation implies that the agent will re-initiate the training stage of the learning process. It is assumed that the new data will not enable the agent to change its causal mechanisms, although the new evidence might allow an agent to use knowledge based reasoning to pinpoint a particular condition that needs to be changed. For retraining, the agent will start to collect additional training instances about the use of the expectation. Whenever the expectation is supposed to be used the values of the conditions will be recorded together with the value of the assertion resulting from the design. The retraining will generate an updated expectation.

The overall review process is can be repeated for a pre-defined number of times. If the expectation does not reach a stable status the agent will drop the expectation.

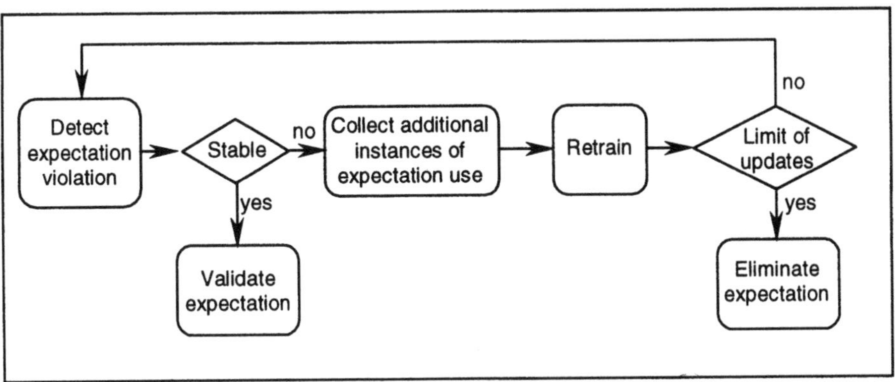

Figure 7. Monitoring expectation validity

Several causes can prevent an expectation from being accepted. The causal mechanisms can lack sufficient coverage to include important discriminating conditions in the candidate set. Another possibility stems from the fact that several expectation learning processes can proceed simultaneously in several of the agents, thus changing their decisions and their behavior. If one of the changing elements associated with an agent is included among the conditions of an expectation that is developed by another agent, it is likely that this expectations will take a longer time to 'stabilize', or may lead to it being eliminated.

6. THE AGENT ARCHITECTURE

The multi-agent architecture that we use models a group of designers. Agents act as design specialists and as group members. There are no agent hierarchies or relations between the agents that create rigid 'links' between them. However, the types of interactions between agents are predetermined, and they essentially represent the rules that create the group behavior. The interactions result dynamically, at run-time, and originate in the problem the system attempts to solve. The agents have complete autonomy in organizing their actions, with regard to the decisions they take as design specialists, or to their interactions with the rest of the group.

The agent model evolved from the Single Function Agent (SiFA) paradigm (Dunskus et al. 1995), and includes specialized, knowledge-based design agents with precise functionality. Each agent has a predefined function in the design process. The agent types we see as most important are:

- *Designers* – agents that are responsible for taking design decisions, such as selecting values for design parameters, or creating links between design components in a configuration process.
- *Critics* – agents that criticize design aspects, such as design parameter values, or weak properties of component configurations. Beyond revealing undesirable properties of the design, critics may point out constraints or quality requirements that are not met by the design aspect on which they focus.
- *Praisers* – are meant to praise design aspects that rate particularly highly from a given point of view. Positive evaluations are important when designers have to decide which parts of the design need to be revised and which ones should preferably remain unchanged.
- *Estimators* – produce estimates of design aspects, such as parameters, or component types, that are needed in design decisions, but are unavailable at that point in the design process. The unavailability is often caused by cyclic dependencies and design constraints, where computations cannot be ordered such that all the needed elements are computed in previous design steps.

The agent function types are not necessarily limited to the ones previously described. The final application domain and the scale of the multi-agent system are the factors that ultimately decide the agent types to be included in the system.

All design agents have a restricted area of influence called a "target". The target represents the design elements that are the object of an agent's functionality. In parametric design problems an agent's target can be as narrow as a single design parameter. Several agents, of various functionalities, can have overlapping targets. For example, a component material can be decided by a designer agent, and can be criticized by two different critics.

Design agents can be classified on a third dimension – their domain of specialization. Agents typically group knowledge and heuristics that allow them to reason in a particular domain. For example, two critics that target the material of a component can have different domains of specialization, such as cost or reliability.

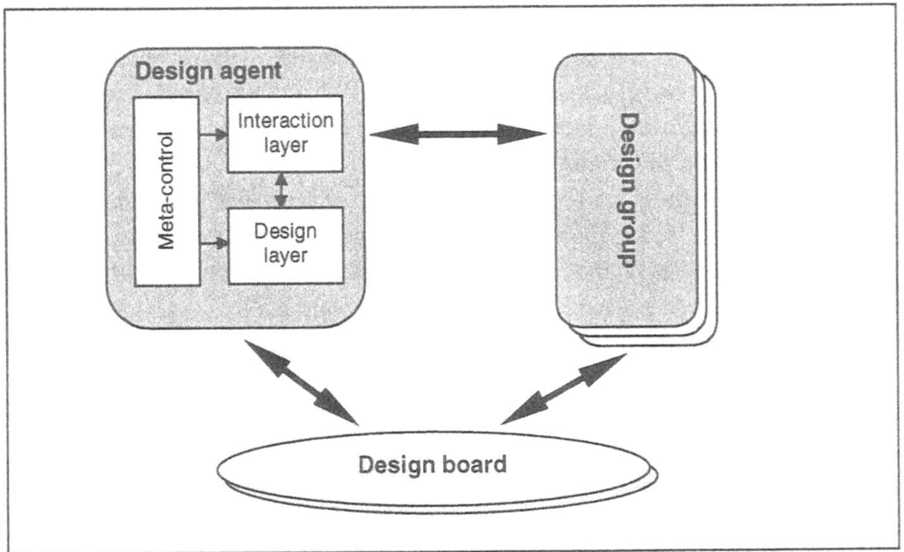

Figure 8. High-level representation of the multi-agent design system architecture

The description given so far covers one of the two main components that make up a design agent – the design layer. The knowledge incorporated at this level gives the agent the ability to function as an independent design specialist. A second layer – the interaction layer – allows the agent to be part of the design group. The interaction layer includes the knowledge that is necessary to communicate, coordinate and reach agreements with other group members (figure 8):

- *Coordination:* Agents act on a task-centered basis. An agent takes on, or 'assumes' a task if it decides it can achieve the requirements of the task. Once an agent has acquired a task, the scheduling of the task and its execution are entirely decided by that agent. An agent can delay the execution of a task if it does not have the necessary resources to proceed (parameter values, critiques of a given decision, etc.). Agent coordination is generated by the computational needs that arise during task execution. The coordination module searches for and acquires the information needed for the agent's computations. The availability of such information can be determined from the current design state or by querying other agents.
- *Conflict resolution:* Conflicts occur mainly due to constraint violations. Previous design decisions may have left no choices for subsequent design aspects that depend on these decisions. The agents that have over-

constrained the design and the agent that cannot proceed as a result of these constraints have to agree on a set of values that allows them all to accomplish their respective tasks. Previous work on single function agents has looked extensively into conflict classification (Dunskus et al. 1995), conflict detection (Berker and Brown 1996), and conflict resolution (Brown, Dunskus, and Grecu 1994). The conflict resolution strategies that were successfully tested in the SiFA environment are reimplemented in the current agent model.

- *Communication* is implemented using a speech act framework with KQML (Finin et al. 1992). Messages include performatives defining the permissible actions that an agent can attempt in communicating with another agent (e.g., 'ask', 'evaluate', 'reply' etc.). The communication is direct, i.e., it doesn't use any intermediary facilitation or mediation agents.

The multi-agent design system is implemented in the CLIPS rule-based environment (Giarratano and Riley 1998). The machine-learning components are based on source code for wrapper techniques and inductive learning included in the MLC++ machine learning library (SGI 1996).

7. THE EVALUATION METHODOLOGY

Given the flexibility in learning that is made possible in our approach, and the potential complexity of the MADS, it is clear that careful attention needs to be given to the evaluation of the impact of learning on the design system (Grecu and Brown 1998b). A number of issues need to be considered for the evaluation.

The first issue focuses on the sets of features in the design environment that are 'perceived' by the agents, that is, the observable world of each agent. The learning result will significantly depend on the features available to the agents. The features in the design environment that are visible to an agent will determine the subset that eventually gets selected by the learning component to represent new expectations.

The causal mechanisms for selecting candidate conditions represent a second major validation topic. Causal mechanisms strongly bias the learning process. A large set of initial candidate conditions will transfer part of the learning bias toward the covariational analysis, and relies on the latter's ability to filter out conditions in a domain-independent way. On the other hand, a restrictive, low-level set of causal mechanisms, that cope with very narrow situations, may forfeit the chance to develop an expectation, given that critical information may be omitted from the very beginning.

The covariational analysis has three factors that influence the final definition of the expectation. The learning algorithm used has to suit the types of features selected by the causal mechanisms, and its selection depends of the size of the training set that is being provided. Second, the candidate conditions can be generated and refined using several techniques, such as hill-climbing. And, finally, various criteria of relevance can be used, including the accuracy and the size of the feature subset. All of the three factors need an estimate and an analysis of adequacy for the class of design problems that are being approached.

The expectation validation process itself has several parameters open to validation. The amount of training instances that are acquired before the expectation is revised determines the 'granularity' of the expectation revision. It has to be coordinated with the number of times expectation revisions are accepted, such that the decision to eliminate an expectation corresponds to the learning limits of the agent with respect to the design environment, and not to weak stabilization criteria.

Although not directly included in the learning process itself, but nevertheless of considerable impact, are the criteria that determine whether and when an agent decides to acquire an expectation. This directly influences the number of learning processes that will be active. It is also critical in preventing an agent from acquiring irrelevant knowledge that would impede on its decision making rather than enhancing it.

A problem directly related to the number of expectations that are simultaneously learned is the potential interference between learning processes, as described in section 5.3. The focus here lies on the differences between a set of expectations learned and revised sequentially, and the same set of expectations learned concurrently, with a lower rate of stabilization.

Finally, learning needs to be evaluated with respect to the objectives of the design problem. The evaluation has to answer whether design aspects have been improved, and/or whether the design process has become more efficient, for example, by generating fewer conflicts, or less backtracking cases.

8. CONCLUSIONS

There are several important aspects of the approach to guiding learning in MADS that have been presented here. The first, and most general idea, is that learning is distributed throughout the MADS, and that learning can occur independently and concurrently.

The second is that the learning activity is temporary, in the sense that learning is active at a particular location in the MADS until the learning result has been validated or eliminated.

The third important aspect is that learning processes shift around the system at run time in response to the agents' information needs. These patterns of activating learning processes are affected by the design problems approached and by their requirements. In addition, given the same design problems, it is clear that the learned expectations will be different depending on the agents that are present in the system.

The manipulation of the expectation learning parameters discussed in the last two sections offers the possibility of experimentation with learning in a MADS. The use of wrappers strongly supports the flexibility of the learning methodology, and allows Machine Learning experiments to be carried out to determine the effect of different algorithms.

We believe that learning in MADS is an important and necessary area of investigation that will ensure the effectiveness and efficiency of future design systems. The approach we have described for guiding learning in multi-agent design systems provides the flexibility needed to take advantage of the power of learning and to dynamically target it to areas that need it in the MADS. We are experimenting with our approach and details of its performance will be described in future articles.

REFERENCES

Berker, I., and D.C. Brown (1996). Conflict and negotiations in single function agent based design systems. *Concurrent Engineering: Research and Applications*. Special issue on Multi-Agent Systems in Concurrent Engineering, D.C. Brown, S. Lander, and C. Petrie (eds.) (1):17-3.

Brown, D.C., B. Dunskus, and D. Grecu (1994). Using Single Function Agents to Investigate Negotiations. AAAI-94 Workshop on Models of Conflict Management in Cooperative Problem Solving, Seattle, WA.

Cherniak, C. (1986). *Minimal Rationality*. Cambridge, MA: The MIT Press.

Dunskus, B.V., D.L. Grecu, D.C. Brown, and I. Berker (1995). Using Single Function Agents to Investigate Conflict. *Artificial Intelligence for Engineering Design, Analysis and Manufacturing*. Special issue on Conflict Management in Design, I. Smith (ed.). 9:299-312.

Etzioni, A. (1964). *Modern Organizations*. Englewood Cliffs, NJ: Prentice Hall.

Finin, T., J. Weber, G. Wiederhold, M. Genesereth, R. Fritzson, J. McGuire, D. McKay, C. Shapiro, W. Pelavin, and S. Beck. (1992). Specification of the KQML Agent Communication Language: Enterprise Integratrion Technologies, Inc.

Gennari, J.H., P. Langley, and D. Fisher. (1989). Models of incremental concept formation. *Artificial Intelligence* 40:11-61.

Giarratano, J.C., and G. Riley. 1998. *CLIPS Reference Manual*: PWS Publishing Co.

Grecu, D.L., and D.C. Brown (1998). Dimensions of Learning in Design. *Artificial Intelligence for Engineering Design, Analysis and Manufacturing*. Special issue on Machine Learning in Design, A.H.B. Duffy, D.C. Brown, and A.K. Goel (eds.) 12 (April):117-122.

Grecu, D.L., and D.C. Brown (1998). Evaluating the Impact of Distributed Learning in Real-World Design Problems. Workshop on Machine Learning in Design (5th International Conference on Artificial Intelligence in Design), Lisbon, Portugal.

Hilton, D.J. (1990). Conversational Processes and Causal Explanation. *Psychological Bulletin* 107 (1):65-81.

Kohavi, R., and G.H. John (1998). Wrappers for Feature Subset Selection. *Artificial Intelligence* 97 (1-2):273-324.

Koslowski, B. (1996). *Theory and Evidence: The Development of Scientific Reasoning*. Edited by L. Gleitman, S. Carey, E. Newport and E. Spelke, *Learning, Development, and Conceptual Change*. Cambridge, MA and London, UK: The MIT Press.

Lander, S. (1998). Issues in Multiagent Design Systems. *IEEE Expert*:18-26.

Liu, H., and R. Setiono (1998). Incremental Feature Selection. *Applied Intelligence*.

Russell, S., and E. Wefald (1991). *Do the Right Thing - Studies in Limited Rationality*. Cambridge, MA: The MIT Press.

SGI (1996). MLC++ Utilities: Silicon Graphics.

Shultz, T.R., G.W. Fisher, C.C. Pratt, and S. Rulf (1986). Selection of Causal Rules. *Child Development* 57:143-152.

Tversky, A., and D. Kahneman (1974). Judgment under uncertainty: heuristics and biases. *Science* 185:1124-1131.

14

A KICAD Tool For Pro-Active Exploration Support To 'Design Synthesis For Multi-X'

Jonathan.C. Borg[1], Xiu-TianYan[2] & Neal.P. Juster[2]
[1]*Department of Manufcturing Engineering, University of Malta,Malta*
[2]*Department of Design, Manufacture and Engineering Management, University of Strathclyde, U.K.*

Key words: Concurrent engineering, DFX, artefact life exploration, decisions, design reuse

Abstract: Designers are now expected to 'generate' life-oriented design solutions. This transition to *'Design Synthesis for Multi-X (DFΣX)'* reflects an increase in demands being put on designers. This paper reports on the development and implementation of a Knowledge Intensive CAD (KICAD) tool aimed at pro-actively supporting designers in foreseeing and exploring multiple life-cycle consequences co-evolving during mechanical artefact design decision making. A phenomena model describing 'how' consequences are generated highlights the necessity of designers engaging in concurrent synthesis. This understanding is exploited by a 'Knowledge of Consequences' approach to DFΣX on which the KICAD implementation is based. The paper includes an outline of the KICAD's knowledge model, system requirements and architecture. The application of a prototype named FORESEE to pro-actively supporting 'life-oriented' exploration is demonstrated via a thermoplastic component design scenario. An evaluation of the prototype revealed strengths and limitations that highlight future research challenges for developing KICAD tools aimed at supporting DFΣX.

1. INTRODUCTION

Industry is increasingly becoming concerned with delivering products that cater for a *host* of total life-cycle values (Ishii, 1995). Focusing on 'function' during design leads to products that are "not being designed for..." (Duffy et al., 1993) a number of 'X-abilities'. Thus design in industry is increasingly concerned with product life issues such as design for manufacturab*ility* with the result that "the number of *'ilities'* are growing" (Brown, 1996). Designers are now expected to generate solutions that cater for more total life issues, this manifesting itself in a transition to what is termed *'Design Synthesis for Multi-X (DFΣX)'*. As a result of the options encountered in the solution space, the design process is decision intensive as reflected by for instance (Medland, 1997).

The *reality* is that all design decisions have a consequence, *intended* or *unintended*, good or bad (Borg and Yan, 1998). Moreover, design decisions can have a propagation effect that spans multiple life-phases (Borg and MacCallum, 1996). Design decisions are known to influence the performance of other life-cycle phases in terms of measures such as cost and time (Olesen, 1992). Decisions which seem good for one phase can lead to problems and high costs in another. Due to human mental processing limitations, designers are frequently unaware of *life-cycle consequences (LCC)*, resulting from their decisions, these being (Borg and Yan, 1998):

- life phase behaviour of the artefact
- life phase behaviour of the life-phase systems
- new decision spaces
- new life cycle constraints.

Although designers have a number of manual and computer based approaches at their disposal, as argued in the review found in (Borg and Yan, 1998), designers are still not adequately supported during early design in foreseeing unintended life-cycle consequences co-evolving with their solution, this necessary for life-oriented exploration purposes. These tools/methods including DFX guidelines, FMEA, constraint networks and expert systems:

a) provide an insight into life cycle consequences rather late in the design process, this separate from the synthesis activity, thus not readily supporting exploration;
b) provide a narrow and segmented insight into consequences associated with a solution;
c) provide a generic insight rather than problem/company specific insight.

These limitations suggest that any tool assisting designers, as from the early stages of design, to have an insight into consequences co-evolving across *multiple* life phases is highly desirable i.e. a tool supporting a DFΣX approach. This paper presents initial results of research into the development, implementation and evaluation of such a KICAD tool, aimed at pro-actively supporting artefact life exploration to promote 'Design Synthesis for Multi-X' of mechanical components.

The development of the KICAD tool is based on the design tool development framework proposed by (Duffy and Andreasen, 1995) who state that computational tools should be based on *information models* derived from models of the *reality*, termed *phenomena models*. The specific phenomena concerned with in this research is that design decisions give rise to life-cycle consequences. A phenomena model aims to explain through observations made *how* the phenomena is caused in the *reality*. The *knowledge model* is concerned with *what* elements should form part of the knowledge structure and with *how* these elements should be related to each other and organized, in order to result in codified knowledge. The *computer model* encompasses existing or new techniques to realize and manipulate the knowledge model for supporting the design reality.

2. CONSEQUENCE PHENOMENA MODEL

To provide support allowing designers to foresee co-evolving LCCs, it is necessary to understand *how* LCCs are generated from decision commitments. Based on research case-study observations and building on decision making models, a phenomena model (Borg and Yan, 1998) describing how LCCs are generated from two fundamentally different conditions is being introduced in this section. For explanations in the remaining paper sections, the notation in Table (1) will be employed.

Table 1. Notation

Symbol	Meaning	Symbol	Meaning
{ }	a set	⌊a⌋	a class e.g. ⌊Ferrous materials⌋
$a \Leftarrow b$	'a' has properties 'b'	M	a material e.g. M = ductile cast-iron
$a \wedge b$	'a' and 'b'	F	a form feature e.g. F= slot
$a \vee b$	'a' or 'b'	F_a	an assembly feature e.g. F_a= snap-fit
$a \subset b$	'a' is a subset of 'b'	P	a technical process e.g. P = milling
a => b	'a' results in 'b'	D{O}	Decision proposal concerning a set of options {O} e.g. diameter value ?
a •→ b	'a' kind_of 'b'	$d_E\{O\}$	an explicit synthesis decision commitment i.e. selected option
a → b	'a' part_of 'b'	S	a space of decision proposals e.g. S={what diameter? ∧ what depth? }
¬	'not'	<phase>_i	life-phase 'i' e.g. $\text{<phase>}_{disposal}$
a >---b	'a' is suitable for 'b'	[k]	a model of 'k' e.g. [component]

In this paper, a decision is assumed to exist due to a selection between a number of *alternatives* (or options). Strictly speaking, without alternatives, there would be no decision (Holtzman, 1988). In the case of mechanical artefacts, the designer encounters alternatives due to degrees of freedom concerning manipulable parameters which (Tjalve, 1979) states are *structure, form, material, dimensions, surface quality*. Together, these completely describe a product - they are the variables that can be manipulated by the designer. Key activities that *re-occur* during design are synthesis, analysis and evaluation (Blessing, 1994; Roozenburg and Eekels, 1995). This paper argues that during synthesis, designers make what are termed *synthesis decision commitments* (Borg and Yan, 1998) these being:

> A commitment that is reflected in the evolving solution model - e.g. type of material, type of assembly feature or a parameter value.

Synthesis decision commitments change the state of the artefact solution – the solution becomes either more *concrete* (a circular opening is added) or *detailed* (the radius of the opening is specified). Irrespective of the designer's intention, it is consequences associated with these commitments with which designers should therefore be concerned in a 'Design Synthesis for Multi-X' approach. Synthesis decision commitments concern those characteristics which the designer has direct control of. Viewing an artefact's structure from a constructional perspective, it is composed of several levels (product, sub-assembly, component, component element) that evolve from synthesis decision commitments. These reflect characteristics defined by the designer during synthesis, termed in this paper *Product Design Elements (PDE)*, since irrespective of the product structure abstraction level they belong to, they will eventually form part of the final artefact design solution. In the case of components, PDEs include reusable component elements such as form features (Shah and Mantyla, 1995), assembly features, material and surface textures. Of relevance to artefact life exploration is that during its life, a component encounters what are termed in this paper *Life Cycle Phase Elements (LCPE),* examples being fabrication, assembly, servicing and disposal systems. Viewed as technical systems (Hubka and Eder, 1988), LCPEs can be decomposed into various sub-systems.

2.1 Non-interacting consequences

Individual elements (PDEs or LCPEs) present in an *artefact life model**, introduced by synthesis decision commitments can give rise to unintended consequences. In this case, a LCC is generated by one specific element commitment. This means that given the set $\{O_1\}$ of alternatives (could be a set of PDEs or a set of LCPEs) in Figure 1a, the option selected by the designer, in this case, o_1^1, becomes *'part of'* the evolving artefact life model. This introduces its associated consequence of the ***n***on-***i***nteracting type (LCC_{ni}), shown as 'x' in Figure 1a. Formally, this can be stated as:

* An artefact life model <life model> consists of an artefact and life-phase system compositional models

$$(d_E\{O_1\} = o_1^1) \Rightarrow (LCC_{ni} = \text{'x'}). \quad (1)$$

A typical example is when a snap-fit (o_1^1) is selected from a set of assembly features $\{O_1\}$, resulting in the consequence (x) 'weak bond', formally stated as:

$$(d_E\{\text{snap-fit} .. \vee .. \vee \text{ screw}\} = \text{snap-fit}) \Rightarrow (LCC_{ni} = \text{'weak bond'}). \quad (2)$$

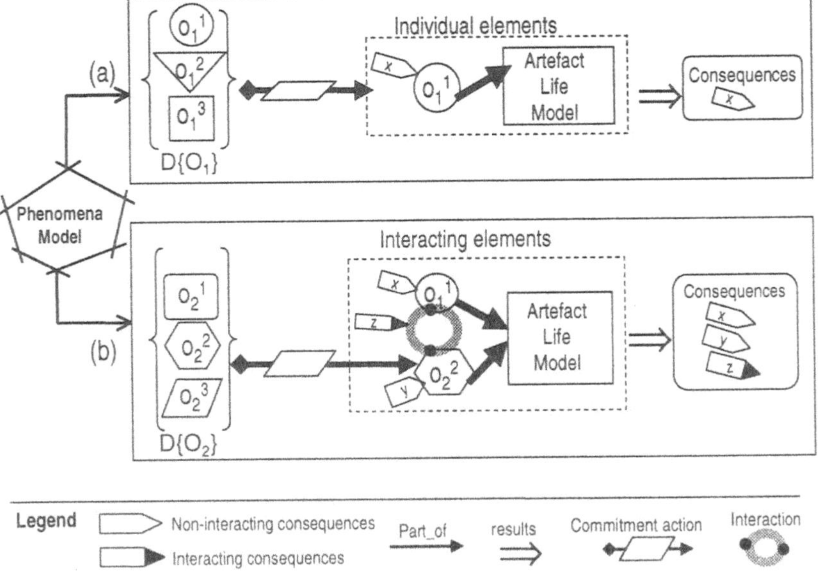

Figure 1. LCC generation phenomena model

2.2 Interacting consequences

Interacting type LCCs depend upon the interaction between a set of ***'n'*** life synthesis commitments where $n > 1$. Considering Figure 1b, as the solution synthesis activity proceeds, the designer makes another decision commitment concerning a different set of elements $\{O_2\}$. Assuming that in this case, the designer commits option o_2^2, this introduces its associated consequence of the non-interacting type i.e. 'y', formally:

$$(d_E\{O_2\} = o_2^2) \Rightarrow (LCC_{ni} = \text{'y'}). \quad (3)$$

An example concerning a set $\{O_2\}$ of LCPEs is the commitment of an injection moulding process system (o_2^2), this resulting in consequence (y) that a 'mould is required', formally:

$(d_E\{P\}$ = Injection Moulding) => (LCC_{ni} = 'mould is required'). (4)

The elements committed i.e. o_1^1 and o_2^2 can sometimes *interact* to give rise to a consequence 'z', this being termed an *interacting* consequence (LCC_i), formally:

$$(d_E\{O_1\}= o_1^1) \wedge (d_E\{O_2\} = o_2^2) \Rightarrow (LCC_i = \text{'z'}). \quad (5)$$

A typical example is the formation of *sink mark defects* during the realization phase, this based on the interaction between the following specific set of component life synthesis commitments:

$(d_E\{F_a\}$=snap-fit) $\wedge(d_E\{M\}$=STYRON)$\wedge((d_E\{P\}$ = Injection Moulding**) → <phase>$_{realization}$)=>(LCC_i='sink mark defect'). (6)

3. A 'KNOWLEDGE OF CONSEQUENCES' APPROACH FRAMEWORK

The phenomena model highlights that for generating a life-oriented component design solution, *concurrent 'artefact'* and *'life-phase system' synthesis* (Andreasen et al., 1996) is necessary if designers are to 'Design Synthesis for Multi-X' . Otherwise, consequences resulting from the interaction of solution specific commitments will be difficult to reveal and cater for during synthesis. Also, the phenomena model contributes an understanding to *how* consequences are generated. This understanding provides the basis to *what* should be captured and modelled to causally relate synthesis decision commitments and LCCs. This causality is useful for:

a) *foreseeing consequences*: depending on commitments made, modelled LCCs co-evolving with the solution, can be revealed during synthesis;
b) *solution synthesis guidance*: it provides a means to search for elements that need to be committed to result in an intended consequences; e.g. what assembly feature results in a sub-assembly that is easy to dis-assemble in the disposal phase?
c) *LCC avoidance/relaxation:* designers can be pro-actively made aware of LCCs and their *source* commitments; this knowledge provides guidance to *what* commitments can be *explored* to avoid/relax a detected LCC.

** The phase is being explicitly modelled to avoid confusion to which life phase the explicit synthesis decision commitment is made

This understanding can be exploited to reveal LCCs co-evolving with the solution, thereby allowing designers to explore the co-evolving artefact life solution and problem space. The argument is that for 'Design for Multi-X', synthesis decision making will be better accomplished by reasoning with knowledge of co-evolving LCCs.

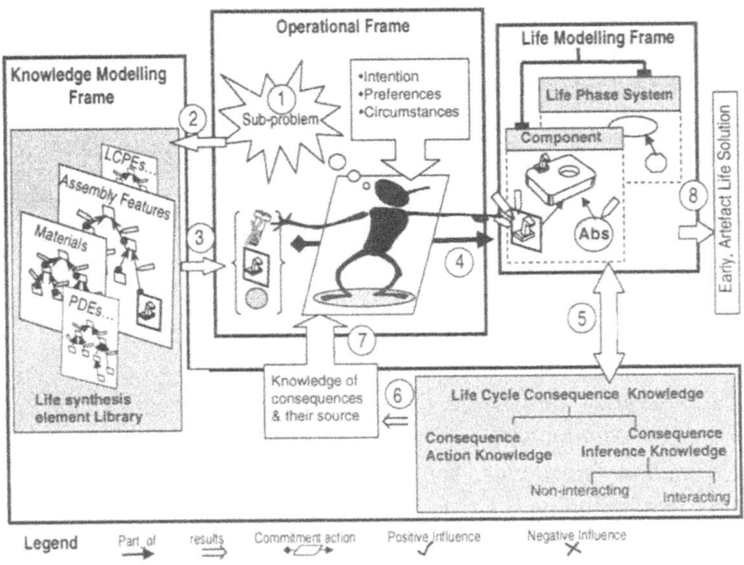

Figure 2. 'KC' Approach Framework

Using these principles, a ***'Knowledge of life-cycle Consequences' (KC) approach framework***, to component 'Design Synthesis for Multi-X' based on the following three frames (Figure 2) has been developed.

1. Operational frame: this concerns the operating principles of the approach. Basically, it assumes that many well-developed solution concepts (PDEs) and well-known life cycle phase elements (LCPEs) are reused during synthesis and encountered during the total life of an artefact. A fundamental operating principle is that a designer is engaged in concurrent synthesis - the *artefact life model* is *what* the designer generates and models during component life design synthesis. For this purpose, when a design sub-problem is encountered (step 1), the designer can interact with a synthesis elements library to search (step 2) for a set of suitable elements (step 3). Based on designer intentions, preferences and circumstances, the designer commits (step 4) elements to evolve the artefact life model. This evolving model is monitored (step 5) by consequence inference knowledge which infers (step 6) any co-evolving LCCs. Relevant consequence action knowledge infers actions that need

to be carried out, such as changes in performance measures of appropriate life-phase metrics to allow designers to monitor the artefact life behaviour. Collectively, this inferred knowledge is utilized (step 7) for exploring the avoidance/relaxation of the LCCs detected.

2. *Artefact life modelling frame:* due to the need of concurrent synthesis, designers need to handle both artefact and life-phase system models. This frame therefore comprises a set of domain specific *synthesis elements* (PDEs and LCPEs) linked with *part_of relationships* describing the evolving compositional *artefact* and *life-phase system* models from a pre-set synthesis viewpoint (e.g. constructional);
3. *Knowledge modelling frame:* this concerns the description of:

a) *a synthesis element library*, consisting of various models of synthesis elements (PDEs and LCPEs) reused during the design and life of a mechanical artefact domain. In the case of components, this includes models of form features, assembly features, materials and LCPEs such as fabrication systems and assembly systems;

b) *life-cycle consequence knowledge*, consisting of:

- *LCC inference knowledge* for revealing non-interacting and interacting LCCs co-evolving with synthesis decision commitments;
- *LCC action knowledge*, for performing actions specific to an inferred LCC, this including LCC to performance mapping, concurrent synthesis patterns and guidance/explanation to LCC avoidance/relaxation (see Section 4.3).

4. A KNOWLEDGE MODEL

A *KICAD* tool provides a means of how captured knowledge can be reused in new design situations, at fast processing speeds, this providing a sensible solution to adopting the 'KC' approach framework. KICAD tools require a knowledge model. As reflected by the phenomena model, LCCs co-evolve with *concretization* (e.g. adding a hole) and *detailing* (e.g. specifying the diameter) synthesis decision commitments being made to the evolving artefact life solution. Modelling LCC knowledge is concerned with the description of *causal relationships* between the evolving *artefact life model* and the resulting *LCCs*, the latter mapped as fluctuations in performance measures across multiple life-phases. This is schematically illustrated in Figure (3).

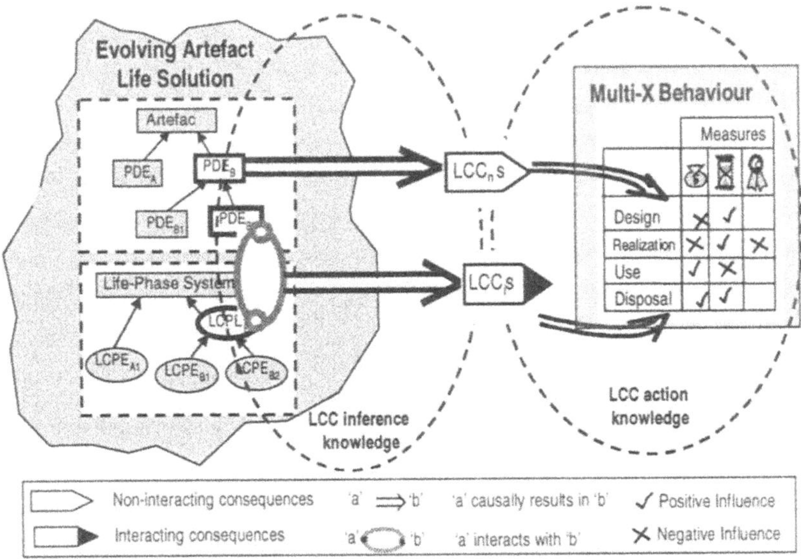

Figure 3. Relationships embodying LCC knowledge

4.1 LCC_{ni} inference knowledge

Consequence 'x' in relationship (1) is a piece of knowledge that can be associated with the synthesis commitment option o_1^{1}. That is, knowledge of LCC_{ni}s can be modelled as:

$$(d_E\{O\}) \Leftarrow \{(LCC)_{ni}\} \tag{7}$$

read as:
A synthesis commitment $d_E\{O\}$ has ($\Leftarrow$) an associated set $\{(LCC)_{ni}\}$ of non-interacting life-cycle consequences.

The associated knowledge will depend on the specific commitment e.g. using the notation {a} to represent a set of assembly characteristics, a LCC_{ni} knowledge model for a screw PDE is:

$$(F_a\text{=screw}) \Leftarrow (\{a\} = \{\text{assembly slow} \wedge \text{requires hole} \wedge \text{dis-assembly easy}\}). \tag{8}$$

Through the commitment of this screw model to the evolving artefact solution, it can be inferred that a screw-joint dis-assembling activity (e.g. in the disposal phase) is *easy* because:

$(d_E\{F_a\} = \text{screw}) \Rightarrow ([\text{screw}] \Leftarrow \{\text{assembly slow} \wedge \text{requires hole} \wedge \text{dis-assembly } \textit{easy}\}) \rightarrow [\text{artefact}]$. (9)

4.2 LCC_i inference knowledge

Causal relationship (5) depicts that it is the *interacting relationship (IR)* between elements o_1^1 and o_2^2 (i.e. the synthesis decision commitments) which causes the interacting life-cycle consequence 'z'. A specific interacting relationship $(IR)_j$ between a set of elements is a *LCC-specific* conjunctive set of $d_E\{O\}_j$ ($j \geq 2$) synthesis commitments formally:

$$(IR)_j = \{d_E\{O\}_1 \wedge d_E\{O\}_2 \wedge \ldots d_E\{O\}_j\}. \quad (10)$$

Then a specific LCC_i is modelled by causally relating it to a specific interacting relationship, formally:

$$(IR)_j \Leftarrow \{(LCC_j)_i\} \quad (11)$$

read as:

An interacting life-cycle consequence $(LCC_j)_i$ is associated with an interacting relationship $(IR)_j$ concerning a consequence-specific conjunctive set of synthesis commitments.

A specific example is the piece of knowledge concerning the formation of *weld line defects* in thermoplastic components:

$$((d_E\{F\}=\text{hole}) \wedge (d_E\{M\}=\text{STYRON}) \wedge ((d_E\{P\}=\text{Injection Moulding}) \rightarrow \langle\text{phase}\rangle_{\text{realization}}))) \Leftarrow \{(LCC)_i = \text{'component can have a weld line defect'}\}. \quad (12)$$

Therefore, if at any time during synthesis, an interacting relationship $(IR)_j$ is a sub-set of the evolving artefact life compositional model, <life model>, then the associated interacting life-cycle consequence $(LCC_j)_i$ can be inferred, formally:

$$(IR)_j \subseteq \langle\text{life model}\rangle \Rightarrow (LCC_j)_i. \quad (13)$$

For example, through (12) and (13), it can be inferred that a component made from STYRON and having a hole form feature, which is going to be injection moulded is likely to have a weld line defect, even though the solution may still be incompletely defined.

4.3 Consequence action knowledge

Performance mapping knowledge:

An action that can result due to a LCC is a change (δ) to a *performance measure* (PM) e.g. time, of a transformation process [P], formally:

$$(LCC_{ni}) \Rightarrow (\delta PM)P \quad \text{or} \quad (LCC_i) \Rightarrow \delta(PM)P. \tag{14}$$

Through (14), a *change (δ)* caused in the respective performance measure can be causally related to the respective LCC. Changes in performance measure values are modelled *relative* to values resulting from other possibilities (e.g. 'assembly fast) and on a range –10 to +10. For example, for the LCC_{ni} = 'Assembly slow' generated with the screw in (8):

$$((LCC_{ni}) = \text{'Assembly slow'}) \Rightarrow (\text{Quality}=-5)(P=\text{assembly}) \wedge (\text{Time}=+5)(P=\text{assembly}) \wedge (\text{Cost}=+5)(P=\text{assembly}). \tag{15}$$

Such fluctuations in performance measures may be propagated to other life-cycle phases since the transformation in a $<\text{Phase}>_i$ is the result of a set of transformations by different processes $\{P_j\}$ forming *part of* that phase. A specific measure e.g. $(PM)_x$ of a phase is thus given by:

$$(PM)_x<\text{Phase}>_i = \Sigma(PM)_x P_j. \tag{16}$$

Relationships (14) and (16) therefore allow *relative* performance measures for different life-phases to be calculated and used as a means by which a designer can foresee and monitor the virtual behaviour of the artefact's life due to consequences co-evolving with the solution.

Concurrent synthesis knowledge:

A type of LCC is a decision space 'S' with a set of decision proposals D{O}. In some circumstances, an option set {O} can have an associated default commitment. For instance although there exists a set of how circular holes can be generated, in the case of injection moulding, the default is to use a core-pin in a mould tool. Such a LCC results in a *concurrent synthesis pattern* as once modelled, it provides a means to automatically evolve a specific *[model]* forming *part of* the artefact life model:

If (LCC)=> (D{O}) with a default commitment o'), then ($d_E\{O\}$ = o')→[model]. (16b)

Having inferred a LCC (e.g. the formation of a weld line defect), action knowledge providing an *explanation* of the LCC and *guidance* to its avoidance/relaxation is also required. By exploiting the phenomena of LCCs, knowledge of which commitment(s) give rise to a detected consequence can be made explicit. This provides designers with a list of commitments that can be explored. Guidance knowledge is very LCC specific.

4.4 Knowledge structuring

The generic models in (7) and (11) are useful to generate a LCC knowledge base. However, for *relevant* knowledge to be revealed and utilized at the *right time*, with both *least* (Guan and MacCallum, 1995) and *specific* synthesis decision commitments, a knowledge base needs to be structured, this being also necessary for knowledge management and scaling issues.

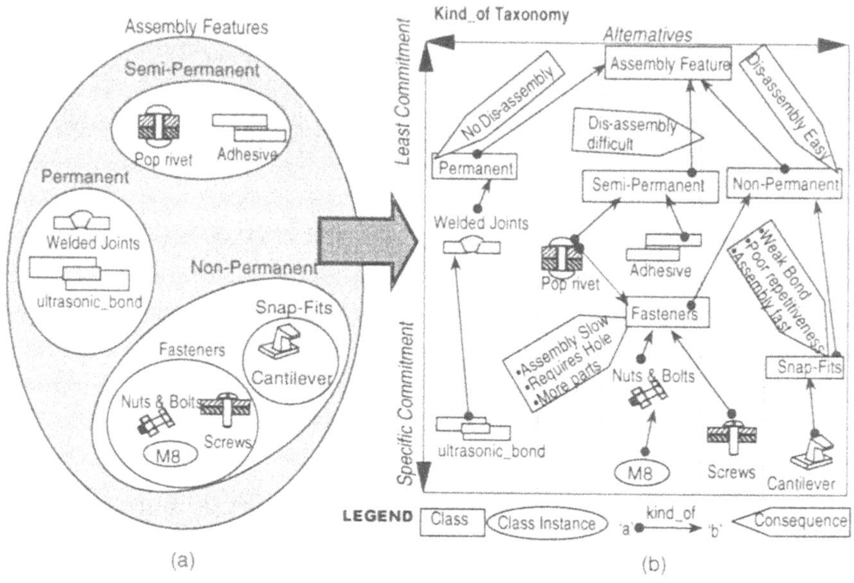

Figure 4. LCC knowledge structuring via Kind_of taxonomies

4.4.1 LCC_{ni} knowledge structuring

Rationalization mechanisms (Kerr, 1993) can be employed to structure a synthesis elements library. For example, Figure 4a demonstrates a (non-exhaustive) set of assembly features organized into sub-sets by their joint permanence characteristic. Such a class rationalisation process enables synthesis elements to be organized into *kind_of* taxonomies as illustrated in

Figure 4b and Figure 5. A *kind_of* taxonomy allows elements (or concepts) at the top of the hierarchy to be more abstract than those lower down. For example, we can say that bolt *M8* •→ *⌊Nuts&Bolts⌋* This also means that reusable concepts can be organized into classes and sub-classes. Such a *kind_of* taxonomy allows designers to explore *alternative* synthesis elements (e.g. a pop-rivet versus an M8 bolt) and make commitments at the desired *level of detail* (e.g. an M8 bolt versus simply a ⌊Fasteners⌋). The significance of these taxonomies is that LCC_{ni} knowledge can be associated to different abstraction levels in the taxonomy as illustrated in Figure 4b. For example, based on (7),

⌊Non-Permanent⌋ ⇐ ($(LCC)_{ni}$ = 'Dis-assembly Easy') (17)

whilst at a more specific level in the taxonomy:

⌊Fasteners⌋ ⇐ ($(LCC)_{ni}$ = 'Assembly slow' ∧ 'Requires hole'∧ 'More parts') (18)

⌊Snap-Fits⌋ ⇐ ($(LCC)_{ni}$ = 'Weak Bond' ∧ 'Assembly fast' ∧ 'Poor repetitiveness') (19).

This concept of associating LCC_{ni} knowledge with relevant classes reduces the duplication of common knowledge, thereby making it attractive from a knowledge scaling point of view. For example, there is no need to explicitly associate *'Requires hole'* with instance M8, as this piece of knowledge will be inherited from (18) since *M8* •→*⌊Fasteners⌋* *Kind_of* taxonomies can also exploit *union inheritance* (Walters and Nielsen, 1988), this useful in situations where a class or instance has more than one parent. An example is ⌊Snap-Fits⌋, this being both an assembly feature and a protruding form feature:

⌊Snap-Fits⌋•→⌊Non-Permanent⌋) ∧ (⌊Snap-Fits⌋•→⌊Protruding⌋) (20)

⌊Pop rivet⌋ in Figure 4b is an example of a class having 2 parents within the same taxonomy:

(⌊Pop rivet⌋•→⌊Semi-Permanent⌋) ∧ (⌊Pop rivet⌋•→⌊Fasteners⌋). (21)

4.4.2 LCC_i knowledge structuring

Building on relationships (10) and (11), LCC_i knowledge models can be generalized by defining interacting relationships (IR)j as sets of class-based commitments, formally:

$$(IR)_j = \{(d_E\{O\}_1 \bullet\!\!\rightarrow \lfloor \text{class} \rfloor_1) \wedge \ldots (d_E\{O\}_j \bullet\!\!\rightarrow \lfloor \text{class} \rfloor_j). \qquad (22)$$

Figure 5 illustrates an example of sink marks in thermoplastic components, formally stated:

$$((d_E\{F\} \bullet\!\!\rightarrow \lfloor \text{Protruding} \rfloor) \wedge (d_E\{M\} \bullet\!\!\rightarrow \lfloor \text{Thermoplastics} \rfloor) \wedge (d_E\{P\} \bullet\!\!\rightarrow \lfloor \text{Solidification\_based} \rfloor)) \Leftarrow ((\ (LCC)_i = \text{'sink mark defect'}) \rightarrow [\text{component}]\ ). \qquad (23)$$

As structured in (23), interacting relationships forming between commitments of sub-classes and instances can be also detected during synthesis. For example, 23 is equally applicable to a component made from STYRON (a *kind of* ⌊Thermoplastics⌋ material) having a snap-fit (from 20, this also a *kind of* ⌊Protruding⌋ form feature) that is going to be injection moulded (a *kind of* ⌊Solidification_based⌋ fabrication process).

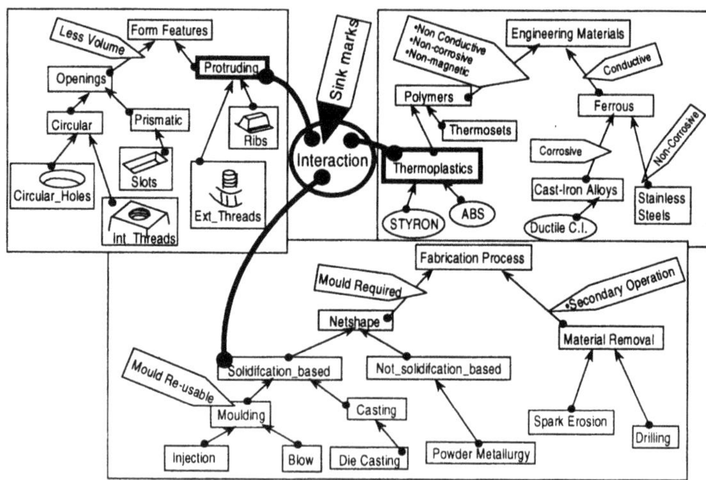

Figure 5. Example of LCC_i knowledge structuring principle

5. KICAD SYSTEM REQUIREMENTS

Based on the previous discussions, key requirements of a KICAD tool aimed at supporting designers to foresee and explore LCCs co-evolving with the solution are:

a) *supports a flexible synthesis sequence*: designers should not be constrained to make synthesis decision commitments in a fixed sequence;
b) *supports concurrent 'artefact' and 'life-phase' synthesis and modelling*: this due to the phenomena of interacting LCCs;
c) *supports artefact life concepts/solutions re-use:* The system should provide designers with a library comprising a set of well developed synthesis elements including PDEs (such as materials) and LCPEs (such as assembly systems and mould tools) that can be reused to model both artefact and life-phase systems;
d) *supports static and dynamic concept models:* certain synthesis elements do not change in behaviour with a change in time or environmental conditions e.g. a model of a circular hole form feature. However, certain concepts can change and thus need to be modelled in a way that reflects their dynamic nature. For example, a material's property such as stiffness, changes with different temperatures. For DFΣX such changes need to be foreseen if they are to be taken into consideration;
e) *supports the evolution of solutions with both least and specific commitments*: this is necessary to allow designers to foresee and explore LCCs as from early (rather than late) design. That is the tool should also support least synthesis decision commitments;
f) *supports the handling of both inaccurate and incomplete models:* it should be possible to foresee and explore LCCs of inaccurate models (e.g. component has an 'opening') and incomplete models (e.g. component has a 'hole' with unspecified parameter values);
g) *provides pro-active exploration support:* to cater for human mental processing limitations, the tool should pro-actively support the designer through:
   - *guidance in the retrieval of relevant and feasible option sets*: e.g. the tool should help designers retrieve assembly features that result in a non-permanent bond;
   - *the timely attraction to co-evolving LCCs:* i.e. revealing LCCs co-evolving with synthesis decision commitments being made;
   - *explanation of LCCs revealed:* suitable and relevant explanations need to be provided if a designer is to be motivated in avoiding/relaxing detected LCCs that relate to artefact life issues about which a designer may not be knowledgeable;

- *LCC avoidance:* the distinction between *interacting* and *non-interacting* LCCs should be exploited to *pro-actively guide* the designer's reasoning to those commitments which could be explored in order to avoid/relax a specific LCC detected;

h) *provides knowledge management facilities:* to avoid that captured knowledge faces obsolescence, the tool should support the updating of LCC knowledge;

i) *maintains truth:* of causal relationships (Yan and Sharpe, 1995) since component life exploration involves both decision commitment and retraction, this necessary for:
   - *consequences* - retracting a synthesis commitment should be associated with the retraction of causally related non-interacting and interacting consequences.
   - *performance measures* - the retraction of a consequence should result in an update of the values of the relevant performance measures influenced by that consequence;
   - *component and life-phase models*: a change to a component model (e.g. a different thermoplastic material) may require life-phase model updating (e.g. mould dimensions);

j) *supports the concurrent monitoring of multiple life phase behaviour:* to overcome a problem with current tools that provide a narrow and segmented insight into LCCs, it is necessary that the behaviour of multiple life-phases in terms of performance measures be concurrently estimated and monitored;

k) *automatically maintains a design session history* of synthesis decision commitments, retractions and the related fluctuations in life-phase behaviour. This is significant for design review meetings, for learning and for communicating the design intent. Automating this record keeping task avoids wasting the time and effort of a designer;

l) *provides a suitable user interface* that allows designers to *provide* and *retrieve* information to/from the system to support them in concurrent artefact life synthesis and exploration.

6. PROTOTYPE IMPLEMENTATION

A KICAD prototype, named FORESEE, has been implemented in the Windows95 environment of CLIPS (Giarratano and Riley, 1994), this providing multiple knowledge representation schemes, necessary for the codification of the established knowledge model. The domain selected concerns the conceptual design of thermoplastic components as these provide a suitable case for artefact life exploration due to alternative PDEs and LCPEs such as form, assembly features and fabrication systems. The implementation employs knowledge compiled from *public* sources and *private* expertise acquired through discussions with various artefact life actors involved in the domain. The *library access module* in the system architecture (Figure 6), allows the designer to search for synthesis elements that result in intended consequences. The *knowledge manager* provides utilities to dynamically add/modify classes/instances of synthesis elements stored in the library.

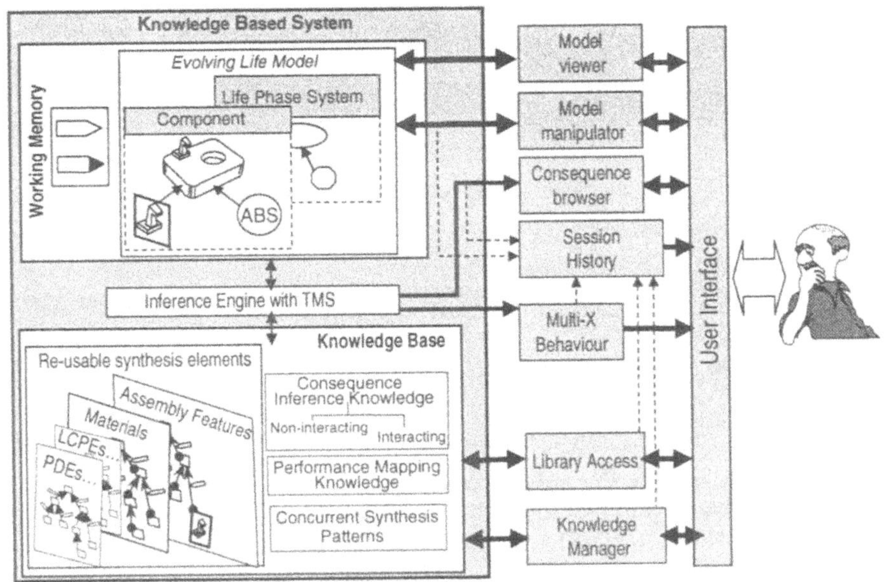

Figure 6. FORESEE's system architecture

The *model manipulator* provides functions that allow the designer to add/detail/refine elements to the *models* being concurrently synthesized, these represented internally in the *working memory* of the *knowledge based system*. A compositional hierarchy of an evolving model is displayed in the *user interface* (Figure 7) via the *model viewer*. The *inference engine* employs *LCC inference knowledge* to reveal LCCs co-evolving with the solution and *LCC action knowledge* to enable the KICAD tool to take a pro-active role in component DFΣX. The LCCs detected are displayed in the hypermedia (Html) based *consequence browser* this allowing a LCC to be individually browsed to reveal details about its meaning, its source commitment(s) and guidance to its avoidance. The *multi-X behaviour module* employs *performance mapping knowledge* to estimate and display fluctuations in performance measures as a result of consequences inferred. The *session history module* automatically maintains the design history.

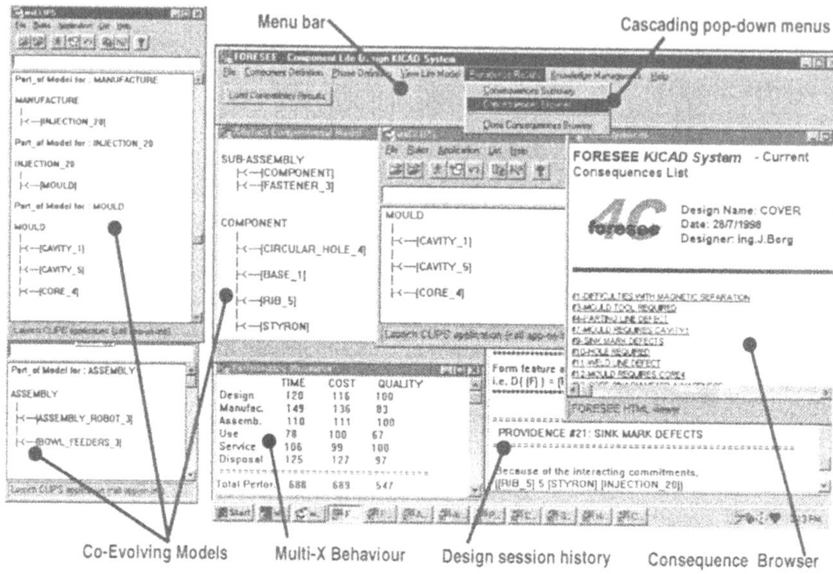

Figure 7. FORESEE's user interface

6.1 Knowledge representation

To codify the established knowledge model, a hybrid knowledge representation scheme has been employed. Models of different classes of synthesis elements captured in the knowledge base are represented in frames (Walters and Nielsen, 1988). Each frame has a number of slots particular to the element modelled. *Kind_of* taxonomies are represented through semantic networks. For this purpose, each frame has a slot 'parent' allowing *kind_of* relationships to be specified. For example, STYRON, a *kind_of* thermoplastic material will have the slot 'parent' defined as 'Thermoplastics' as in Figure 8. Frames also have a *'part of'* slot whose value is specified during synthesis, when instances of that frame are being created and related to other elements in the compositional model. For example, the 'Circular_Hole' frame in Figure 8 has 'Component' specified as a value of the *'part_of'* slot. Based on (7), LCC_{ni} knowledge associated with a class of elements is represented in frame slots. For example, the 'Screw' frame in Figure 8 has the value 'Requires hole' in the *Characteristics* slot.

$$\begin{array}{ll} \text{IF} & ((M \bullet\!\!\rightarrow \lfloor \text{Thermoplastic} \rfloor) \rightarrow [\text{component}]) \\ \text{AND} & ((F \bullet\!\!\rightarrow \lfloor \text{Protruding} \rfloor) \rightarrow [\text{component}]) \\ \text{AND} & ((P \bullet\!\!\rightarrow \lfloor \text{Solidification\_based} \rfloor) \rightarrow \langle \text{phase} \rangle_{\text{realization}}) \\ \text{THEN} & (LCC)_i = (\text{'sink mark defect'} \rightarrow [\text{component}]). \end{array} \quad (24)$$

LCC_i knowledge is represented in FORESEE with frame-based production rules (Walters and Nielsen, 1988) as these support the LCC_i structuring concept presented in (22), an example given in (24).

Performance mapping knowledge is represented as a function executed when a LCC-specific production rule is triggered. The function will cause a specific relative fluctuation (e.g. +5) in a specific performance measure (e.g. time) of a specific phase (e.g. realization). An example such a representation is in (25) :

IF (LCC)$_i$ = ('sink mark defect' → [component]) (25)

THEN ((Quality)<phase>$_{use}$ = -9)

AND ((Time)<phase>$_{realization}$ = +5)

AND ((Cost)<phase>$_{realization}$ = +4).

Concurrent synthesis patterns: these are represented in FORESEE as specific functions that cause the necessary manipulation (add/delete/modify) of a specific element forming part of the evolving artefact life model when a LCC-specific production rule is triggered. An example of this representation is given in (26):

IF (LCC_{ni} = 'Requires_hole') (26)

THEN ((d_E{F}= Circular_Hole)→[component]).

7. A DESIGN SCENARIO WITH FORESEE

To demonstrate the effectiveness and applicability of the 'KC' approach through interaction with the FORESEE prototype, this section considers a small design scenario involved during component synthesis. The scenario considers the conceptual design for a component intended to act as a cover for electronic circuitry housed in an enclosure. The requirements known at this early design stage are that 9000 such covers are required, the cover needs to be non-corrosive, lightweight and to allow frequent servicing of the electronic circuitry. The scenario concerns qualitative commitments. As design progresses, quantitative commitments can also be made, such as the specification of parameter values, which through more specific knowledge can evolve further consequences. To help the reader visualize the commitment steps involved, *part_of* relationships in Figures 8, 9 and 10 have an associated alphabetic symbol e.g. *(a)* in Figure 8 that will be referred to in the text. Further, the figures do not portray screen dumps but an internal representation of FORESEE, by displaying PDE/LCPE models, taxonomies and the evolving solution. We consider the state, early in design, when a base form feature forms *part_of (a)* the component (Figure 8) to which other PDEs are being added. At this stage, no specific dimensions of the base have been specified.

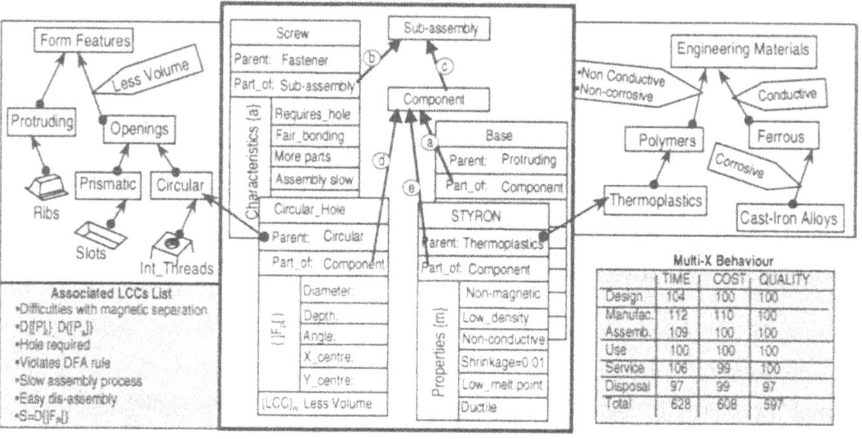

Figure 8. Consequences co-evolving with component solution

Search for intended consequence – easy dis-assembly:

To satisfy the servicing requirements, the designer uses the library access module (Figure 6) and searches for PDEs that result in a non-permanent bond, this giving rise to a decision proposal with a set of feasible options:

$$D\{F_a\}=\{\text{Fastener} \vee \text{screw} \vee \text{snap-fit} \vee \text{pop rivet} \vee \text{nuts\&bolt}\} \quad (27).$$

The designer commits *(b)* a 'screw', which from the taxonomy in Figure 4b has a set of LCC_{ni} as reflected in (17) and (18). The LCC_{ni} 'More parts' results *(c)* in a sub-assembly. Through performance mapping knowledge, these consequences influence performance measures of different processes involved in different life phases. For example from (15), 'Assembly slow' influences those phases that include an assembly process, these being the 'use phase' due to a service activity and the 'realization phase'. The measures are estimated and reported in the 'Multi-X Behaviour' window. From (26), the consequence *'Requires_hole'* introduced by the screw model results in the addition of a hole *(d)* to the component model. As shown in Figure 8, the model of the Circular_Hole, a *kind_of* ⌊circular⌋ form feature, gives rise to a decision space 'S', concerning feature parameters, formally:

$$(d_E\{F\}= \text{Circular\_hole}) \Rightarrow S=\{\text{Diameter?} \wedge \text{Depth?} \wedge \text{Angle?} \wedge \text{X\_centre?} \wedge \text{Y\_centre?}\}. \quad (28)$$

Search for intended consequence – suitable material:

At this early stage, the designer proceeds without specifying hole parameter values but interacts with FORESEE to search for materials that have a *low_density* and are *non-corrosive*. This gives rise to a decision proposal concerning feasible alternatives:

D{M} = {least_thermosplastic ∨ STYRON ∨ ABS ∨ Bakalite ∨ Aluminium}. (29)

In this scenario, the designer explores committing *(e)* STYRON, a *kind_of*⌊Thermoplastic⌋ as in Figure 8. The model of this material brings a set of inherited material properties {m} including the unintended property *'Non-magnetic'*.

Disposal phase consequence detection:

With the component still incompletely and imprecisely defined, FORESEE works in the background, independently from the designer through LCC inference knowledge to reveal that difficulties will be encountered during the component's disposal phase – specifically selecting the component with magnetic separation is not possible. Relevant performance mapping knowledge updates the multi-X behaviour (Figure 8).

Foreseeing compatible technical processes and associated LCCs:

Through the compatibility relationship in (30) and based on the formalism of a technical process model, FORESEE infers a set of technical processes {P} compatible with the selected STYRON material, this given in (31)

({t} ⊂ {m}) => (P >---- M) (30)

read as:

if the set of process technological properties {t} are a sub-set of the material properties {m}, then the process P is suitable for material M.

D{P} = {injection_moulding ∨ milling ∨ twist_drilling ∨ blow_moulding}. (31)

Realization phase system concurrent synthesis:

From the options in (31), the designer explores committing an injection moulding process *(f)*. From (4), this introduces a LCC_{ni} that a 'mould is required', this added *(h)* by the KICAD tool to the injection moulding system as in Figure 9. This generates its own LCC_{ni} such as the 'component can have a parting line defect'. Through the concurrent synthesis pattern in (32), a core-pin is added *(i)* to the mould tool as illustrated in Figure 9.

$$(d_E\{LCPE\}=\text{mould tool}) \wedge (d_E\{F\}=\text{circular\_hole}) \Rightarrow (LCC_i = [\text{core-pin}] \rightarrow [\text{mould tool}]). \quad (32)$$

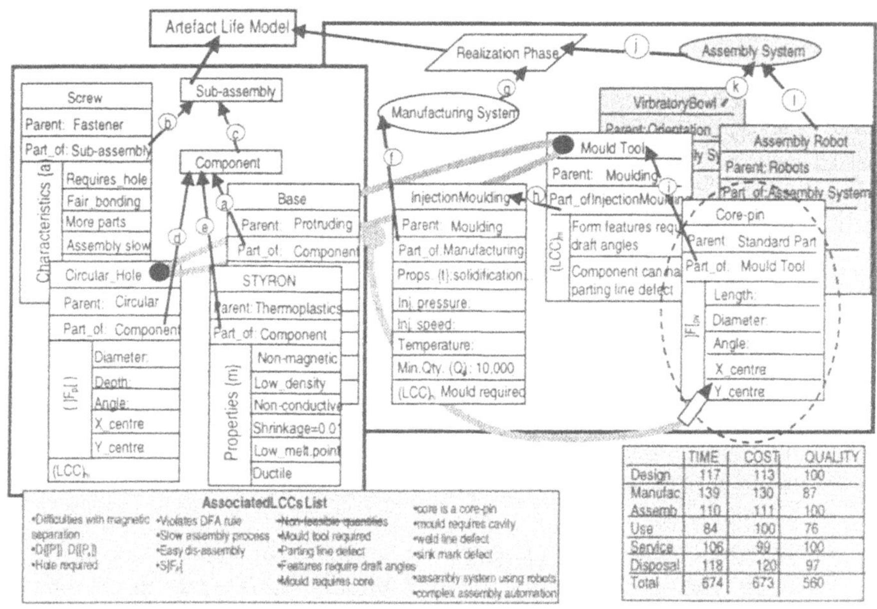

Figure 9. Consequence evolution with realization phase synthesis

The incomplete atefact life model in Figure 9, results in a number of other LCCs. From (12), the 'component can have a weld line defect'. The model of the injection moulding process includes knowledge of the minimum economic quantity (Q_e) this being 10,000. This value interacts with the required quantity Q, which is 9000. Through a piece of captured knowledge, this results in 'non-feasible quantities.' To avoid this LCC, the designer increases Q to 10,100 justified by catering for spare covers.

Assembly system concurrent synthesis:

The newly specified quantity (Q=10,100) triggers a piece of company specific knowledge that recommends assembly automation when $Q>9,500$. The designer accepts this recommendation, which through (33) results in *(j)*. Through concurrent synthesis knowledge, the screw assembly feature interacts with this new state of the assembly system, to evolve the assembly system as in (34), illustrated by *(k)* and *(l)* in Figure 9. The latter LCPEs co-evolve new consequences that influence different performance measures, such as cost of assembly.

$$([\text{automated\_assembly}] \rightarrow [\text{Assembly System}]) \rightarrow \langle \text{phase} \rangle_{\text{realization}}. \quad (33)$$

$$(([\text{Vibratory Bowl}] \wedge [\text{Assembly Robot}]) \rightarrow [\text{Assembly System}]) \rightarrow \langle \text{phase} \rangle_{\text{realization}}. \quad (34)$$

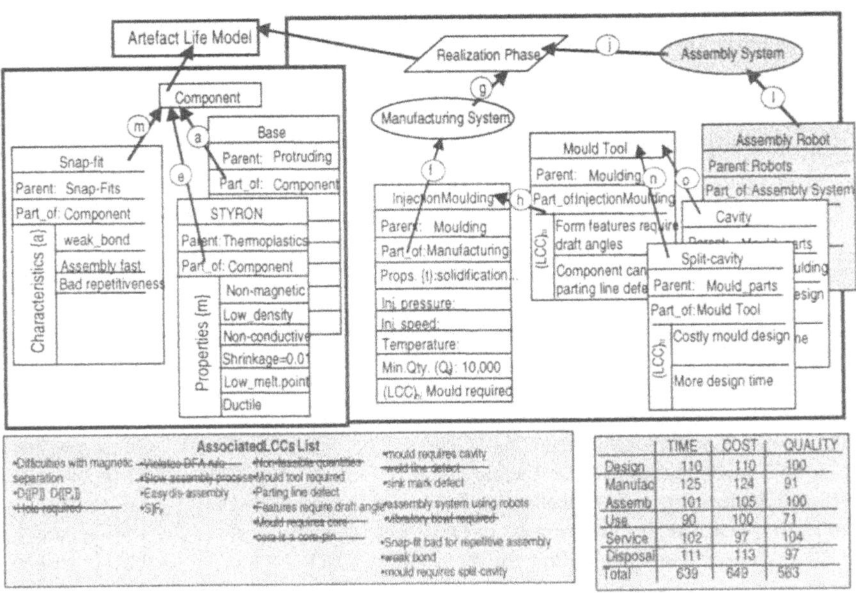

Figure 10. Consequences resulting with alternative, snap-fit partial solution

Exploration of alternative assembly feature:

With a number of LCCs detected (Figure 9) for this incomplete artefact life solution, the designer explores retracting *(b)* the screw and from the alternatives in (27), opts to commit *(m)* a *snap-fit* (Figure 20). From (20), this also a ⌊Protruding⌋ form feature, introduces its own LCCs such as from (23) the formation of sink mark defects. This alternative partial solution avoids certain consequences (e.g. violates DFA rule, hole required, mould requires core, vibratory bowl required, weld line defect) but generates others e.g. snap-fit bad for repetitive assembly, weak-bond, mould requires split-cavity (Figure 10). The designer can compare the multi-X behaviour of this snap-fit based partial solution with that of the screw based partial solution in Figure 9. In this case, the overall behaviour of the snap-fit partial solution is relatively better. The decision of which alternative partial solution to select and proceed with is still entirely controlled by the designer.

8. EVALUATION

To acquire an unbiased assessment of the KICAD based 'Knowledge of Consequences' approach to component 'Design Synthesis for Multi-X', formal demonstrations via FORESEE were carried out in the U.K. with 9 academic researchers, 7 practicing/consulting designers and 7 post-graduate students. The case-study demonstrated was similar to that presented in section 7. Following the demonstration, evaluators were individually questioned during a structured interview. The results, partially listed in Table (2), broadly reflect that FORESEE addresses limitations with current tools in that it:

- provides a *multiple* and *interacting* insight into LCCs co-evolving with an incomplete and imprecise solution *during* the synthesis activity;
- it motivates and supports 'artefact' and 'life-phase system' *exploration*, this leading to a more 'life-oriented' conscious commitment of decisions;
- provides a *solution specific* rather than a generic insight of LCCs.

Table 2. Partial Evaluation Results

Evaluation criteria	%Yes	%No	%Other
Made aware of LCCs with an incomplete solution	96	0	4 (not sure)
Made aware of LCCs with an imprecise solution	74	9	17
Made aware of multiple and interacting LCCs	64	4	32 (segmented)
Made aware with component life specific LCCs	45	24	31 (not sure)
Provided advice on avoiding/relaxing LCCs	45	13	42 (not sure)
Motivated to explore due to awareness of LCCs	87	0	13 (not sure)
LCCs awareness assists committing decisions more consciously	83	0	17 (not sure)
Usefulness of 'KC' approach in practice	91	0	9 (not entirely)

Major issues revealed concerning the KICAD prototype facilitating the 'KC' approach are:

- the problem of practically acquiring, maintaining and evolving the relevant LCC knowledge whose source is *public, private, internal* and *external* to an organization;
- it mainly caters for synthesis at the component level and from a construction viewpoint;
- FORESEE only handles one 'component life solution' at a time, this making it difficulty to rapidly compare LCCs co-evolving with alternative partial solutions;
- some felt the simultaneous report of LCCs propagating across multiple life phases disturbs their ability to focus on individual issues;
- FORESEE lacks to display a graphical representation of the evolving solution, this not in correlation with the way practicing designers traditionally visualize early solution concepts;

- the FORESEE user interface (Figure 7) is difficult to manipulate - users need to laboriously learn the *language* of the system in order to avoid inputting errors and not get lost in using FORESEE.

9. DISCUSSION

A benefit of designing with FORESEE is that it provides designers with a synthesis elements library consisting of reusable PDEs and LCPEs models, this allowing 'artefact' and 'life-phase system' compositional models to be constructed through the artefact life modelling frame. In this sense, the overall framework of the 'KC' approach extends the concept of 'feature based design' to early 'artefact life' design. As demonstrated, LCC knowledge plays a significant role in the support provided by FORESEE. Through the embedded LCC inference knowledge, FORESEE reveals the LCCs co-evolving with the underlying compositional models. Thus a key frame in the developed framework is that concerning LCC knowledge modelling. This frame helps in the acquisition and codification of LCC knowledge, as it identifies *what* needs to be modelled for an application domain i.e. models of reusable synthesis elements, consequence inference knowledge and consequence action knowledge. In an attempt to reduce knowledge duplication, different synthesis elements are organized into *kind_of* taxonomies, with relevant LCC knowledge associated to different abstraction levels in these taxonomies. Through such structuring, the degree of abstraction of each chunk of LCC knowledge is intensified by being more generic. This allows a designer to foresee and explore LCCs co-evolving with either *specific* or *least* synthesis decision commitments. However, exploiting these advantages requires the vigorous generalisation and abstraction of synthesis elements and LCC knowledge. Thus, experimentation with FORESEE highlighted a number of future research challenges. Union inheritance employed in the established structure reduces knowledge duplication. However, it requires the knowledge engineer to validate the codified knowledge because LCC inherited can be conflicting. For instance, the ⌊Pop rivet⌋ class in Figure (4b) inherits knowledge that it results in both 'Dis-assembly easy' and 'Dis-assembly difficult.' Also, while *kind_of* taxonomies do contribute to controlling the scaling up of LCC knowledge, extending FORESEE to practical applications requires evolving and maintaining the integrity of a large knowledge base. Although no substantial effort has been made yet in this direction, this would involve:

- modelling more synthesis elements to support solution synthesis at different artefact abstraction levels (e.g. sub-assembly) and from different viewpoints (e.g. functional), not merely constructional;

- organizing the resultant extended set of synthesis elements into relevant taxonomies, this perhaps requiring other rationalization mechanisms and not solely *kind_of* relationships;
- laboriously capturing, codifying and validating for the extended set of synthesis elements, more LCC inference and LCC action knowledge;

Additionally, knowledge modelling requires further work in order to:

- generate a structure with a *customizable* knowledge perspective, this for supporting say the exploration of LCCs associated with bought-in items (e.g. fasteners and standard mould parts) furnished by different suppliers;
- identify and associate *certainty factors* with LCCs, currently modelled as being dertministic;
- identify the *type* and *magnitude* of performance measures e.g. can quality be measured?

Also, improving FORESEE's functionality includes developing:

- knowledge management utilities that allow distributed artefact life actors to dynamically update/customize both LCCni and LCCi knowledge they encounter, in the right format;
- a non-textual display representation of an early artefact life compositional model – a form of 'artefact life sketch';
- a means allowing designers to simultaneously manipulate multiple 'artefact life models'.

10. CONCLUSION

This paper reported on the development and implementation of a KICAD prototype, FORESEE, based on the 'Knowledge of life-cycle Consequences' approach framework to component DFΣX. The approach is founded on a phenomena model describing *how* LCCs are generated, this reflecting the necessity of designers engaging in concurrent 'artefact' and 'life-phase system' synthesis so that both *non-interacting* and *interacting* consequences co-evolving with the design solution can be revealed. The broadly positive evaluation results indicate that the concept of revealing life cycle consequences co-evolving with a solution, supports designers in exploring design opportunities and avoiding/relaxing unintended consequences. This demonstrates that a significance of the 'KC' approach framework is that it contributes to the effective development of KICAD tools aimed at providing designers *during* synthesis, pro-active exploration support so as to generate 'life-oriented' component design solutions.

ACKNOWLEDGEMENTS

The authors thank Prof.M.M.Andreasen of the Technical University of Denmark and Dr.Ken J.MacCallum, Bell College of Technology (U.K.) for discussions on material presented in this paper. The first author also thanks the University of Malta for funding research visits to the University of Strathclyde (UK) and The Technical University of Denmark (DK).

REFERENCES

Andreasen, M. M., A. H. B. Duffy, K. J. MacCallum, J. Bowen and T. Storm (1996). "The Design Co-ordination Framework: key elements for effective product development". *The Design Productivity Debate.* A. H. B. Duffy. London, Springer-Verlag: pp. 151-172.

Blessing, L. M. (1994). "A Process-Based Approach To Computer Supported Engineering Design". *Ph.D.*, Enschede, University of Twente.

Borg, J. and K. J. MacCallum (1996). "Structuring Knowledge of Life-Cycle Consequences for Supporting Concurrent Design Exploration"; *IFIP TC5 WG5.2, International Conference on Knowledge Intensive CAD*,Vol. 2, Carnegie Mellon University, Pittsburgh, PA, USA, Chapman & Hall, pp. 208-223.

Borg, J. and X. T. Yan (1998). "Design Decision Consequences: Key to 'Design For Multi-X ' Support"; *Proceedings, 2nd International Symposium 'Tools and Methods For Concurrent Engineering'*, Manchester, UK, pp. 169-184.

Brown, D. (1996). "Which way to KIC?"; *IFIP TC5 WG5.2, International Conference on Knowledge Intensive CAD*,Vol. 2, Carnegie Mellon University, Pittsburgh, PA, USA, Chapman & Hall, pp. 291-295.

Duffy, A. H. B. and M. M. Andreasen (1995). "Enhancing the Evolution of Design Science"; *International Conference on Engineering Design,* Praha, pp. 29-35.

Duffy, A. H. B., M. M. Andreasen, K. J. MacCallum and L. N. Reijers (1993). "Design Co-ordination for Concurrent Engineering." *Journal of Engineering Design* 4(4): pp. 251-265.

Giarratano, J. C. and G. D. Riley (1994). *Expert Systems: Principles and Programming.* USA, PWS.

Guan, X. and K. J. MacCallum (1995). "Handling of positional information in a system for supporting early geometric design"; *AI System Support for Conceptual Design,* Ambleside, UK, Springer-Verlag, pp. 55-70.

Holtzman, S. (1988). *Intelligent decision systems.* Reading Mass., Addison-Wesley.

Hubka, V. and E. Eder (1988). *Theory of technical systems: A total concept theory for engineering design.* Berlin/Heidelberg, Springer-Verlag.

Ishii, K. (1995). "Life-Cycle Engineering Design." *Transactions of the ASME 117*: pp. 42-47.

Kerr, S. M. (1993). "The Importance of Manipulating Past Design Knowledge by Group Rationalisation". *Internal Report,* Glasgow, CAD Centre, DMEM, University of Strathclyde.

Medland, T. (1997). "A decision directed design approach." *Engineering Designer* (May): pp. 4-7.

Olesen, J. (1992). "Concurrent Development in Manufacturing - based on dispositional mechanisms". *Ph.D.*, Institute for Engineering Design Lyngby, The Technical University of Denmark.

Roozenburg, N. F. M. and J. Eekels (1995). *Product Design: Fundamentals and Methods.* Wilshire, John Wiley & Sons Ltd.

Shah, J. J. and M. Mantyla (1995). *Parametric and Feature-based CAD/CAM.* New York, John Wiley & Sons, Inc.

Tjalve, E. (1979). *A Short Course in Industrial Design.* London, Newnes-Butterworths.

Walters, J. R. and N. R. Nielsen (1988). *Crafting Knowledge Based Systems - Expert Systems Made Realistic.* New York, John Wiley & Sons.

Yan, X. T. and J. E. E. Sharpe (1995). "Reasoning and Truth Maintenance of Causal Structures in Interdisciplinary Product Modelling and Simulation.". *International Workshop on Engineering Design: AI System Support for Conceptual Design.* England, Springer: pp. 403-425.

Author index

Keyword Index

www.ingramcontent.com/pod-product-compliance
Ingram Content Group UK Ltd.
Pitfield, Milton Keynes, MK11 3LW, UK
UKHW020102200726
13856UKWH00002B/335

* 9 7 8 1 4 7 5 7 5 6 3 5 7 *